FAMILY NURSE PRACTITIONER

Certification Review

FAMILY NURSE PRACTITIONER

Certification Review

JoAnn Zerwekh, EdD, RN, FNP, CS
University of Phoenix
Carondelet Health Network Community Services
Tucson, Arizona
Nursing Education Consultants
Dallas, Texas

Jo Carol Claborn, MS, RN, CNS
El Centro College
Nursing Education Consultants
Dallas, Texas

W.B. SAUNDERS COMPANY
A Division of Harcourt Brace & Company
Philadelphia London Toronto Montreal Sydney Tokyo

W.B. SAUNDERS COMPANY
A Division of Harcourt Brace & Company

The Curtis Center
Independence Square West
Philadelphia, Pennsylvania 19106

Library of Congress Cataloging-in-Publication Data

Zerwekh, JoAnn Graham.
    Family nurse practitioner certification review / JoAnn Zerwekh, Jo
Carol Claborn.
        p.   cm.
    ISBN 0-7216-7743-6
    1. Family nursing—Examinations, questions, etc.   2. Nurse
practitioners—Examinations, questions, etc.   I. Claborn, Jo Carol.
II. Title.
    [DNLM: 1. Nursing Care examination questions.   2. Family Practice
examination questions.   3. Nurse Practitioners examination
questions.   WY 18.2Z58f   1999]
RT120.F34Z47   1999
610.73'076—dc21
DNLM/DLC   98-34772

FAMILY NURSE PRACTITIONER CERTIFICATION REVIEW   ISBN 0-7216-7743-6

Printed in the United States of America

Last digit is the print number: 9   8   7   6   5   4   3   2   1

To Tom, my soul mate,
who brings a smile to my face and
a warm glow in my heart.
                              JoAnn

To Robert, my friend and partner,
whose love and patience keeps me going.
                              Jo

Series Contributors

Susan E. Chaney, EdD, MS, BSN
Professor, Family Nurse Practitioner
  Coordinator
Texas Woman's University
Family Nurse Practitioner
Homeless Outreach Medical Services
Parkland Health and Hospital System
Dallas, Texas

Cynthia Churgin, RN, FNP, CNM
Casa Blanca Medical Group
Mesa, Arizona

Sharon I. Decker, RN, CS, MSN,
  CCRN
Professor of Clinical Nursing
Director, Clinical Simulation Center
Texas Tech University Health Sciences
  Center
Lubbock, Texas

Nicolette Estrada, RN, MS, FNP-C
Chief Research Coordinator
Carl T. Hayden VA Medical Center
Phoenix, Arizona

Mary Jo Gagan, RNCS, FNP, PhD
Assistant Professor
University of Arizona College of Nursing
Nurse Practitioner
Campus Health
University of Arizona College of Nursing
Tucson, Arizona

Ela-Joy Lehrman, MS, MAEd, PhD
Program Manager for Nursing, Counseling,
  and General Studies
University of Phoenix
Tucson, Arizona

Beverly McCoy, BSN, MS, FNP
Clinical Director/Family Nurse Practitioner
Breaking the Circle Children's Health Care
Arizona State University
College of Nursing
Tempe, Arizona

Jacquelyn McGlamery, BSN, FNP
Family Nurse Practitioner
Sierra Tucson
Tucson, Arizona

Loretta Manning, RNC, MSN, GNP
Educational Consultant, Sylvia Rayfield &
  Associates
Executive Director, I CAN, Inc. Publishing
Atlanta, Georgia

Kathleen T. Ogle, RN, MS, CFNP
Instructor
Bowie State University
Department of Nursing
Bowie, Maryland;
Family Nurse Practitioner
Maryland Primary Care Physicians
Arnold, Maryland

Alice B. Pappas, BSN, MSN, PhD
Associate Dean for Academic Affairs
Baylor University School of Nursing
Dallas Texas

Jodi Pelusi, RN, MS, FNP
University of Phoenix
Phoenix, Arizona

Patricia J. Pinckard, MS, ANP
Adult Nurse Practitioner
Occupational Health
Desert Samaritan Medical Center
Mesa, Arizona

Sylvia M. Root, EdD, RNC, FNP
Associate Professor
Arizona State University
Tempe, Arizona

Patricia Scully, RN, MS, JD
Nurse Attorney Consultant
Tucson, Arizona

Patricia A. Shannon, RNC, MS, CPNP
Faculty, University of Phoenix;
Director of Nurses and Nurse Practitioners
North Valley Pediatrics PC
Phoenix, Arizona;
Adjunct Faculty
Arizona State University
Tempe, Arizona;
President/Consultant
Pediatric Nursing . . . PLUS
Phoenix, Arizona

Linda Stevenson, RN, PhD
Baylor University School of Nursing
Dallas, Texas

Gail Tucker, RN, MS, FNP
BMT Nurse Practitioner
Good Samaritan Regional Medical Center;
City of Hope/Samaritan Bone Marrow
    Transplant
Phoenix, Arizona

Gayle P. Varnell, RN, PhD, CPNP
Assistant Professor
Nurse Practitioner Program Coordinator
The University of Texas at Tyler
Tyler, Texas

John Walter, RN, BS, CPNP
Guest Lecturer
Family Nurse Practitioner Program
University of Arizona College of Nursing;
Pediatric Nurse Practitioner
University Physicians
Tucson, Arizona

Pamela Becker Weilitz, AD, BSN,
    MSN(R)
Assistant Clinical Professor, Graduate
    Program
St. Louis University School of Nursing;
Adult Nurse Practitioner
Washington University School of Medicine
University Care
St. Louis, Missouri

Margaret "Pegi" Yancy, RN, MS,
    OGNP
Faculty Associate
Arizona State University
Tempe, Arizona;
Women's Health Nurse Practitioner
Department of Reproductive Medicine
St. Joseph's Hospital and Medical Center
Phoenix, Arizona

Preface

With the dawn of the role of the nurse practitioner, there is an increasing need for additional reference information and study materials for the certification examinations. Nurse practitioners are playing a vital role in the changing health care delivery system in the United States. The numbers of candidates for the certification examinations is rapidly increasing as more nursing programs implement the nurse practitioner curriculum in their graduate programs. *Family Nurse Practitioner Certification Review* has been developed to assist the advanced practice nurse to prepare for the FNP certification examination. Extensive efforts have been made to include current information that is representative of the content based on the blueprints for the certification exams. This book of questions is not intended to be an exhaustive review of the content, but an adjunct to the review process. Over 1,300 review questions are included in all.

Test taking strategies are included in Chapter 1. As a candidate prepares for the examination, it is vitally important to be familiar with and to practice good testing strategies. Testing strategies can prevent the candidate from making mistakes and selecting the wrong answer. As the review process begins, a review of the testing strategies chapter and the practice of good testing strategies is critical. With many years experience in the field of testing, we have consistently identified the importance practice testing plays in the review process. Practice questions give the candidate an opportunity to review questions written from different perspectives. To enhance the review process, answers with complete rationales are provided at the end of each chapter. Not only does the candidate increase their knowledge of the subject area, but with more practice, testing skills become fine tuned. Good testing skills make the candidate more comfortable and help to decrease the stress associated with certification exams.

This book also includes chapters reviewing important concepts related to Growth and Development and Health Promotion and Maintenance. These chapters provide questions that test information related to growth and development, general health supervision, and health maintenance. The clinical chapters are developed using a systems approach, i.e., cardiovascular, respiratory, endocrine, etc. In each of these chapters, the test questions are divided into three areas: Physical Examination and Diagnostic Tests, Disorders, and Pharmacology. This format assists the candidate to easily locate specific questions. The last three chapters in the text are on Theory and Research; Issues and Trends; and Legal and Ethical aspects of nurse practitioner practice. The test questions in these chapters focus on professional competencies inherent in the role and function of the FNP.

Our thanks to the many nurse practitioners across the country who provided questions and insight into the role of the nurse practitioner. We wish to thank Robin Carter, our editor at W.B. Saunders, for her support and suggestions in our preparation of the manuscript. Thank you also goes to all the nurse practitioners who took time from their busy schedules to review the questions for content and clarity.

Acknowledgments

We are continually grateful for the contributions and efforts of our test item contributors who provided their expertise and knowledge for this nurse practitioner certification review series.

We thank the manuscript reviewers for their suggestions and insights as we tackled this large project:

Harvey Baker, RNCS, ARNP
Oswego Family Medical Clinic
Oswego, Kansas

Susan Appel, RN, MN, CCRN, CS
Carolinas College of Health
  Sciences
Charlotte, North Carolina

Genell Lee, BSN, MSN, JD
Hauth & Lee, LLC
Birmingham, Alabama

Stephanie A. Batalo, RN, BSN,
  MSN, FNP
Trinity Health System
Steubenville, Ohio

Dorothy J. Stuppy, RN, PhD
University of Texas at Arlington
Arlington, Texas

Lynette M. Wachholz, MN, RN,
  ARNP, IBCLC
The Everett Clinic
Everett, Washington

We thank the staff at W.B. Saunders Company: Robin Carter, Senior Editor, and Marie Pelcin and Ross Landy, editorial assistants for their calmness and patience. Joan Sinclair, who managed the book's production. It was such a pleasure to work with you again on another publication. Berta Steiner for copyediting and typesetting the manuscript. What a job to keep track of thousands of questions!

Last, but certainly not least, we want to thank: Our children, Tyler and Ashley Zerwekh, Jaelyn Claborn, Michael Brown, and Kim Aultman, for teasing their mothers about writing 5 books!! Our parents, Charles Graham and Hazel Cooper, for their continued support and encouragement. Tom Gaglione and Robert Claborn for their encouragement, support, and love. We love you all.

Contents

Test-Taking Strategies

Testing Strategies

Knowing how to take an examination is a skill that is developed through practice and experience. Being able to take an examination effectively is almost as important as the basic knowledge required to answer the question. Everyone has taken an examination only to find in the review of the exam that questions were missed due to inadequate testing skills. Nurse practitioner programs provide the graduate student with a comprehensive base of knowledge; how you utilize this knowledge will determine your success on a certification examination. The certification examination is an objective test that covers knowledge, understanding, and application of professional nursing theory and practice. When you register for the examination, you will receive a "Candidate Handbook" or information materials from the Certification Board administering the examination. This handbook will have helpful information to assist you in preparing, such as important registration information, test content outline, sample test questions, and in some cases a bibliography. This important information can assist you in your review process.

Read the information in this chapter carefully and make sure you understand the strategies discussed. This chapter is designed to help you identify problem areas in testing skills and learn how to use strategy and judgment in selecting correct answers. It is important for you to practice testing skills if you are going to be able to utilize these skills on the certification examination.

Question Characteristics

A. Multiple-choice questions.
   1. Scene or scenario—establishes the setting of the question. Not all questions will have a scenario; if a scenario is included, consider the appropriateness of the answer to the information provided.
   2. Stem—states the question that is being asked.
   3. Options—there are four options from which to choose an answer.
      a. Distractors—designed to distract you from the correct answer.
      b. Correct answer—correctly answers the question asked in the stem.
      c. There are only four options in any item; there are no combinations of options to consider.
      d. There is only one correct response; no partial credit is given for another answer.
B. Questions are derived from clinical situations common in the practice setting.

Strategies for Multiple-Choice Questions

1. Cover the options with your hand or a piece of scratch paper.* This strategy makes you focus on the content of the question and prevents your eyes from "darting" to look at the distractors. If you peruse the distractors before you completely understand the question, key words in the distractors will influence your interpretation of the question.

2. Do not read extra meaning into the question. The question is asking for specific information; if it appears to be simple "common sense," then assume it is simple. Do not look for a hidden meaning in what appears to be an easy question.

EXAMPLE:

The nurse practitioner understands that the most common form of facial paralysis in the adult client is:

1. Facial nerve fasciitis.
2. Trigeminal neuralgia.
3. Bell's palsy.
4. Herpes zoster.

The correct answer is Option #3. Be careful not to "read into" the question and add pain to the facial paralysis symptom. The most common form of facial paralysis is Bell's palsy, which is a disorder affecting the facial nerve and characterized by muscle flaccidity of the affected side of the face. Trigeminal neuralgia is a disorder of cranial nerve V characterized by an abrupt onset of pain in the lower and upper jaw, cheek, and lips. Herpes zoster affects the dermatomes and does not cause a paralysis, but pain is possible with postherpetic neuralgia.

EXAMPLE:

When administering skin tests to an immunocompromised client, the nurse practitioner must consider:

1. The importance of not applying more than one skin test at a time.
2. The skin test may react more aggressively than expected.

3. The use of a known allergen for the client and utilize it as a control.
4. The immunocompromised client should not be skin tested.

The correct answer is Option #3. Do not read into the question and make it more difficult by trying to make the client sicker (i.e., full-blown acquired immunodeficiency syndrome [AIDS]). It is important to remember to apply controls when skin testing the immunocompromised client. Ask clients what diseases they believe they have immunity to, such as measles. Apply the "known" allergen and the skin test to be tested. If the client is unable to mount an immune response at all, the known allergen will not react. By not applying the controls, the nurse practitioner may assume a skin test is negative, when in fact the client's immune system is unable to respond.

3. Read the stem correctly. Make sure you understand exactly what information the question is asking.

EXAMPLE:

The nurse practitioner would refer to a pediatric cardiologist for work-up and evaluation within 1–2 weeks, a child with:

1. Signs of exercise intolerance, dyspnea, and elevated pulse.
2. Poor feeding, increased cyanosis with crying, and dizziness.
3. Nonfunctional heart murmur, respiratory crackles, and retarded growth and development.
4. Systolic ejection murmur, grade II, which disappears on sitting.

The question asks you to determine which child's symptoms would require a referral to a pediatric cardiologist within the next 1–2 weeks. Options #1, #2, and #3 are considered unstable and acute and should be immediately referred to a pediatric cardiologist. Children with a murmur need to be further evaluated, but it is not considered emergency as long as they are asymptomatic, have normal activity and exercise, and are growing normally.

4. Before considering the options, formulate in your mind possible answers to the question. If none of the options fit in the pool of answers you anticipated, go back and re-evaluate the question. Assess each of the options with regard to your pool of possible answers.

---

*This testing strategy of covering the distractors is from Phoebe K. Helm, Ed.D.

E X A M P L E :

A mother who is 3 days postpartum has been complaining of soreness and fullness in her breasts and that she wants to stop breast-feeding her infant until her breasts feel better. The nurse practitioner:

1. Shows the client how to apply a breast binder to decrease the discomfort and the production of milk.
2. Tells the client that breast fullness may be a sign of infection and to stop breast-feeding.
3. Suggests to the client that she decrease her fluid intake for the next 24 hours to temporarily suppress lactation.
4. Explains to the client that the breast discomfort is normal and that the infant's sucking will promote the flow of milk.

Formulate in your mind possible answers to the question. Think to yourself, "Is it normal to have fullness and soreness in the breasts during the first 3 days of lactation?" If you are unsure, go back and reassess the question. In this instance, Option #4 is correct. Initially, breast soreness may occur for about 2–3 minutes during each feeding until the let-down reflex is established.

5. Identify what type of response the question is asking. A positive stem requires identification of three false items and one positive as the correct answer.

E X A M P L E :

Clients who believe they have been exposed to human immunodeficiency virus (HIV) should have an HIV antibody test how soon after the exposure?

1. The next day and 2 months later.
2. 6 months after exposure and again at 12 months.
3. 6 to 12 weeks after exposure and again at 6 months.
4. 4 weeks and 12 weeks.

The correct answer is Option #3. This question requires you to identify three incorrect responses and one correct response. The HIV antibody develops between 6 and 12 weeks after exposure. Because of the variability of antibody development, it is recommended that the test be repeated in 6 months to confirm the findings.

6. Identify questions that require identification of something the practitioner should not or would not do (i.e., unsafe action, contraindication, inappropriate action).

E X A M P L E :

The nurse practitioner is prescribing astemizole (Hismanal) for a geriatric client's allergy problems. When considering the client's current medications, which medication would be a contraindication to the administration of astemizole (Hismanal)?

1. Erythromycin ethylsuccinate (E.E.S.).
2. Verapamil (Calan).
3. Propanolol (Inderal).
4. Captopril (Captoten).

The correct answer is Option #1. Macrolides and Hismanal should not be administered concurrently. The nurse practitioner is required to identify a medication that should not be ordered.

7. Questions may also be analytical. These questions may ask the nurse practitioner to identify findings, statements, and the like, that are consistent/inconsistent with the client's presenting problem and/or differentiate between them.

E X A M P L E :

A child is being evaluated for attention deficit hyperactivity disorder (ADHD). Which test is helpful in evaluating the difference between ADHD and a learning disability?

1. Standardized IQ achievement test.
2. Denver Developmental Screening Test.
3. Audiological and visual testing.
4. Complete neurologic examination.

Before you examine the options in this question, it is important to think about the differences between ADHD and learning disabilities. The correct answer is Option #1. Children with learning disabilities and ADHD are often impulsive, inattentive, and overactive. Usually, children with ADHD do not have lower IQ achievement scores; however, children with a learning disability usually demonstrate a level of educational achievement substantially below that of the IQ.

8. Identify key words that affect your understanding of the question. Make sure you understand exactly what information the question is asking. Be aware of questions in which the stem includes words such as *except, contraindicated, avoid, least, not applicable,* and *does not occur.* These words change the direction of the question. It may help to rephrase the question in your own words in order to better understand what information is being requested.

EXAMPLE:

Clients with arteriosclerotic heart disease (ASHD) go through several stages before becoming severely compromised. Which **does not occur** in the early stages of ASHD?

1. Decreased urine output.
2. Dyspnea on exercise.
3. Anginal pain relieved by rest.
4. Increased serum triglyceride levels.

Rephrase the question: In early stages of ASHD, which of the following does not occur? It is important that you identify the key point "early stages of ASHD" and the key words "does not occur." If you miss these essential points, you do not understand the question, and chances are you will not choose the correct answer. The correct answer is Option #1: a decrease in urine output occurs when cardiac disease is advanced enough to cause a severe decrease in cardiac output and renal perfusion.

9. As you read the options, eliminate those you know are not correct. This will help narrow the field of choice. When you select an answer or eliminate a distractor, you should have a specific reason for doing so.

EXAMPLE:

A 45-year-old female complains of knee pain when kneeling and a "clicking" noise when walking up steps. On exam, there is a slight knee effusion and tenderness when palpating the patella against the condyles. The diagnosis for this client is:

1. Anterior cruciate tear. (*No, the client generally cannot bear weight on the extremity without it buckling or giving way.*)
2. Dislocated patella. (*No, there would be considerable effusion and locking of the knee in flexion.*)
3. Chondromalacia patella. (*Yes, there is clicking and anterior knee pain around or under the kneecap aggravated by knee extensor stress.*)

4. Tendinitis. (*No, there would be no clicking sound with movement.*)

After systematically evaluating the options, Option #3 is the correct answer.

10. Identify similarities in the distractors. Frequently, three distractors will contain similar information, and one will be different. The different one may be the correct answer.

EXAMPLE:

An elderly client is to be encouraged to increase her intake of protein. The addition of which of these foods to 100 ml of milk will provide the greatest amount of protein?

1. 50 ml light cream and 2 tbsp corn syrup.
2. 30 gm powdered skim milk and one egg.
3. 1 small scoop (90 gm) ice cream and 1 tbsp chocolate syrup.
4. 2 egg yolks and 1 tbsp sugar.

Options #1, #3, and #4 all contain a simple sugar. The correct answer, Option #2, has more protein. Notice that three of the options are similar; the one that is different may be the correct answer. This strategy is not a substitute for basic knowledge but may help you figure out the answer.

11. Select the most comprehensive answer. All of the options may be correct, but **one** will include the other three options or need to be considered first.

EXAMPLE:

A new mother tells the nurse practitioner that her infant was born HIV-positive. She asks the nurse practitioner how long her baby has to live. The nurse practitioner's response would be based on the knowledge that:

1. The antibodies present in the baby's blood may reflect the antibodies received from the mother at the time of birth.
2. If antibodies are present at birth, the baby has AIDS in an active form.
3. Since the baby is HIV-positive, the child will develop full-blown AIDS within 3 years.
4. The antibodies detected at birth indicate presence of the HIV; the test does not indicate when the child will develop AIDS.

The correct answer is Option #4. It is important to give the mother as much hope as possible but still be realistic about the condition. There is no way to tell when or if the child will convert to active AIDS. Many infants seroconvert to HIV-negative status.

12. Select the best answer that is most specific to what the question asks. All of the options may be correct, but **one** is more specific or essential.

E X A M P L E :

When a child comes in for a health maintenance clinic visit, what is essential for the nurse practitioner to do?

1. Order routine laboratory tests.
2. Perform vision and auditory screening.
3. Plot height and weight on charts.
4. Review immunization record.

It is absolutely essential that the immunization record be reviewed. The other options are important but are not essential for a health maintenance visit. Recognize key words that identify the question that is asking for a priority of care—first, initial, best, most. The correct answer is Option #4; the other alternatives may be correct but should be prioritized.

13. Watch questions in which the options contain several items to consider. After you are sure you understand what information the question is requesting, evaluate each part of the distractor. Is it appropriate to what the question is asking? If an option contains one incorrect item, the entire option is incorrect. All of the items listed in the selection must be correct, if it is to be the answer to the question.

E X A M P L E :

Diagnostic studies used in the differential diagnosis of systemic lupus erythematosus (SLE) include:

1. Complete blood count (CBC), SMA-12, and erythrocyte sedimentation rate (ESR).
2. Chest x-ray and coagulation profile.
3. Antinuclear antibodies (ANA), ESR, and C-reactive protein.
4. CBC, urinalysis (UA), and chest x-ray.

The correct answer is Option #3. In a methodical evaluation of the items in the options, you can eliminate items in options #1, #2, and #4.

Although all of the tests included in the answer may be included in a complete physical examination, the laboratory test specific to the diagnosis of SLE includes the ANA, ESR, and C-reactive protein. During flares, the ESR and C-reactive protein are elevated. The ANA titer in a client with SLE is positive at a 1:80 ratio.

14. Be alert to relevant information contained in previous questions. Sometimes, as you are answering questions, you will find information similar to the question being tested. Previous questions may assist you in identifying relevant information in the current question.

E X A M P L E :

The American College of Physicians (ACP) recommends that healthy adults receive a tetanus-diphtheria (Td) booster vaccination:

1. Every 5 years.
2. At age 75.
3. At age 65.
4. Every 10 years.

The ACP recommends that adults receive a Td booster every 10 years or a single booster at age 50 for clients who have completed full pediatric series, including teenage and young adult boosters. The correct answer to this question is Option #4. In another question involving immunizations, you read the following question.

E X A M P L E :

In taking the history of an alert, older adult, the nurse practitioner determines the client is an avid gardener and spends a great deal of time outside. He had a pneumococcal vaccination last year and states he cannot remember when he had a tetanus vaccination. A health maintenance recommendation for this client would be to obtain:

1. Pneumococcal vaccine.
2. Tetanus vaccine.
3. Hepatitis B vaccine.
4. No recommendation.

The correct answer is Option #2. A clue to the answer to this question may be found in the previous question. Older adults who enjoy gardening and outdoor activities should have a Td booster once every 10 years, as the ACP recommends this practice. Some professionals advocate high risk populations (e.g., gardeners, construction workers, or others who spend a lot of time outdoors) to have a Td booster every 5 years.

15. Multiple-choice mathematical computations may be included in the exam. Mathematical computations may include calculations of IM, PO, and IV dosages; calculations of pediatric dosage; determining creatinine clearance; and conversion of units of measurement.

E X A M P L E :

The nurse practitioner is ordering amoxicillin (Amoxil) for a child with otitis media. The child weighs 22 lbs. How would the order be written?

1. Amoxicillin 250 mg/5 ml Sig: 5 ml PO tid × 10 days.
2. Amoxicillin 500 mg Sig: 1 tab PO tid × 3 days.
3. Amoxicillin 350 mg/5 ml Sig: 5 ml PO bid × 14 days.
4. Amoxicillin 125 mg/5 ml Sig: 5 ml PO tid × 10 days.

First, you must convert the lb to kg, which is 2.2 lb/kg. This child weighs 10 kg. The dose for amoxicillin is 30–50 mg/kg/day for a child. 10 kg × 40 mg/kg/day = 400 mg/day. Amoxicillin is supplied in 125 mg/5 ml and 250 mg/5 ml. The correct dose for this child would be the 125 mg/5 ml. The answer closest to that dosage is Option #4.

16. Evaluate priority questions carefully. Frequently all of the answers are appropriate to the situation. You need to decide which of the actions you should do first.

E X A M P L E :

While attending a rural public school, a 7-year-old child was bitten on the hand by a raccoon. At the rural clinic, the nurse practitioner cleansed the wound. The next action is:

1. Administer tetanus antitoxin.
2. Contact local animal control authorities.
3. Administer rabies immune globulin (RIG) and human diploid cell vaccine (HDCV).

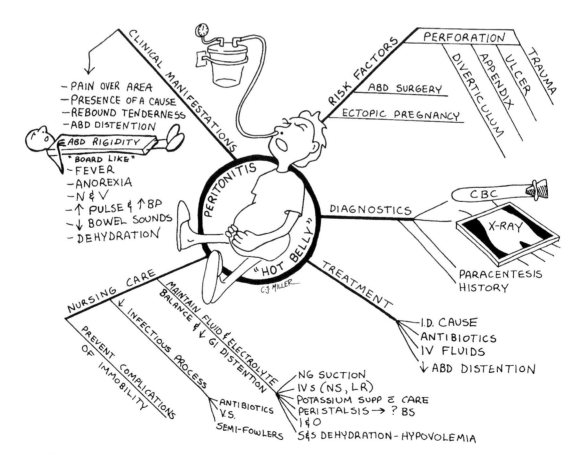

FIGURE 1–1 PERITONITIS "HOT BELLY"
From Zerwekh J, Claborn J, Miller CJ: Memory Notebook of Nursing, Vol II. Dallas, TX: Nursing Education Consultants Publishing, Inc, 1997, p. 85, with permission.

4. Teach the family how to do hourly soaks to the hand using normal saline and peroxide.

The correct answer is Option #3. Any type of animal bite that might be associated with an animal that may potentially harbor rabies (skunks, bats, raccoons, foxes, coyotes, rats) should be treated with both active and passive rabies immunization. The priority action is to prevent rabies. Tetanus antitoxin would be indicated if the child was not current on the immunization. Animal authorities would be called after the initial treatment to locate the animal and sacrifice it, so that the brain can be examined for rabies.

Techniques to Increase Critical Thinking Skills

Memory aids and mindmapping are tools that assist in drawing associations from other ideas with the use of visual images. Mnemonics are words, phrases, or other techniques that help you re-member information. Imagery is a tool that helps you identify a problem and visualize a mental picture. Learning content utilizing these techniques will assist you to recall information more effectively.

Mindmapping™ is a method of organizing important information that is in sharp contrast to the traditional outline format. A thought or concept is written in the center of the page, and images and color are added to information as ideas begin to flow from the center focus (see Fig. 1–1).

Acronyms help you to recall information via word association or arrangements of letters to recall specific information. Examples of these are the BRAT diet (see Fig. 1–2), 6-Ps of dyspnea (see Fig. 1–3), the 5-Ps of circulatory assessment (see Fig. 1–4), and the ABCs of malignant melanoma (see Fig. 1–5).

Acrostics are catchy phrases in which the first letter of each word stands for something to recall. For example, in remembering the use of canes and walkers (Fig. 1–6) think of "Wandering Wilma's Always Late" (**W**alker **W**ith **A**ffected **L**eg). Everyone remembers the cranial nerve mnemonic (see Fig. 1–7).

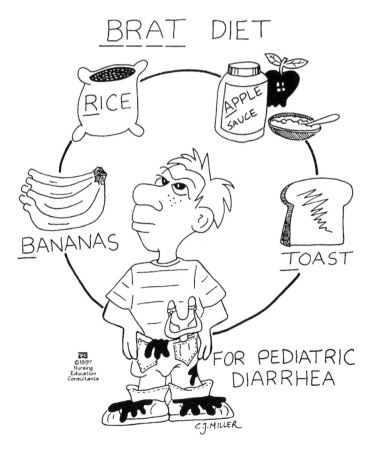

FIGURE 1–2 BRAT DIET
From Zerwekh J, Claborn J, Miller CJ: Memory Notebook of Nursing, Vol II. Dallas, TX: Nursing Education Consultants Publishing, Inc, 1997, p. 17, with permission.

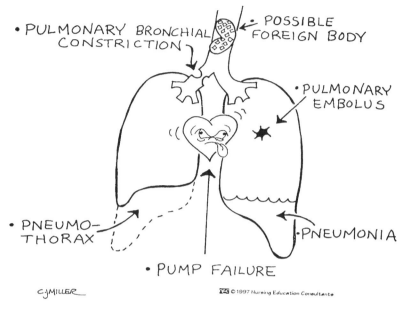

FIGURE 1–3 6-Ps OF DYSPNEA
From Zerwekh J, Claborn J, Miller CJ: Memory Notebook of Nursing, Vol II. Dallas, TX: Nursing Education Consultants Publishing, Inc, 1997, p. 22, with permission.

Memory aids or images are pictures or caricatures that help you to recall information more effectively (see Fig. 1–8).

Rhymes are phrases or words spoken in a rhythmic or musical manner that increase recall. A helpful musical rhyme for hypoglycemia versus hyperglycemia is "hot and dry, sugar high; cold and clammy, need some candy" (see Fig. 1–9). Another rhyme, "fingers, nose, penis, toes," identifies the areas where lidocaine with epinephrine is contraindicated as a local anesthetic. Or, "two is too much," may help you remember toxic levels of the following three drugs, which have a narrow margin of safety—lithium, digoxin, theophylline (see Fig. 1–10). *Note: These are just examples. There are entire books on these helpful aids (see the list of references).*

Testing Skills for Paper-and-Pencil Tests

1. Go through the exam and mark all the answers that you know are correct. This ensures you have adequate time to answer the questions you know. Go back and evaluate those questions for which you did not readily recognize the answer.

2. Do not indiscriminately change answers. If you go back and change an answer, you should have a specific reason for doing so. Sometimes you remember information and realize you answered the question incorrectly. Frequently, test-takers "talk themselves out of" the correct answer and change it to an incorrect one.

3. After you have completed the exam, go back and check your booklet and make sure all of the questions are answered. Answer all of the questions, even if you must guess.

Testing Skills that Apply to Both Paper-and-Pencil Tests and Computer Testing

1. Listen carefully to the instructions given at the beginning of the examination. Make sure you understand all of the information given and exactly how to mark your answers, and/or how to use the keyboard.

2. Watch your timing. Do not spend too much time on one question. It is very important that you practice your timing on the sample exams. When you begin to take a paper-and-

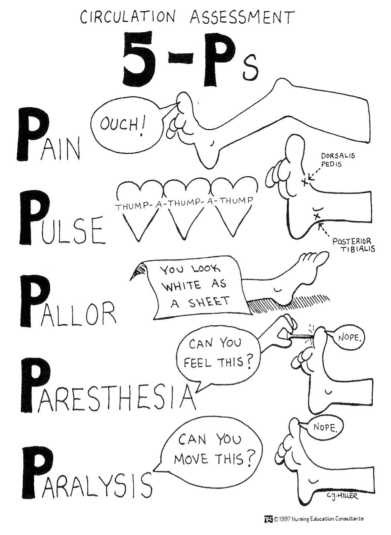

FIGURE 1–4 CIRCULATION ASSESSMENT: THE 5-Ps
From Zerwekh J, Claborn J, Miller CJ: Memory Notebook of Nursing, Vol II. Dallas, TX: Nursing Education Consultants Publishing, Inc, 1997, p. 27, with permission.

pencil test, plan on finishing within the first three fourths of the allocated time. It is not necessary to review all of the questions after you have completed the test. Do it right the first time and there is no need to review the entire test again. Go back and answer the questions that you left blank. Watch your timing on computer tests—make use of a computer clock, if it is available.

3. Be aware of your "first hunch." It is frequently the correct answer. Sometimes information is processed by the brain without you being aware of it. If something about an answer "feels right" or you have a "gut-level feeling," pay attention to it.

4. Eliminate distractors that assume the client "would not understand," or "is ignorant" of the situation, or those that "protect them from worry." For example, "The client should not be told she has cancer because it would upset her too much."

5. Be aware of distractors that contain the words *always* and *never*.

6. There is no pattern of correct answers. Both computer and paper-and-pencil examinations are compiled by a computer and the position of the correct answers is selected at random.

Decrease Anxiety

Your activities on the day of the examination strongly influence your level of anxiety. By carefully planning ahead, you will be able to eliminate some anxiety-provoking situations. If you are a diabetic or have special needs, contact the certi-

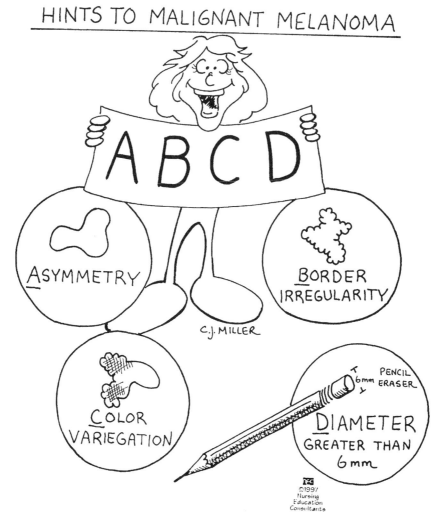

FIGURE 1–5   HINTS TO MALIGNANT MELANOMA (ABCD)
From Zerwekh J, Claborn J, Miller CJ: Memory Notebook of Nursing, Vol II. Dallas, TX: Nursing Education Consultants Publishing, Inc, 1997, p. 137, with permission.

fication agency ahead of time to make arrangements to have food or other accommodations that you might require.

1. Visit the examination site prior to the day of the exam. Evaluate travel time, parking, and time to get to the designated area. Get an early start to allow extra time.

2. If you have to travel some distance to the examination site, try to spend the night in the immediate vicinity.

3. Do something pleasant the evening prior to the examination. This is not the time to "crash study."

4. Anxiety is contagious. If those around you are extremely anxious, avoid contact with them prior to the examination.

5. Make your meal before the test a light, healthy one.

6. Avoid eating highly spiced or different foods. This is not the time for a gastrointestinal upset.

7. Wear comfortable clothes. This is not a good time to wear tight clothing or new shoes.

8. Wear clothing of moderate weight. It is difficult to control the temperature to keep everyone comfortable. Take a sweater or wear layered clothes that can be removed if you get too warm.

9. Wear soft-soled shoes; this decreases the noise in the testing area.

10. Make sure you have the papers that are required to gain admission to the exam

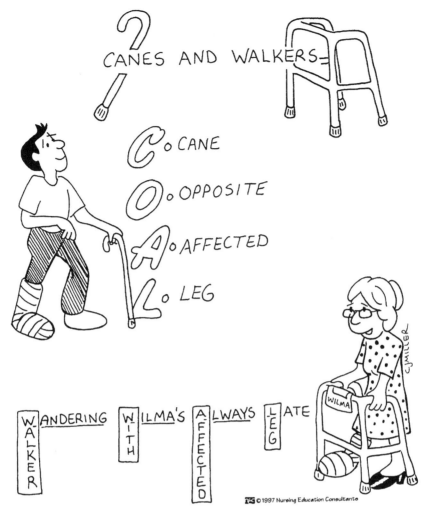

FIGURE 1–6   CANES and WALKERS
From Zerwekh J, Claborn J, Miller CJ: Memory Notebook of Nursing, Vol II. Dallas, TX: Nursing Education Consultants Publishing, Inc, 1997, p. 8, with permission.

site. Do not forget your reading glasses, if you wear them.

11. Do not take study material to the exam site. You cannot take it into the exam area and it is too late to study.

12. Do not panic when you encounter content with which you are unfamiliar in a question. Use good test-taking strategies, select an answer, and continue. Remember, you are not going to know all of the right answers.

13. Reaffirm to yourself that you know the material. It is not time for any self-defeating behavior or negative self-talk. **YOU WILL PASS!!** Build your confidence by visualizing yourself in 6 months working in the area you desire. Create that mental picture of where you want to be and who you want to be—certified nurse practitioner. Use your past successes to bring positive energy and "vibes" to your certification. **WE KNOW YOU CAN DO IT!**

Study Habits

Enhancing Study Skills

- Decide on a study schedule—write it down and stick with it.
- Divide the review material into segments—pediatrics, well woman, geriatric, and so forth.

CRANIAL NERVE MNEMONIC

| S = Sensory | M = Motor | B = Both |

O	Olfactory	O	On	S	Some
O	Optic	O	Old	S	Say
O	Oculomotor	O	Olympus'	M	Marry
T	Trochlear	T	Tiny	M	Money
T	Trigeminal	T	Tops	B	But
A	Abducens	A	A	M	My
F	Facial	F	Finn	B	Brother
A	Acoustic	A	And	S	Says
G	Glossopharyngeal	G	German	B	Bad
V	Vagus nerve	V	Viewed	B	Business
S	Spinal	S	Some	M	Marry
H	Hypoglossal	H	Hops	M	Money

© 1994 Nursing Education Consultants

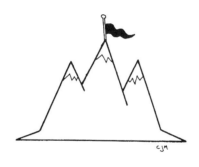

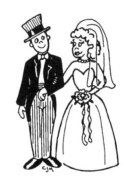

FIGURE 1–7   CRANIAL NERVE
MNEMONIC
From Zerwekh J, Claborn J, Miller CJ:
Memory Notebook of Nursing, Vol II. Dallas,
TX: Nursing Education Consultants
Publishing, Inc, 1997, p. 91, with permission.

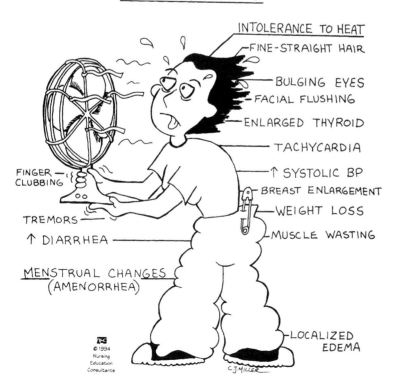

FIGURE 1–8   HYPERTHYROIDISM
From Zerwekh J, Claborn J, Miller CJ: Memory
Notebook of Nursing, Vol II. Dallas, TX: Nursing
Education Consultants Publishing, Inc, 1997, p. 46,
with permission.

BLOOD SUGAR MNEMONIC

Hot & Dry = Sugar High

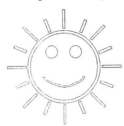

Cold & Clammy = Need Some Candy

FIGURE 1–9 BLOOD SUGAR MNEMONIC
From Zerwekh J, Claborn J, Miller CJ: Memory Notebook of Nursing, Vol II. Dallas, TX: Nursing Education Consultants Publishing, Inc, 1997, p. 50, with permission.

- Prioritize the segments; review first the areas in which you feel you are deficient and/or weak.
- Identify areas that will require additional review.
- Establish a realistic schedule—study in short segments or "bursts." Avoid marathon sessions.
- Plan on achieving your study goal several days prior to the examination.
- Do not study when you are tired or when there are frequent distractions or interruptions.
- Review general concepts of practice from a variety of resources.

Group Study

- Keep the group limited to four or five people.
- Group members should be mature and serious about studying.
- The group should agree on the planned study schedule.

- If the group makes you anxious or you do not feel it meets your study needs, do not continue to participate.

Testing Practice

- Include testing practice in your schedule.
- Select about 50 questions for a practice testing session of 1 hour. This will allow you to evaluate the pace of the exam (i.e., approximately a question per minute).
- Try to answer the questions as if you were taking the real examination. Do not look up the right answer immediately after answering the question.
- Utilize the testing strategies described in this chapter.
- Evaluate the practice exams for problem areas: testing skills and knowledge base.
- Evaluate the questions you answer incorrectly. Review the rationale for the right answer and understand why you missed it.

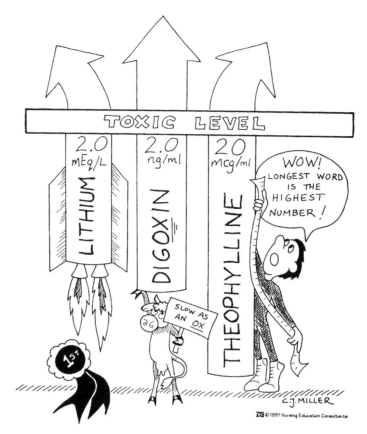

FIGURE 1–10   TOXIC LEVELS OF LITHIUM, DIGOXIN, AND THEOPHYLLINE
From Zerwekh J, Claborn J, Miller CJ: Memory Notebook of Nursing, Vol II. Dallas, TX: Nursing Education Consultants Publishing, Inc, 1997, p. 43, with permission.

• Utilize the questions at a later point to review the information again.

References

Beitz J: Unleashing the power of memory: The mighty mnemonic. *Nurse Educator*, 22(2), 25–28, 1997.

Bloomingfield R: Mnemonics, Rhetorics, and Poetics for Medics. Salem NC: Harbinger Medical Press, 1982.

Rayfield S, Manning L: Nursing Made Insanely Easy. Shreveport, LA: ICAN, Inc. Publishing, 1997.

Zerwekh J, Claborn J: Test-taking strategies. In NCLEX-RN℠: A Comprehensive Study Guide, 3rd ed. Dallas, TX: Nursing Education Consultants Publishing, Inc, 1997.

Zerwekh J, Claborn J, Miller CJ: Memory Notebook of Nursing, Vol I. Dallas, TX: Nursing Education Consultants Publishing, Inc, 1994.

Zerwekh J, Claborn J, Miller CJ: Memory Notebook of Nursing, Vol II. Dallas, TX: Nursing Education Consultants Publishing, Inc, 1997.

Growth & Development

Physical Assessment

1. The following is the sequence recommended for well-child examinations up to the age of 5:

   1. 2 weeks, 2 months, 4 months, 6 months, 1 year, 15 months, 18 months, and every year from age 2–5.

   2. 2 months, 4 months, 6 months, 9 months, and annually from years 1–5.

   3. 2 weeks, 2 months, 4 months, 6 months, 9 months, 12 months, 15 months, 18 months, and annually years 2–5.

   4. The same intervals recommended for immunizations.

2. An appropriate treatment for overweight children under 8 years of age would include:

   1. Administer an appetite suppressant.

   2. Eliminate all carbohydrates in the diet.

   3. Plan a program of activity and exercise.

   4. Use vitamin therapy and herbal teas.

3. The nurse practitioner is seeing a 2-week-old newborn on the first clinic visit. She notes dysmorphic facial features. The nurse practitioner's evaluation includes:

   1. Ordering a chromosome analysis.

   2. Complete postnatal history.

   3. Detailed physical examination and perinatal history.

   4. Avoiding discussion with parents until diagnostic studies are completed.

4. An 18-month-old's feet turned inward. The mother is concerned; however, the child is unaware of it. The differential diagnosis includes all **except**:

   1. Femoral anteversion.

   2. Metatarsus adductus.

   3. Legg-Calvé-Perthes disease.

   4. Adducted great toe.

5. The characteristics of an innocent heart murmur in children include:

   1. Asymptomatic, loud diastolic rumble, grade I–V.

   2. Midsystolic, no thrill, and asymptomatic.

   3. Asymptomatic with an S_4 heard at left lower sternal border.

   4. May disappear on sitting and following any type of physical activity.

6. The nurse practitioner is examining a 6-month-old-infant. What would be the anticipated findings on examining the infant's fontanels?

   1. Both anterior and posterior should be open.

   2. The anterior should be open, the posterior closed.

   3. Both anterior and posterior should be closed.

   4. The anterior should be closed, the posterior open.

7. Genu varum up to 20 degrees is normal until age:

   1. 18 years old.

   2. 5 years old.

   3. 18 months old.

   4. 6 months old.

8. When approaching a toddler to complete a cardiac assessment, the nurse practitioner would:

   1. Allow the toddler to handle the stethoscope while the history is being taken.

   2. Explain in detail what you are going to do and get the toddler involved.

   3. Keep the child warm and covered to minimize discomfort.

   4. Approach the child by cheerfully calling his name out.

9. In performing a physical examination, the nurse practitioner first allows the child to touch the medical equipment and then begins by examining the extremities. This sequence would be most appropriate to use for what age client?

   1. Infant.

   2. Toddler.

   3. School-age child.

   4. Adolescent.

10. An appropriate test to check for color perception in a preschooler would be:

    1. Ishihara's test.

    2. Bruchner's test.

    3. Hirschberg's test.

    4. Jaeger's test.

11. When assessing the cranial nerves in a young child, the nurse practitioner should:

    1. Obtain help from the parents to enlist the child's cooperation.

    2. Defer assessing the cranial nerve until the child is older.

    3. Modify the technique of examination based on the child's developmental level.

    4. Expect minimal variations among age groups.

12. The nurse practitioner understands the following about the Denver Developmental Screening Test Revised (DDST-R or Denver II):

    1. It is a measurement of intelligence (IQ).

    2. It screens personal/social, fine and gross motor, and language.

    3. It is conducted when the examiner pronounces words and the child repeats.

    4. It is used for ages 0–36 months.

13. Genu valgum is considered normal from:

    1. 1–2 years old.

    2. 2–6 years old.

    3. 8–10 years old.

    4. 12–16 years old.

14. An African-American mother and her newborn are seen by the nurse practitioner for a well-baby visit. The mother is responsive to the baby's cries, and the baby comforts easily and makes frequent eye contact with the mother. Upon examination, the nurse practitioner notes the following: height and weight are at the 75th percentile on growth charts, there is a strong sucking reflex, and there is a large blue-black macular lesion over the lumbosacral area. The nurse practitioner should:

    1. Contact a social worker and report the mother to Child Protective Services immediately.

    2. Refer the mother and infant to a dermatologist.

    3. Recognize that the blue-black spot is a Mongolian spot, and counsel the mother that no treatment is necessary.

    4. Prescribe clotrimazole cream 1% (Mycelex) bid for 4 weeks.

15. The plantar fat pad, which makes a young child appear to have pes planus, is normal until age:

    1. 1–2 years old.

    2. 2–3 years old.

    3. 2–6 years old.

    4. 6–8 years old.

16. Growth hormone secretion tests along with a history and physical exam have indicated a positive diagnosis for delayed puberty. The next step for the nurse practitioner is to:

    1. Treat with hormone replacement.

    2. Refer to pediatric endocrinologist.

    3. Treat with hormone stimulation therapy.

    4. Refer for possible pituitary tumor.

17. During the physical examination of a 13-year-old female, it is developmentally important that the nurse practitioner:

    1. Maintain a comfortable silence.

    2. Verbally affirm normalcy.

    3. Discuss only the major areas of abnormality.

    4. Verbally address problems of sexually transmitted diseases.

18. At a school clinic, a 14-year-old girl comes in complaining of dizziness midmorning and a second episode in class that morning. The practitioner should question the adolescent regarding diet/nutrition, drug use, and:

    1. Asthma.

    2. Pregnancy.

    3. Heart disease.

    4. Stress.

19. The nurse practitioner understands that sulfa medications are not recommended for children less than which age?

    1. 18 months.

    2. 12 months.

    3. 6 months.

    4. 2 months.

Growth & Development

20. The major influence on the timing of puberty is:

    1. Exposure to light.

    2. Genetics.

    3. General health.

    4. Nutrition.

21. A 14-year-old girl is seen in the clinic by the nurse practitioner because she has not achieved menarche. Examination reveals axillary and pubic hair and breast buds with increased size of areola. Based on these findings the most appropriate intervention would be:

    1. Bone age studies.

    2. Labs for luteinizing hormone (LH) and follicle-stimulating hormone (FSH) levels.

    3. Chromosome analysis to rule out Turner's syndrome.

    4. Reassurance that she is developing normally.

22. A 13-year-old male is seen by the nurse practitioner for a sports physical. The genital exam reveals straight dark pubic hair at the base of the penis and testicular enlargement. Using the Tanner scale, the nurse practitioner would record these findings as:

    1. Tanner stage I.
    2. Tanner stage II.
    3. Tanner stage III.
    4. Tanner stage IV.

23. An 11-year-old girl who has just begun to show signs of breast development asks the nurse practitioner when she will start having periods like her friends? The nurse practitioner's response is based on the knowledge that:

    1. The average age of menarche is 12.8 years.
    2. Most girls will have a growth spurt following the onset of menarche.
    3. Menarche usually occurs about 3–6 months after the onset of breast development.
    4. Menarche usually occurs about 18–24 months after the onset of breast development.

24. A teenage girl with curly pubic hair on the mons pubis and breast enlargement without secondary contour would be classified on the Tanner scale as:

    1. Tanner stage I.
    2. Tanner stage II.
    3. Tanner stage III.
    4. Tanner stage IV.

25. A mother of a 2-year-old brings her child to see the nurse practitioner because he has been irritable and has a small "knot" under his left ear. The child has no history of fever, upper respiratory infection, or pulling at his ears. The most likely reason for these symptoms is:

    1. Otitis media.
    2. Teething.
    3. Tonsillitis.
    4. Otitis externa.

26. A routine well-child visit for a healthy full-term infant should include a hemoglobin and hematocrit at:

    1. 1 month of age.
    2. 4 months of age.
    3. 6–9 months of age.
    4. 1 year of age.

27. The mother of a 3-month-old infant is concerned because her baby seems to sleep most of the time. The nurse practitioner's response is based on the knowledge that a 3-month-old infant usually spends:

    1. 10 hours in 24 sleeping.
    2. 15–16 hours in 24 sleeping.
    3. 18–19 hours in 24 sleeping.
    4. Most of the 24 hours sleeping, waking only to eat.

28. What advice should the nurse practitioner give a mother who reports during a routine well-child exam that her 5-month-old (weight, 15 lb) who was sleeping all night at 3 months of age is now waking up in the middle of the night hungry. A diet history reveals that the infant is taking six 6-oz bottles of formula in a 24-hour period and has 2 tbsp of rice cereal in the morning.

    1. Increase the amount of formula at each feeding to 8 oz.
    2. Take the child off formula and switch to homogenized milk.
    3. Decrease the amount of formula to 32 oz in 24 hours and add fruits, cereals, and juices.
    4. Continue the same amount of formula and introduce a variety of baby foods.

29. The father of a 12-year-old male tells the nurse practitioner that he is afraid that his son is getting "fat." The child is at the 50th percentile for height and the 75th percentile for weight on the growth chart. The most appropriate response would be:

    1. Reassure the father that the son is not "fat."
    2. Assess family for presence of obesity.

3. Suggest a low-calorie, low-fat diet.

4. Explain that this is typical of the growth pattern of boys at this age.

30. A mother asks the nurse practitioner if an infant walker will help her 6-month-old to learn to walk faster. The nurse practitioner's response is based on the knowledge that:

    1. Infant walkers help to strengthen the infant's extremities and prepare them to walk.

    2. Infants who are placed in walkers usually walk about 1 month earlier than other infants.

    3. Infant walkers are dangerous and should not be recommended for use.

    4. There have been very few injuries related to the use of infant mobile walkers.

31. The mother of a 6-month-old infant tells the nurse practitioner that the baby was spitting up his formula so she put him on goat milk. The nurse practitioner is concerned because goat milk places the infant at risk of developing:

    1. Rickets.

    2. Scurvy.

    3. Folic acid deficiency.

    4. Botulism.

32. A 1-year-old reaches for the nurse practitioner's stethoscope with his left hand and the father says, "It looks like he is going to be a lefty just like his old man!" The nurse's response is based on the knowledge that:

    1. Male infants usually have the same hand preference as their fathers.

    2. Hand preference is well established by 9 months of age.

    3. Children will not demonstrate a hand preference until about age 6.

    4. Children usually develop handedness by 18–24 months.

33. A mother is concerned that her 7-month-old breast-fed infant is not getting enough to eat. The infant weighed 7 lb 8 oz at birth and was 19 inches long. At 6 months of age, he weighed 15 lb and was 25 inches long. He now weighs 15 lb and is 25½ inches long. The nurse practitioner's response is based on the knowledge that:

    1. Infants should gain 2–4 oz/wk and ½ inch in height a month during the first six months of life.

    2. Infants should triple their birth weight by 6 months of age.

    3. Infants should gain 3–4 oz/wk and ½ inch in height a month from 6–12 months of age.

    4. Infants should gain 1–2 oz/wk and 1 inch in height a month from 6–12 months of age.

34. A child will be able to do which of the following fine motor skills first?

    1. Imitate a circle.

    2. Copy a square.

    3. Copy a triangle.

    4. Copy a diamond.

35. The nurse practitioner would expect a child to follow a one-step command given without a gesture and using only four to six individual words at what age?

    1. 7 months.

    2. 9 months.

    3. 14 months.

    4. 20 months.

36. The nurse practitioner knows that language is the best single measure of normal cognitive development in early childhood. At what age do children begin to combine two words together?

    1. 8–10 months.

    2. 10–12 months.

    3. 12–15 months.

    4. 14–23 months.

37. A mother of 2-year-old twins is concerned that the twins do not talk very much and seem to have their own "private" language. The nurse practitioner should:

    1. Tell the mother to spend some individual time with the twins so that they learn language skills.

    2. Perform a pure tone audiometry.

    3. Tell the mother that this is normal for twins or siblings that are close in age.

    4. Refer to a speech pathologist for further testing.

38. The nurse practitioner notices that a 9-month-old infant who was born 2 months prematurely only reaches for an object with his left hand. The nurse would:

    1. Record these findings as normal for a premature infant.

    2. Refer the infant for further evaluation.

    3. Order a muscle biopsy to rule out muscular dystrophy.

    4. Make a note on the chart that the child will probably be left-handed.

39. The mother of a 6-month-old infant tells the nurse practitioner that her infant is now taking homogenized milk instead of an iron-fortified infant formula. The nurse practitioner's response would be based on the knowledge that:

    1. Homogenized milk has the same solute load as formula and is a safe alternative to iron-fortified formula if vitamin supplements are given.

    2. There is an increased incidence of occult gastrointestinal bleeding and the development of iron deficiency anemia in infants fed homogenized milk before 1 year of age.

    3. Once the infant is taking solid foods regularly, there is no need to continue offering iron-fortified formula.

    4. Homogenized milk has too high of a fat content and needs to be diluted 2:1 with water.

40. The development of the male sexual characteristics in utero is dependent on:

    1. Estrogen.

    2. Progesterone.

    3. Prolactin.

    4. Testosterone.

41. The production of sperm usually begins during the:

    1. Eighth week of gestation.

    2. Beginning of puberty.

    3. End of puberty.

    4. Eighth month of gestation.

42. What is true about the developmental process of sperm or spermatozoa?

    1. Each mature sperm contains 23 chromosomes.

    2. Sperm become motile immediately at maturation.

    3. Spermatogenesis takes place in the prostate.

    4. Higher than body temperature contributes to sperm production.

43. What is produced by the testes?

    1. Alkaline phosphate.

    2. Gonadotropin.

    3. Testosterone only.

    4. Acid phosphate.

44. Which statement is correct concerning healthy sexual developmental tasks?

    1. At 9 years of age, children are less self-conscious and readily expose themselves to younger children or parents of the opposite sex.

    2. At 16 years of age, adolescents are significantly influenced by the media in terms of sexual content and conduct.

    3. At 4 years of age, children distinguish organs associated with each sex and demonstrate increased sexual curiosity.

    4. At 5 years of age, children begin to have concerns about body image and begin to investigate their own sexual organs.

45. The nurse practitioner understands the following about birth defects and growth and development problems in mother's with prenatal alcohol exposure:

 1. If alcohol is ingested late in the pregnancy, there is a higher incidence of postmaturity syndrome.

 2. The practice of drinking alcohol while eating a meal significantly reduces the risk of fully expressed fetal alcohol syndrome.

 3. If alcohol is ingested in large amounts early in the pregnancy, there is an increased incidence of fully expressed clinical features.

 4. Growth retardation is associated with early trimester alcohol consumption and postmaturity syndrome.

46. In response to a young adult male's question concerning the production of sperm, the nurse practitioner knows that sperm is produced in the:

 1. Epididymis.

 2. Vas deferens.

 3. Prostate.

 4. Seminiferous tubules.

47. An adolescent female with breast budding and sparse, straight, lightly pigmented pubic hair along medial border of labia is at which Tanner Stage of Sexual Maturity?

 1. Stage I.

 2. Stage II.

 3. Stage III.

 4. Stage IV.

48. Precocious puberty is defined as:

 1. Onset of puberty before age 8 in females and 9 in males.

 2. Onset of puberty before age 5 in females and 7 in males.

 3. Onset of puberty before age 10 in females and 12 in males.

 4. Onset of puberty for either sex before older siblings enter puberty.

49. The mother of a 5-month-old infant brings her child to the clinic because the infant awakens frequently at night and cries. The nurse practitioner understands that the most common cause of night awakening in healthy infants is:

 1. Night terrors and nightmares.

 2. Separation anxiety.

 3. Trained night crying.

 4. Hunger pain and wet diaper.

50. A 10-day-old breast-fed infant is brought to the clinic because the mother is concerned about the infant's "yellow-orange" color. History and findings are as follows: Mother's blood type AB-positive, infant's blood type B-negative, total bilirubin 15 mg/dl. The nurse practitioner understands that this is most likely due to:

 1. Hemolytic jaundice.

 2. Breast-fed jaundice.

 3. Obstructive jaundice.

 4. Physiologic jaundice.

51. A new mother presents to the clinic inquiring about when she should start feeding her 2-month-old infant solid foods. The nurse practitioner should recommend that the mother:

 1. Start the infant on meat and eggs now.

 2. Wait until the infant is 1 year old before introducing solid foods.

 3. Start the infant on cereals now.

 4. Introduce one new food at a time when the infant is 4–6 months old, based on the readiness of the child.

Aging

52. As an individual ages, which physiologic change would affect responses to pharmacologic agents?

 1. Increased gastric emptying.

 2. Increased glomerular filtration rate.

 3. Decreased percentage of body fat.

 4. Decreased albumin concentration.

53. The number one cause of accidental death in clients older than 65 years of age is:

    1. Motor vehicle accidents.
    2. Poisoning.
    3. Falls.
    4. Drowning.

54. The nurse practitioner selects which assessment tool to evaluate balance and gait problems in the elderly?

    1. Lawton & Brody Balance and Coordination Scale.
    2. Tinetti Balance and Gait Evaluation.
    3. Instrumental Activities of Daily Living Scale.
    4. Index of Independence of Activities of Daily Living.

55. The nurse practitioner is assessing the nutritional status of an elderly client. The nurse practitioner identifies the common physiological changes in the gastrointestinal (GI) system to be:

    1. Increased peristalsis.
    2. Decreased absorption of iron.
    3. Maintenance of normal fat metabolism.
    4. Increased drug metabolism.

56. What are the normal physiologic changes in the thyroid gland that occur with aging?

    1. Hypertrophy with a decrease in the triiodothyronine (T3) and thyroxine (T4).
    2. Normal size with an increase in thyroid-stimulating hormone (TSH) and a decrease in T_4.
    3. Atrophy of the gland with a decrease in TSH, T_3, and T_4.
    4. Increase in nodularity with normal TSH and T_4.

57. The aging process causes what normal physiological changes in the heart?

    1. Heart size stays the same, and the valves thicken and become rigid secondary to fibrosis and sclerosis.
    2. Cardiomegaly occurs along with prolapse of the mitral valve and regurgitation.
    3. Dilatation of the right ventricle with sclerosis of pulmonic and tricuspid valves.
    4. Hypertrophy of the right ventricle with decreasing capacity and compromised efficiency of the coronary arteries.

58. Which pulmonary physiologic change is commonly associated with the aging process?

    1. Increased cough response.
    2. Decrease in vital capacity.
    3. Decreased anteroposterior (AP) diameter of thorax.
    4. Increase in residual P_{CO_2}.

59. Which of these clinical findings would indicate a deviation from the normal age-related changes in the neurologic system and may have some diagnostic significance for the older client?

    1. Decreased sense of touch.
    2. Increased tolerance to pain.
    3. Decreased short-term memory.
    4. Decreased ability to maintain balance.

60. During a teaching session, the nurse practitioner instructs the client regarding normal skin lesions in the older population. These would include:

    1. Seborrheic dermatitis.
    2. Senile keratosis.
    3. Senile lentigines.
    4. Squamous cell.

61. Which assessment is a normal physiologic change of the respiratory system that occurs with aging?

    1. Decreased residual lung volume (RV).
    2. Hyperresonance.
    3. Increased forced vital capacity (FVC).
    4. Increased tactile fremitus.

62. The nurse practitioner indicates an understanding of the normal aging process with which documentation of the GI system in the physical examination?

    1. Increase in the size of the liver (16 cm).

    2. Absent bowel sounds.

    3. Femoral bruit.

    4. Increased adipose tissue.

63. During the physical examination of an older client, the nurse practitioner indicates an understanding of deviations in the neurologic system from the normal aging processs with which clinical finding?

    1. Decrease in short-term memory.

    2. Decrease in deep tendon and superficial reflexes.

    3. Decreased sense of touch.

    4. Positive Romberg's sign.

64. Which functional assessment tool should the nurse practitioner use to evaluate the safety for a cerebrovascular accident (CVA) client planning to return to his home environment?

    1. OARS ADL Scale.

    2. Bennet Social Isolation Scales.

    3. Mini Mental State Examination.

    4. Norton Scale.

65. The nurse practitioner understands which factor is most influential in the driving ability of an older adult?

    1. Ability to coordinate the transmissions.

    2. Acuity of vision.

3. Comprehension of the details of the road rules.

4. Reaction times.

66. As an individual ages, which physiologic change would affect sleep?

    1. Decreased rapid-eye-movement (REM) sleep.

    2. Increased delta or stage IV sleep.

    3. Decreased nocturnal awakenings.

    4. Decreased sleep latency.

67. When treating an infection in the older adult, the nurse practitioner must consider:

    1. Thymus-derived immunity is increased.

    2. Immune function declines with age.

    3. Immune function increases with age.

    4. Antibody production increases.

68. The diminished immunity of the older adult can be attributed to a decline in:

    1. B-cell function.

    2. T-cell production.

    3. B-cell production.

    4. T-cell function.

69. Which physiologic factor of aging contributes to incontinence in the elderly?

    1. Decreased vascularity of the bladder mucosa.

    2. Increased urethral closing pressure.

    3. Increased ability to concentrate urine.

    4. Decreased bladder capacity.

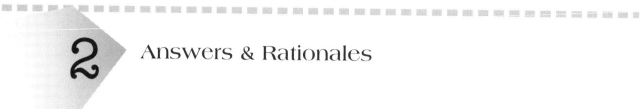

Answers & Rationales

Physical Assessment

1. **(3)** These are the recommended health evaluation intervals for children to obtain regular assessment information regarding growth and development and to administer recommended immunizations.

2. **(3)** An approach with a well-balanced diet, activity, and exercise are necessary for weight reduction. This allows for a slow approach to weight loss that incorporates healthy behavior habits.

3. **(3)** The first and most important part of all data gathering starts with a detailed history and physical examination. A detailed, objective description of the dysmorphic features is essential for comparison to textbook descriptions, and so forth. Although chromosome analysis will probably be ordered, it is not done initially. Parents should be included in the discussion of findings and be kept informed of the progress throughout all the evaluation process.

4. **(3)** In-toeing is a common problem and can result from femoral anteversion, adduction of the great toe, medial tibial torsion, and metatarsus adductus. Legg-Calvé-Perthes disease is commonly seen in older children (ages 4–8 years) with loss of hip medial rotation.

5. **(2)** Characteristics of innocent murmurs include: midsystolic, asymptomatic, less than a grade III, loudest in pulmonic area (2–3 left intercostal space at the left sternal border [LSB]), no radiation to other areas, may disappear on sitting, may intensify with fever, activity, anemia, and stress. Any S_4 sound is considered pathologic in children, as well as adults.

6. **(2)** The posterior fontanel is usually closed by 2 months of age; the anterior fontanel closes around 24 months of age.

7. **(3)** Genu varum (bow legs) of 20 degrees is normal up to the age of 18 months.

8. **(1)** Toddlers like to make the first move (i.e., let them move closer and initiate eye contact first, don't call out their name—it may frighten them). Allowing them to handle the stethoscope will decrease their fear. Option #2 is more appropriate when assessing a school-age child.

9. **(2)** Allow a toddler to explore the instruments and start with the extremities. Save the most invasive examination (of the head) for last. In infants, auscultate the heart and lungs while the infant is quiet and then proceed to do a head-to-toe assessment. In the school-age and adolescent, a head-to-toe sequence is preferred.

10. **(1)** Ishihara's—tests for color perception; Bruchner's—tests for the red reflex; Hirschberg's—tests corneal light reflex; Jaeger's—tests near vision.

11. **(3)** Assessing cranial nerves can be a challenging task for the nurse practitioner; consequently, she should employ techniques that take into consideration the child's developmental level.

12. **(2)** The DDST-R is used for infants through age 5½ years. It is interpreted as normal, suspect, or untestable and measures personal/social area, fine and gross motor skills, and language. Option #3 is the Denver Articulation Screening Exam (DASE) and Option #4 refers to the age group used for the Early Language Milestone Scale (ELM).

13. **(2)** Genu valgum (knock knee) is considered normal from the age of 2 to the age of 6.

14. **(3)** Mongolian spot are commonly found in African-American, Hispanic, Native American, and Oriental infants. These spots are benign, and tend to fade and disappear by age 3, requiring no intervention/treatment. Abuse is not suspected because signs of a healthy mother–infant relationship are noted, namely, mother and infant respond positively to one another, and the baby is thriving.

15. **(2)** The plantar fat pad is normal to the age of 2–3 years old.

16. **(2)** Once the tentative diagnosis is made, the nurse practitioner should refer to a pediatric endocrinologist for further work-up. It is beyond the scope of the practitioner's practice to treat at this point.

17. **(2)** Early adolescence is a time when the child undergoing great physical changes continually wonders if they are normal. Verbal affirmation of areas of normalcy during the exam can decrease anxiety.

18. **(2)** Although all areas would be assessed, pregnancy is a common reason for midmorning syncope in adolescents—associated with altered nutrition.

19. **(4)** Newborns and infants up to age 2 months may develop kernicterus as sulfas displace bilirubin from the plasma proteins.

Growth & Development

20. **(2)** Genetics is the primary determinant of the timing of puberty. Other factors including geographic location, exposure to light, nutritional status, and health status all play a role, but genetics is the major influence.

21. **(4)** Menarche usually occurs about 18–24 months after the onset of breast development. Bone age and labs are not necessary, since development is within the normal limits. The findings are not indicative of a chromosomal abnormality; therefore, chromosome analysis is unnecessary.

22. **(2)**

Stage	Pubic Hair
I	None
II	Countable; straight; increased pigmentation and length
III	Darker; begins to curl; increased quantity
IV	Increased quantity; coarser texture; covers most of pubic area
V	Adult distribution; spread to medial thighs and lower abdomen

	Genital Development
I	Prepubertal
II	Testicular enlargement; slight rugation of scrotum
III	Further testicular enlargement; penile lengthening begins
IV	Testicular enlargement continues; increased rugation of scrotum; increased penile length
V	Adult

23. **(4)** Menarche usually occurs about 18–24 months after the onset of breast development. The average age of menarche is 12.8 years, but that is not what the nurse practitioner should base her response on. Most girls have a growth spurt at Tanner stage IV.

24. **(3)**

Stage	Pubic Hair
I	None
II	Countable; straight; increased pigmentation and length
III	Darker; begins to curl; increased quantity on mons pubis
IV	Increased quantity; coarser texture; labia and mons well covered
V	Adult distribution; with feminine triangle and spread to medial thighs

	Breast Development
I	None
II	Breast bud present; increased areolar size
III	Further enlargement of breast; no secondary contour
IV	Areolar area forms secondary mound on breast contour
V	Mature; areolar area of part of breast contour; nipple project

25. **(2)** At approximately 20 months of age, the lower second molars erupt and at 24 months of age the upper second molars erupt. With a history of irritability and lymph node enlargement without fever or other symptoms, it is the most likely cause of discomfort.

26. **(3)** It is important in a healthy infant to check the hemoglobin and hematocrit between 6 and 9 months of age when the maternal hemoglobin stores have been depleted. Before 4 months of age, the infant has not depleted his hemoglobin stores. One would not want to wait until 1 year of age to check hemoglobin.

27. **(2)** Normally 3-month-old infants sleep 15–16 hours in a 24-hour period.

28. **(3)** Consumption of 32 oz of formula per day is usually an indicator of the need for solids. Formula is recommended for the first year of life. Nutritional requirements are 110–120 cal/kg/day. Introduction of solids usually occurs between 4 and 6 months of age.

29. **(4)** It is normal for boys at this age to appear heavier before they get their "growth spurt." Reassuring the father, although appropriate, is not the best response. Since the findings are within normal limits, it would not be necessary to assess the family for the presence of obesity. Low-calorie, low-fat diets are contraindicated for the growing child.

30. **(3)** The American Academy of Pediatrics Committee on Injury and Poison Control made a statement in *Pediatrics* 95:778–780 recommending a ban on the manufacture and sale of mobile infant walkers. Infant walkers may delay crawling. Up to 35% of infants who use walkers sustain an injury requiring medical attention. Stairs are a very real danger and have caused deaths.

31. **(3)** Goat milk can cause folic acid deficiency, which can lead to megaloblastic anemia. Rickets is caused by the lack of vitamin D. Scurvy is caused by a lack of ascorbic acid in the diet. Botulism is food poisoning caused by an endotoxin produced by the bacillus *Clostridium botulinum*. Most botulism occurs after eating improperly canned or cooked foods. Infants have been known to develop botulism from raw honey that is placed on their pacifiers.

32. **(4)** Children usually develop handedness by 18–24 months. The hand preference is usually fixed after 5 years of age.

33. **(3)** Infants should gain 3–4 oz/wk and ½ inch in height a month from 6–12 months of age. This child also doubled its birth weight by 6 months of age as expected.

	Weight	Length/Height
0–6 months	6–8 oz/wk (doubles birth weight by 5–7 months)	1 in/mo
6–12 months	3–4 oz/wk (triples birth weight by 1 year)	½ in/mo

34. **(1)** A child should be able to imitate a circle at 30 months, copy a square at 4 years, copy a triangle at 5 years, and copy a diamond at 6 years.

35. **(3)** A child should be expected to follow a one-step command given without a gesture and using only four to six individual words between 10.5 and 16.5 months of age.

36. **(4)** Two-word combinations are expected at 14–23 months of age.

37. **(3)** It is normal for twins or sibling close in age to develop a "private" language understood only by them. Although it is important for the mother to spend individual time with each child, that is not what the question is asking. Pure-tone audiometry is done after age 3. There is no need for a referral to a speech pathologist at this time.

38. **(2)** The infant should be referred for further evaluation. Handedness before 1 year of age may be an early sign of cerebral palsy. The history of prematurity could be an indication of anoxia at birth and would warrant further investigation. The earlier a child is diagnosed; the earlier intervention can be started.

39. **(2)** Homogenized milk does not have the same solute load as formula and is not a safe alternative to iron-fortified formula even if vitamin supplements are given. The solute load of whole milk is too hard on the infant's immature kidneys. The infant needs to continue taking iron-fortified formula for the first year of life if at all possible. There is an increased incidence of occult gastrointestinal bleeding and the development of iron deficiency anemia in infants fed homogenized milk before 1 year of age.

40. **(4)** The most important sex hormone, during embryonic development, is the primary male sex hormone, testosterone. Testosterone is produced by the gonads of the genetic male embryo causing the male gonads to develop into two testes, which produce sperm. The other hormones are female hormones. Estrogen, the major female hormone, is produced by the ovaries (ovarian follicle and corpus luteum) and cortices of the adrenal glands and placenta during pregnancy. Progesterone, the second major female hormone, is produced by the corpus luteum. Prolactin is an anterior pituitary hormone and one of the somatotropic hormones that are secreted by lactotropic cells and target the breast to cause milk production.

41. **(3)** Between the ages of 9 and 12 years the gonads produce more of the sex hormones, which triggers sexual maturation or puberty. Puberty in males begins at approximately age 11 and lasts for 2–3 years, ending with the first ejaculation that contains mature sperm.

42. **(1)** Each mature sperm develops from mitotic division of diploid (46-chromosome) germ cells (spermatogonium) found on the basement membrane of each seminiferous tubule and become primary spermatocytes with 23 chromosomes each. Each of these two cells further divide into two more cells (spermatids) with each having 23 chromosomes. Motility is dependent on the biochemicals in semen and in the female reproductive tract. Sperm production needs a temperature that is less than body temperature by at least 1°–2°F.

43. **(2)** The testes have two functions: the production of gonadotropin (androgens and testosterone) and the production of gametes (sperm). The sperm are produced in the seminiferous tubules of the testes. The androgens and testosterone are produced mainly by Leydig cells of the testes (androgens and testosterone are also produced by the adrenal glands).

44. **(2)** Adolescents are greatly influenced by the media and tend to identify with their parents as sexually functioning people. At age 9, children are more interested in their own body and are quite self-conscious. Option #3 is true for 6-year-olds, not 4-year-olds. Option #4 is true for 10-year-olds.

45. **(3)** Large amounts of alcohol early in the pregnancy have the most devastating effects on the maturing fetus. There is no safe, established dose for alcohol in pregnancy. Food consumption along with alcohol intake does not reduce the risk of defects. Ingesting alcohol in the later months of pregnancy is associated with an increased incidence of premature and small-for-gestational-age neonates.

46. **(4)** Sperm is produced in the seminiferous tubules of the testes.

47. **(2)** Tanner has five stages of sexual maturity for both males and females; stage I for both is preadolescent and stage V for both is mature or adult development. Stages II, III, and IV chronicle development of breasts, pubic hair distribution, penis, and testis. This young female is demonstrating characteristics of Tanner stage II. (See table in rationale for question 24.)

48. **(1)** Precocious puberty is defined as that which begins at age 8 for females and age 9 for males.

49. **(3)** Trained night crying can become a problem in infants who are not allowed to learn to self-quiet. Activities such as rocking to sleep, exciting play activities before bedtime, and picking the infant up as soon as he cries can lead to trained night crying. Separation anxiety occurs in infants after 6 months of age. The majority of infants after 4 months of age are able to sleep through the night. Nightmares and night terrors occur at a later age.

50. **(2)** This is a type of exaggerated physiologic jaundice that occurs frequently in breast-fed babies due to the infant's inadequate caloric intake that occurs prior to her milk coming in. It typically occurs between 7 and 15 days of life, whereas physiologic jaundice occurs most commonly after the third day of life. Hemolytic jaundice occurs in an Rh-negative mother who has an Rh-positive infant that becomes isoimmunized.

51. **(4)** Solid foods are not recommended until the infant is 4–6 months old. Cereals should be introduced first, followed by fruits, vegetables, meats, and eggs. All foods should be introduced based on the readiness of the child.

Aging

52. **(4)** Medications are often protein bound (not fat); albumin decreases with age. A low albumin level decreases the number of protein-binding sites, causing an increase in the amount of free drug in the plasma. Drug overdose may occur in the elderly. Gastric emptying and glomerular filtration rate *decrease* with the aging process.

53. **(3)** Falls are the major cause of morbidity and mortality in the elderly. A fall is often the precipitating event for a cascade of problems leading to death. Complications from falls include fractures, pneumonia, pressure ulcers, pain, and immobility.

54. **(2)** The Tinetti Balance and Gait Evaluation is an activity-based test that asks the client to perform tasks, such as sitting and rising from a chair, turning, and bending it. It requires no more than 15–20 minutes to perform. Another appropriate test for assessment of falls is the timed "Up and Go" test, which assesses balance and gait speed. Lawton and Brody are the authors of the Instrumental Activities of Daily Learning, which assesses complex tasks such as shopping, laundry, food preparation, and so forth. The Index of Independence of Activities of Daily Living helps to identify activities of daily living (ADL) with which the client needs assistance.

55. **(2)** Decreased hydrochloric acid, which occurs with aging, leads to decreased absorption of iron and vitamin B_{12}. Fat absorption would decrease, as would peristalsis and drug metabolism.

56. **(4)** There is usually adequate secretion of TSH and a normal serum concentration of T_4. Aging may produce fibrosis and increased nodularity, but overall the thyroid function remains within normal limits.

57. **(1)** The heart does not increase in size with normal aging. An enlarged heart is a result of cardiac dysfunction. Dilatation of the left ventricle occurs with myocardial infarctions and altered cardiac functioning secondary to cardiac disease, not normal aging. The aging process does cause fibrosis and sclerosis of the cardiac valves; all valves are equally affected.

58. **(2)** A decrease in the vital capacity, along with a 50% increase in residual volume, occurs during the aging process. Other aging changes include a less effective cough, impaired ciliary action, and weaker respiratory muscles. Increased AP diameter is associated with aging and in chronic obstructive pulmonary disease (COPD) clients. PO_2 usually decreases, but PCO_2 usually remains unchanged.

59. **(4)** This may indicate a cerebellar complication. The first three findings are normal age-related changes.

60. **(3)** The senile lentigo is a gray-brown, irregular, macular lesion on sun-exposed areas of the face, arms, and hands that are normal skin lesions. The other lesions are commonly occurring abnormal skin lesions in the older adult.

61. **(2)** A normal age-related change is an increase in the AP diameter that results in hyperresonance. Age-related changes result in an increase in the RV and decrease in the FVC. An increased tactile fremitus is a deviation that is of diagnostic significance.

62. **(4)** Common age-related changes with the GI system include increased adipose tissue, decrease in liver size, reduced motility and peristalsis, decrease in acid secretions and motor activity of stomach, and decrease in the glomerular filtration rate. Absence of bowel sounds after 5 full minutes and bruits are deviations of clinical significance.

63. **(4)** Romberg's sign indicates the inability to maintain balance, which indicates a need for further evaluation. Options #1, #2, and #3 are normal age-related changes. A decrease in short-term memory that affects the functional ability would then be considered a deviation.

64. **(1)** OARS ADL Scale is the more appropriate screening tool for identifying at-risk populations. The Bennet Social Isolation Scale would be appropriate to evaluate the social interactions and resources. The Mini Mental State Examination is used to evaluate memory, orientation, and attention. The Norton Scale is used to evaluate pressure ulcer risk.

65. **(2)** The most age-dependent driving factor is sensory change, and the elderly driving client being assessed for driving capacity should use any corrective devices for optimal performance. While poor hearing alone is generally not a limiting factor for motor vehicle operation, vision assessment has received the greatest emphasis in assessing older drivers. Documenting the best corrected binocular visual acuity, color perception, and dark vision are basic elements in assessing driving visual acuity. The other factors have not been clearly demonstrated as highly applicable from laboratory performance to on-the-road skills for the elderly driver.

66. **(1)** REM sleep begins approximately 120 minutes from sleep onset and recurs in three to four regularly spaced, 10 to 15-minute cycles. REM sleep is associated with skeletal muscle atonia, rapid eye movements, and dreaming. This is decreased with aging. The delta or stage IV is deep sleep and is also decreased with aging. There is an increased nocturnal awakening along with an increased sleep latency. Sleep is generally less efficient in the older client. More time is spent in bed with a decreased time in sleeping.

67. **(2)** Immune function declines with age, making the older adult more susceptible to infection. The older adult has less thymus-derived immunity due to the shrinking of the thymus gland, thus making it more difficult for the older adult to produce antibodies.

68. **(4)** The older adult has a diminished cell-mediated immunity due to a decline in T-cell function. The T cells have a decreased ability to produce cytokines, needed to facilitate B-cell growth and maturation, and a decreased ability to proliferate in response to an antigen.

69. **(4)** A decreased bladder capacity along with the decreased ability to concentrate urine and the decreased urethral closing pressure following menopause lead to incontinence. Other factors are depression, decreased mobility, decreased vision, lack of attention to bladder cues of fullness, and so forth.

Health Promotion & Maintenance

1. The current American Cancer Society dietary recommendations for cancer prevention include:

   1. Maintaining a desirable body weight and eating a variety of foods, including fruits and vegetables and foods that are high in fiber.

   2. Increasing the amount of protein in the diet.

   3. Including a moderate amount of alcohol in the diet.

   4. There are no dietary recommendations for the prevention of cancer.

2. In the presence of dyslipidemia and diabetes, the National Cholesterol Education Program guidelines set the goal for lipid levels as:

   1. LDL <130 mg/dl and triglyceride levels <200 mg/dl.

   2. LDL <160 mg/dl and triglyceride levels <240 mg/dl.

   3. LDL <100 mg/dl and triglyceride levels <180 mg/dl.

   4. LDL <150 mg/dl and triglyceride levels <220 mg/dl.

3. The American Diabetes Association recommends screening adults starting at age 45 with a fasting plasma glucose (FPG) test every:

   1. 1 year.

   2. 3 years.

   3. 5 years.

   4. 10 years.

4. Tertiary prevention activities for an older woman who has had a cerebrovascular accident (CVA) would include:

   1. An annual influenza vaccination.

   2. A physical therapy program.

   3. An annual mammogram.

   4. An annual ophthalmologic examination to evaluate for glaucoma.

5. A client is continuing his recovery at home after an extensive surgery. The practitioner would instruct the client to increase his intake of what foods to promote healing?

   1. Tomatoes, rice, whole bran cereal.

   2. Milk, poultry, yellow vegetables.

   3. Red meat, oranges, green beans.

   4. Liver, corn, eggs.

6. When an older client has an alteration in the sensory/perceptual function of hearing, which plan would be most appropriate for the nurse practitioner to implement during a health promotion session?

   1. Increase the pitch of the voice.

   2. Stand behind the client when speaking.

   3. Speak in a tone that does not include shouting.

   4. Use typical complex sentences to prevent insulting the client.

7. The nurse practitioner demonstrates an understanding of primary prevention of falling among the elderly through which management plan?

   1. Evaluate a need for assistive devices for ambulation after the client has been injured from a fall.

   2. Provide resources to correct hazards contributing to falling in the home environment.

   3. Reinforce the need to use prescribed eyeglasses to prevent further injury from falls.

   4. Provide information about medications, side effects, and interactions.

8. Which of the health promotion screenings should be implemented annually for the elderly client over 65?

   1. Chest x-ray.

   2. Pneumococcal vaccination.

   3. Sigmoidoscopy.

   4. Stool guaiac.

9. While teaching a class to a group of senior citizens, which would be most important for the nurse practitioner to consider during the presentation?

   1. Provide a lot of overhead lighting in order to enhance visualization.

   2. Provide handouts on blue paper with black print.

   3. Review a video narrated by a woman.

   4. Recognize that past life experiences are beneficial in learning new information.

10. The most common occupationally related disease is:

    1. Repetitive motion injury.

    2. Hearing loss.

    3. Lung disease.

    4. Cancer.

11. The newest recommendation from the American Cancer Society for yearly mammography to begin is at age:

    1. 50.

    2. 45.

    3. 60.

    4. 40.

12. A 48-year-old male presents to the clinic after having his cholesterol checked at a health fair. He states that they told him it was >300, and that he needed to see his primary care provider for further testing. Appropriate interventions for the nurse practitioner include:

    1. Prescribing a cholesterol-lowering agent.

    2. Ordering an electrocardiogram (ECG) and an exercise stress test.

    3. Starting the client on an exercise program.

    4. Performing a thorough history and physical and drawing a lipid profile.

13. In teaching a client who is to have a colon-rectal screening, the nurse practitioner should instruct the client to:

   1. Eat at least two servings of rare meat daily prior to collecting samples.

   2. Avoid antibiotics, aspirin, iron, and anti-inflammatory medications.

   3. Take extra vitamin C to avoid a subsequent bladder infection that would make collecting samples difficult.

   4. Eat extra servings of vegetables such as broccoli, cabbage, potatoes, cantaloupe, and turnips to increase the fiber and ensure good samples.

14. The age group that should be targeted to be taught testicular self-examination would include which group?

   1. 10–14 years.

   2. 15–25 years.

   3. 30–40 years.

   4. 45–65 years.

15. The recommended number of servings of the bread/cereal/pasta/rice group is how many servings per day?

   1. 6–11 servings.

   2. 2–4 servings.

   3. 3–5 servings.

   4. 2–3 servings.

16. The age at which a screening mammogram is recommended as part of a woman's periodic health evaluation, if the woman is not at increased risk for breast cancer, is:

   1. 30 years old.

   2. 35 years old.

   3. Before the age of 40.

   4. Before the age of 50.

17. The history collected on a new client who enters a practice is to include:

   1. Interval history, past medical and surgical history, family medical and surgical histories, psychosocial history, usual dietary habits, physical activity, tobacco and other substance use, sexual practices, and a review of systems.

   2. Interval history, past medical history, family medical history, dietary habits, substance use, and sexual practice.

   3. Past medical and surgical histories, family medical history, psychosocial history, physical activity, tobacco and other substance use, and sexual practices.

   4. The history listed on the form provided to clients for completion prior to the physical examination is sufficient and no interview needs to be done.

18. A 50-year-old female presents to the clinic for a first-visit checkup. She states she is in good health and takes no medications. She does not know her family history, as she was adopted. She is 62 inches tall and weighs 175 lb. She is a secretary and admits to a sedentary lifestyle. She does not smoke, and admits to drinking four to five beers per week, along with an occasional glass of wine. Appropriate interventions for the nurse practitioner to recommend in this client's plan of care include:

   1. Immediately starting an exercise plan that includes jogging 2 miles/day.

   2. Recommending vitamin supplements and protein shakes to be included in her diet and eliminating or reducing the amount of alcoholic beverages she drinks on a weekly basis.

   2. Changing her job to one that will increase the amount of exercise she gets.

   4. Having her keep a 24-hour record of her usual dietary intake, doing a physical examination to assess her readiness to begin an exercise program, and discussing dietary changes that are necessary for weight loss.

19. Which group is at greatest risk for an altered immune function related to nutritional status?

   1. Young adults.

   2. Adults

   3. Premature infants.

   4. Older adults.

20. The most common cause of infant deaths worldwide is:

    1. Pneumonia.

    2. Dehydration.

    3. Acquired immunodeficiency syndrome (AIDS).

    4. β-streptococcus infections.

21. The nurse practitioner is discussing lifestyle changes and decreasing risk factors for cardiovascular diseases with a group of geriatric clients. What is most important to include in this discussion?

    1. Decrease smoking, increase vitamin supplements, increase protein intake.

    2. Control hypertension, stop smoking, maintain normal weight, exercise regularly.

    3. Maintain normal levels of serum blood sugar, decrease cholesterol intake.

    4. Get a yearly physical examination, increase fiber in diet, exercise regularly.

22. What lifestyle modifications are most effective in controlling hypertension in the older client?

    1. Maintain normal weight, decrease sodium diet, exercise regularly.

    2. Increase dietary protein, decrease weight, use stress reduction techniques.

    3. Consume high complex carbohydrate, low-sodium diet; decrease stress.

    4. Reduce weight, increase vitamin supplements, and exercise regularly.

23. All of the following are models of worksite health promotion **except**:

    1. Multiphasic health screening.

    2. Health risk appraisal.

    3. Onsite emergent care clinic.

    4. Health fair.

24. When a child comes in for a health maintenance clinic visit, what is essential for the nurse practitioner to do?

    1. Order routine laboratory tests.

    2. Perform vision and auditory screening.

    3. Plot height and weight on charts.

    4. Review immunization record.

25. The nurse practitioner is developing written materials on health care information for parents. Guidelines for developing education materials at an acceptable reading level include all **except**:

    1. Present the most important material first.

    2. Use all capital letters.

    3. Keep sentences short and to the point.

    3. Add visual graphic images to clarify information.

26. In explaining the purpose of primary prevention programs to a group of nursing students, the nurse practitioner relates that primary prevention programs:

    1. Work to lower the incidence of birth defects.

    2. Emphasize early diagnosis and treatment of pediatric anomalies.

    3. Minimize the handicapping effect of mental retardation.

    4. Focus on the prevention of complications and rehabilitation.

27. A healthy 4-month-old infant weighing 13 lb 3 oz has started waking up at night after previously sleeping for 9–11 hours. The infant takes 33 oz of formula in a 24-hour period. The nurse practitioner recommends:

    1. Increase the formula to 38 oz in a 24-hour period.

    2. Start introducing one food item at a time, beginning with vegetables.

    3. Reduce the formula to 28 oz and start small amounts of rice cereal.

    4. Change over to whole milk instead of formula.

28. The nurse practitioner understands that the infant mortality rate is:

    1. The number of infant deaths under 1 year of age per 1000 live births.

    2. The total number of infant deaths per 1000 population.

    3. The number of deaths attributed to specific illnesses.

    4. The monthly newborn death rates per 100 live births.

29. The father (74 inches, onset of puberty age 16) of a 15-year-old male adolescent is concerned that his son is going to be short. Upon physical exam, the nurse practitioner finds: Tanner stage II, height 62 inches, physical exam essentially normal for a well-nourished adolescent. After reviewing his growth records, which indicate a growth pattern of height at the fifth percentile, the most likely diagnosis is:

    1. Constitutional growth delay.

    2. Familial short stature.

    3. Hypopituitarism.

    4. Idiopathic gonadotropin deficiency.

30. Anticipatory guidance for the family of a 9-month-old includes all **except**:

    1. Use of shoes for protection, not support.

    2. Encourage self-feeding.

    3. Baby-proof home; pool and water safety.

    4. Issues of independence and dependence.

31. Anticipatory guidance for the family with a 4-year-old includes:

    1. Avoid fluoride supplements to prevent staining of teeth and dental caries.

    2. Continue to use a car seat until the child weighs 60 lbs or his/her head is higher than the back seat.

    3. Instruct parents to use bottled drinking water when traveling to different parts of the country.

    4. Serve only three regular meals, no snacks to prevent poor nutrition habits developing.

32. In teaching a new mother about fevers, the nurse practitioner knows that:

    1. Fevers of 40°C (104°F) can cause brain damage.

    2. All fevers over 40°C (104°F) are usually of bacterial origin.

    3. Children under 6 months of age are especially susceptible to brain damage from a fever.

    4. High fevers may precipitate convulsions in children between 6 months and 6 years of age.

33. A new mother asks about the differences between human milk and cow's milk. The nurse practitioner explains that:

    1. Human milk has more lipase and linoleic acid.

    2. Human milk has more calcium, phosphorus, sodium, and potassium.

    3. Cow's milk has low protein and casein content.

    4. Cow's milk has high linoleic acid and low saturated fatty acids.

34. The nurse recognizes the following as correct for the frequency and quantity of formula feedings:

    1. 1 month: 9–10 feedings/24 hours of 2–3 oz.

    2. 6 months: 8–10 feeding/24 hours of 4–5 oz.

    3. 10 months: 4–5 feedings/24 hours of 7–8 oz.

    4. 12 months: 6–8 feedings/24 hours of 8–9 oz.

35. According to the American Academy of Pediatrics (AAP), infants may be fed whole cow's milk once they reach:

    1. 6 months of age.

    2. 8 months of age.

    3. 12 months of age.

    4. 18 months of age.

36. A mother states that the iron-fortified formula her 3-month-old infant is on has been causing constipation. The nurse practitioner recommends:

    1. Discontinuing the iron-fortified formula.

    2. Starting the infant on rice cereal.

    3. Adding 1–2 tsp of dark corn syrup to formula.

    4. Avoiding prune, apricot, and pineapple juices.

37. Which of the following describes lactose intolerance?

    1. Children usually exhibit symptoms around 4–6 years of age. Symptoms typically include intestinal dilatation, bloating, increased flatulence, and pain followed eventually by diarrhea.

    2. Infants and toddlers are typically affected. Symptoms occur within 30 minutes after eating milk products or drinking milk and are characterized by an abrupt onset of nausea, vomiting, and diarrhea.

    3. It is the same as cow's milk intolerance.

    4. Its prevalence is highest among the Caucasian population.

38. A routine lab study is returned to the nurse practitioner on a 1-year-old who had a normal yearly exam. The lead level is reported as 15 μg/dl. The nurse practitioner takes which action?

    1. Repeat the test since it may be a false result.

    2. Hospitalize for immediate chelation therapy.

    3. Investigate possible sources of lead and repeat in 6 months.

    4. Repeat the test in 1 year.

39. The recommended time for introduction of solid foods into an infant's diet is:

    1. Age 2 months.

    2. Age 4–6 months.

    3. Age 6–8 months.

    4. Age 3 months.

40. The nurse practitioner is aware that fluoride levels in drinking water should be:

    1. 0.5 ppm in temperate and cold climates.

    2. 1.0 ppm in temperate and 0.5 ppm in cold climates.

    3. 1.0 ppm in temperate and cold climates.

    4. 0.6 ppm in temperate and 1.0 ppm in cold climates.

41. A 20-day-old infant is brought to the clinic by her parents. She has not been eating well and has a temperature of 38.2°C (100.8°F). Upon exam no focal bacterial infection is found, lab indicates a white blood cell (WBC) count of 12,000/mm^3 with 1480 bands/mm^3, urinalysis is normal, and there is no diarrhea noted. Management involves:

    1. Treat at home with antipyretics and fluids.

    2. Hospitalize for a septic work-up.

    3. Treat at home with antipyretics and ampicillin.

    4. Do a urine culture and have the infant return in 24 hours.

42. In teaching the fifth through eighth grade child about health promotion behaviors it is important to remember that:

    1. Girls are more extrinsically motivated.

    2. Both boys and girls are highly influenced by family.

    3. Boys are more extrinsically motivated.

    4. High maternal education levels affect both.

43. In the preparation of reading and education materials for clients and parents the nurse practitioner is aware that the reading level of most adults is at the:

    1. Twelfth-grade level.

    2. Tenth-grade level.

    3. Sixth-grade level.

    4. Fourth-grade level.

44. A child presenting with vague symptoms and a serum lead level of 28 μg/dl would be managed by:

1. Removal of the child from the lead source.

2. Removal of the environmental lead hazard.

3. Chelation therapy treatment.

4. Rescreen and referral to physician.

45. Primary injury prevention teaching for the parents of a 2-month-old includes:

1. Set water heater thermostat at <120°F.

2. Make sure crib rails are no more than 3¼ inches apart.

3. Use a rear-facing car seat until the child is >40 lb.

4. Apply sunscreen for when outside and temperature is 75°F.

46. Discussion of home/folk remedies utilized by the Hispanic family of a child with vague symptoms of weakness, irritability, weight loss, constipation, mild ataxia, and a previous history of elevated lead levels might reveal the use of:

1. White willow bark.

2. Arnica root.

3. Mexican yam root.

4. Azarcon and greta.

47. Anticipatory guidance for the parents of a 26-week-gestation premature infant who is going home after 2 months in the neonatal intensive care unit (NICU) would include the infant's need for:

1. Fluoride supplement due to lack of breast-feeding.

2. Lights to be on 24 hours a day.

3. Decreased handling and stimulation.

4. Bright colors and continuous music for stimulation.

Immunizations

48. The mother of a 2-month-old refuses to have her child vaccinated with the oral trivalent polio vaccine (OPV) because she has read that some children can get polio from the vaccine. The nurse practitioner' best action would be:

1. Respect the mother's choice; do not give the vaccine.

2. Explain the seriousness of polio if the child does not get the vaccine.

3. Offer the IPV-E (inactivated trivalent polio vaccine—enhanced) with an explanation.

4. Give the vaccine, as it is a state law and is required on all infants.

49. Before giving a child the measles-mumps-rubella (MMR) trivalent vaccine, it is recommended to wait how long after cancer chemotherapy has stopped?

1. 30 days.

2. 2 months.

3. 3 months.

4. 6 months.

50. The National Childhood Vaccine Injury Act requires standardized consent forms for the administration of vaccines to children. The content on the form for the medical record includes the vaccine lot number, nurse signature, injection/inoculation site, and:

1. Parental signature.

2. Education provided.

3. Absence of contraindications.

4. Vaccine expiration date.

51. The mother of a 15-year-old who has not had chickenpox is concerned and wants her daughter to be vaccinated. The recommendations are:

1. Not recommended for children over age 12.

2. A one-time dose.

3. Three doses 2 months apart.

4. Two doses 4–8 weeks apart.

52. Consultation with the mother of an 18-month-old who has received no immunizations reveals that the child was exposed to measles 48 hours prior to the visit. At this time the practitioner would:

    1. Discharge the client with care instructions.

    2. Administer live attenuated measles vaccine.

    3. Administer 0.5 ml/kg immunoglobulin G (IgG).

    4. Administer half the regular measles vaccine dose.

53. Which statement describing the polyvalent pneumococcal vaccine is **incorrect**?

    1. It is recommended for those with chronic respiratory illness.

    2. It can be given on the same visit as the influenza vaccine.

    3. It should be given yearly.

    4. It is never recommended for children.

54. The influenza vaccination is recommended annually for high-risk groups. The nurse practitioner knows that the greatest need for this vaccination would be for:

    1. Adults with chronic disease.

    2. Residents of long-term care facilities.

    3. Dialysis clients.

    4. Health care employees.

55. The nurse practitioner understands that the only contraindication to hepatitis B vaccination is:

    1. Pregnancy and lactation.

    2. History of poliomyelitis.

    3. Prior anaphylaxis or severe hypersensitivity.

    4. Mild viral illness.

56. Immunizations and chemoprophylaxis offered routinely to clients who are 65 years of age or older are:

    1. Diphtheria, tetanus toxoid, and pertussis absorbed (DPT); influenza; and Pneumovax.

    2. Td, influenza, and pneumococcal vaccine.

    3. Td and influenza; to those with chronic diseases offer the pneumococcal vaccine.

    4. Influenza and pneumococcal pneumonia and Td to those who have not had one in the last 10 years.

57. The nurse practitioner understands that the following is considered an attenuated live-virus vaccination:

    1. Rubella and measles.

    2. Mumps and hepatitis B.

    3. Poliomyelitis and hepatitis B.

    4. Rubella and rabies.

58. The nurse practitioner understands that children who are at high risk to the measles vaccine are children who have severe allergic reactions to:

    1. Fungi.

    2. Pollen.

    3. Pets.

    4. Food.

59. What type of immunity does a child develop after he has contracted chickenpox?

    1. Actively acquired immunity.

    2. Artificially acquired immunity.

    3. Natural passive immunity.

    4. Naturally acquired active immunity.

60. The nurse practitioner is assessing an 8-month-old infant in an immunization clinic. The nurse practitioner knows that by 8 months the child should have had which immunizations?

    1. Hepatitis B first and second dose, all of the DPT series, and two doses of the polio series.

    2. All of the DPT and polio series, MMR.

3. DPT first and second dose, MMR first dose, all of the hepatitis B series.

4. Varicella, DPT first dose, hepatitis B first dose.

61. In considering client situations, which one requires the use of an inactivated (not live) vaccine?

   1. History of nonspecific allergies.

   2. Immunocompromised adult.

   3. Concurrent antimicrobial therapy.

   4. Mild acute illness.

62. In taking the history of a healthy 50-year-old adult, the nurse practitioner determines the client is an avid gardener and spends a great deal of time enjoying the out-of-doors. A health maintenance recommendation for this client is to obtain a:

   1. Pneumococcal vaccine.

   2. Tetanus vaccine.

   3. Hepatitis B vaccine.

   4. Varicella vaccine.

63. The American College of Physicians (ACP) recommends that healthy adults receive a Td booster vaccination:

   1. Every 5 years.

   2. Every 8 years.

   3. At age 60.

   4. Every 10 years.

64. Which statement most correctly describes tetanus toxoid?

   1. Tetanus toxoid (T) induces more persistent antitoxin antibody titers.

   2. DPT and diphtheria and tetanus toxoids absorbed (DT) are safe to give to adults.

   3. The recommended dose for the adult is 0.75 ml IM.

   4. Tetanus toxoid fluid provides the same antitoxin antibody titers as tetanus toxoid.

65. Immunizations recommended for healthy young adults include:

   1. Measles, rubella, varicella, and hepatitis B.

   2. Pneumovax, influenza, and rubella.

   3. Tetanus, influenza, varicella, Pneumovax, and hepatitis B.

   4. Influenza, hepatitis B, rubella, measles, and tetanus.

66. A 2-month-old infant received his immunizations and 12 hours later the mother calls and says the infant has a fever of 101°F. What is the most likely cause of the fever?

   1. The vaccination for the measles, mumps, and rubella.

   2. The combination of the diphtheria and the polio vaccinations.

   3. The presence of an infection when immunizations were given.

   4. The pertussis immunization.

Answers & Rationales

3

1. **(1)** The American Cancer Society recommends the maintenance of a desirable body weight; research has shown an association between increased deaths from various cancers and varying degrees of being overweight. Another recommendation is to eat a wide variety of foods, consistent with the Food Guide Pyramid put out by the U.S. Department of Agriculture and the U.S. Department of Health and Human Services. A variety of fruits and vegetables should be included in the daily diet (five to nine servings/day), because research has shown that there is an association between lower cancer rates and high fruit and vegetable consumption. High-fiber foods are also recommended; a lower risk of colon cancer is seen in those individuals who consume a high-fiber diet. There are no recommendations to increase the amount of protein in the diet at this time; due to the high consumption of red meat in the American diet, many people are already getting large quantities in their current diets. The American Cancer Society recommends limiting the daily consumption of alcohol to two drinks for males, one drink for females, and no drinks for pregnant females. They also state that ideally, no alcohol should be consumed; regular alcohol consumption has been shown to increase the risk of various cancers.

2. **(1)** The recommendation is low-density lipoprotein (LDL) <130 mg/dl and triglyceride levels <200 mg/dl. All other choices have inaccuracies of goals.

3. **(2)** The American Diabetes Association recommends screening adults starting at the age of 45 every 3 years.

4. **(2)** The physical therapy program will assist her in restoring her optimum level of functioning after a CVA. Option #1 is a primary prevention activity nonspecific to a CVA. Options #3 and #4 are examples of secondary prevention activities nonspecific to a CVA.

5. **(3)** The client needs an increased intake of protein and vitamin C to promote healing. Red meat, citrus fruits, and green vegetables will give the highest amounts of these elements from the selections offered.

6. **(3)** Shouting increases the pitch of the voice. In presbycusis, which is a hearing loss in the elderly, high-pitched consonant sounds are the first to be affected, and the change may occur gradually. The nurse practitioner should face the client when speaking. If there is a need to stand behind the client, then use touch to get the client's attention. Simple sentences should be used in order to facilitate understanding.

7. **(4)** This information will prevent complications that may result in a fall. Options #1 and #2 are appropriate for tertiary prevention. Option #3 is appropriate for secondary prevention, which is to prevent the client from experiencing another fall.

8. **(4)** This evaluation will assist in identifying any problems with bleeding. Option #1 is not necessary. Option #2 is not a screening and would not be administered annually. A sigmoidoscopy is recommended every 3–5 years for clients over 50.

9. **(4)** Using past life experiences applies the concept of adult educational principles.

Overhead lighting may produce an increase in the glare, which can decrease visualization. There is an alteration of color perception (e.g., blue appears green-blue) as an individual ages. As individuals age the ability to hear women's and children's voices decreases, since these are high-pitched voices. This video would not enhance the program if the clients frequently have presbycusis as a result of the normal aging process.

10. **(3)** All of these disorders can be associated with workplace exposure but, currently lung disease is still the most common occupationally related disease. Musculoskeletal injuries are on the rise.

11. **(4)** In the summer of 1997, the National Institutes of Health (NIH) and the American Cancer Society changed the recommendation to begin yearly mammography at age 40.

12. **(4)** The client's history and physical will reveal the presence of any coronary heart disease (CHD) risk factors (i.e., age, family history of CHD, diabetes, current cigarette smoking, blood pressure, height/weight, cardiovascular exam). A lipid profile is also recommended to assess the level of risk—it consists of total cholesterol, high-density lipoprotein (HDL), LDL, and triglyceride levels. It would be prudent to have a precise cholesterol level done, as the previous result was from a screening health fair, and there is no written record of the result. It is also important to assess the level of HDLs and LDLs to see if they are present in normal amounts. These parameters should be assessed first before a cholesterol-lowering agent, ECG, or stress test is ordered. An exercise program is also important, but should only be done after a history and physical and lipid profile results are known; if the lipid profile results or exam is abnormal, stress testing may be appropriate before undertaking a new exercise program.

13. **(2)** Screening for colon-rectal cancer includes annual fecal occult blood screening for individuals over age 50. Avoiding medications that can cause gastrointestinal irritation and bleeding can help avoid false-positive results. Rare meat and vegetables that are high in peroxidase (like the ones listed) will cause false-positive results,

while vitamin C can cause false-negative results.

14. **(2)** The 15- to 25-year age group is most commonly affected by testicular cancer.

15. **(1)** The recommended servings for each of the food groups are as follows:

Food Group	Servings
Bread/cereal/rice/pasta	6–11 servings
Fruit	2–4 servings
Vegetable	3–5 servings
Meat/poultry/fish, dry beans, eggs, nuts	2–3 servings
Fats/oils/sweets	Sparing uses

16. **(3)** A screening mammogram is recommended before the age of 40.

17. **(1)** All of these areas are important to probe in the initial interview of a new client. The history will help determine the necessary components of the physical examination and laboratory or radiologic studies that are ordered and the counseling that is done during the appointment.

18. **(4)** An account of the client's usual intake is necessary, so that problem areas can be identified. Before beginning any exercise program, a physical examination should be done to assess the client's physical condition and to aid in the proper selection of a specific exercise plan. A dietary assessment needs to be completed before recommending vitamin and protein supplements; the client may already be receiving adequate amounts in her diet. A more active job would be ideal; however, most people do not have options regarding their choice of job, so increasing her activity outside of work would be most appropriate.

19. **(4)** The older adult is at greatest risk for altered immune function related to nutrition. The older adult often does not get enough nutrition for a variety of reasons: altered taste, eating alone, ability to prepare meals, malabsorption. Adequate nutrition in the older adult has been shown to improve immune status and antibody response to influenza vaccine.

20. **(2)** Dehydration results in the deaths of more infants worldwide than any other syndrome.

21. **(2)** Hypertension, smoking, and hyperlipidemia are the major risk factors in the development of cardiovascular disease. Controlling hyperglycemia, high dietary fiber intake, and vitamin supplements assist in maintaining a healthy lifestyle; however, they are not as important in preventing cardiovascular disease.

22. **(1)** These three modifications are the most effective in maintaining normal blood pressure.

23. **(3)** Multiphasic health screening is a form of period health surveillance where employees undergo a battery of laboratory or diagnostic tests to determine risk factors and disease detection. A health risk appraisal is often part of a multiphasic health screening and involves a scored questionnaire that determines overall health risks or targets specific risks, such as cardiovascular disease. A health fair or special event may provide basic screening services, have booths or exhibits, and presentations on health-related education. An onsite emergent care clinic is not primary health promotion and prevention as employees seek services for emergent care.

24. **(4)** It is absolutely essential that the immunization record be reviewed. The other options are important but not essential for a health maintenance visit.

25. **(2)** Printed materials must be written to a level of readability so that they can be understood. Do not use all capital letters, as words so written are difficult to read. Also, it is helpful to write in the active versus the passive voice, to use one- and two-syllable words, to avoid complex grammatical structures, and to express only one idea in each sentence.

26. **(1)** Primary prevention programs exist to prevent disease, malfunctioning, or maladaptation from ever occurring. Examples of these types of programs include promoting a healthy diet, the practice of safe sex, the avoidance of alcohol and tobacco use, and so forth. Secondary prevention is early diagnosis and treatment (i.e., screening for tuberculosis or sickle cell disease, breast and testicular self-examination). Tertiary prevention is the prevention of complications and rehabilitation after the disease or condition has already occurred (i.e., cardiac rehabilitation, having a complete blood count [CBC] drawn before chemotherapy).

27. **(3)** If the infant has been satisfied up to this point (by sleeping for long intervals), more than likely he needs additional calories in the form of rice cereal. Adding increased amounts of formula can lead to iron deficiency anemia.

28. **(1)** This is a commonly used ratio, which is calculated as follows:

$$\frac{\text{No. of deaths} <1 \text{ year of age in a year}}{\text{No. of live births in the same year}}$$
$$\times 1000 = \text{Infant mortality rate}$$

29. **(1)** Familial short stature is not indicated here, as the father is of normal height. Hypopituitarism would be associated with other findings: micropenis, small testes, immature facies, and olfactory defects. Gonadotropin deficiency might be a possibility, but when considering all the findings in the situation and based on the history of the father having a pubertal onset at age 16 and achieving an average height, the more likely diagnosis is constitutional growth delay.

30. **(4)** Issues of independence and dependence are usually discussed with the parents of a 2-year-old. All of the other options are appropriate for anticipatory guidance along with talking to the child and avoiding bottle tooth decay (no bottle in the bed).

31. **(2)** Car safety and use of a car seat continues to be a priority for the 4-year-old. Bottled drinking water is not necessary when traveling, unless it is out of the country. A fluoridated dentifrice should be used in a small amount (pea-size) and children under 6 should be supervised so that they do not swallow too much toothpaste which would put them at risk for fluorosis. Three regular meals and two snacks are recommended for the busy 4-year-old. Snacks should be rich in complex carbohydrates and low in fat. Avoid candy, chips, and soft drinks.

32. **(4)** Febrile seizures are benign and do not lead to brain damage. Most febrile illness in children is due to a virus, rather than a bacteria, and is associated with a high fever.

33. **(1)** Cow's milk is not as good of a nutritional source as human milk, because it has more mineral content (calcium, phosphorus, sodium, and potassium), which causes a larger renal solute load. In addition, cow's milk is high in protein, casein, and saturated fat and lower in carbohydrates.

34. **(3)** Usual frequency and quantity of formula feedings are as follows:

    0–1 month: 6–8 feedings/24 hours of 2–4 oz.
    2 months: 4–5 feedings/24 hours of 5 oz.
    3 months: 4–5 feedings/24 hours of 5–6 oz.
    4 months: 4–5 feedings/24 hours of 6–7 oz.
    7–10 months: 3–4 feedings/24 hours of 8 oz.
    11–12 months: 3 feedings/24 hours of 8 oz.

35. **(3)** At 1 year of age, infants may be fed whole cow's milk. The purpose for waiting is that it has been shown that cow's milk is low in iron, linoleic acid, and vitamin E, as well as being high in protein, sodium, and potassium.

36. **(3)** The American Academy of Pediatrics does not recommend low-iron formulas and recommends, if stools are hard, to treat for constipation. Typical treatment includes giving 1–2 tsp of dark corn syrup, including fruit juices (prune, pineapple, apricot), nonstarchy vegetables, water, and avoiding rice cereal.

37. **(1)** These are characteristics of lactose intolerance. Symptoms occur from 2 to as many as 12 hours after milk or milk product ingestion. The prevalence is highest in African-Americans, Native Americans, and Asians. Cow's milk intolerance occurs in infancy and has symptoms of blood in the stools often accompanied by allergies, such as eczema, hives, or asthma.

38. **(3)** While 15 μg/dl is an elevated count (normal level is <10 μg/dl), chelation therapy in children with a normal exam is not usually conducted until the level is >25 μg/dl. It is important at this level to identify the source of the elevation and monitor the child frequently.

39. **(2)** Solid food does not need to be introduced before 4–6 months of age. The first foods introduced are cereals. New foods are introduced one at a time at weekly intervals. In this way, the infant's digestive system can get used to the food and any reaction can be easily detected.

40. **(4)** Levels recommended by the dental association of 0.6 ppm in temperate climates and 1.0 ppm in cold climates are based on the rationale that people in temperate climates drink more fluids. Intake is determined at 1 L/day. Below this level, children need supplements, which cannot be prescribed without knowing the exact fluoride/water concentration.

41. **(2)** Practice guidelines recommend that febrile infants under 28 days, even if they meet low-risk criteria, should have a sepsis evaluation.

42. **(1)** Fifth through eighth grade girls are more motivated by peers and family. Boys are more intrinsically motivated, with family and peers having less influence. Peers are also more influential for girls in the high school years. High maternal education level is not an influential factor for boys.

43. **(3)** The reading level of most American adults is at the sixth grade level.

44. **(4)** Recommendations of the Centers for Disease Control and Prevention (CDC) for a serum lead level >10 μg/dl are for rescreening and referral to a physician. Rescreening is done prior to removal of the child/family from the hazard, although a thorough environmental assessment is essential at the time of rescreening.

45. **(1)** The water heater should not be set over 120°F, to prevent scald burns. Crib rails should be no more than 2³/₈ inches apart; the rear-facing infant seat is applicable to 20 lb or one year of age. Sunscreen should be applied whenever there is sun exposure.

46. **(4)** Azarcon and greta are traditional Hispanic remedies that contain lead, which can lead to increased lead levels and eventual poisoning. The other substances will not cause the symptoms described. The Mexican yam root is utilized for menopausal symptoms and is a source of natural progesterone.

47. **(2)** Premature infants who have spent an extended period of time in the NICU take 6–10 months to be deinstitutionalized to the noise and light. These must be decreased slowly over a period of time.

Immunizations

48. **(3)** IPV-E has been proven to be effective against wild polio and is recommended for use by some health experts. Therefore, individuals refusing OPV can receive IPV-E.

49. **(3)** The MMR is a live virus vaccine and children severely immunosuppressed due to cancer therapy should wait until immunoglobulin levels have increased or they are at increased risk for serious complications and the disease.

50. **(1)** The law calls for the parental signature to be maintained in the clinical record.

51. **(4)** Children over the age of 13 who have not had chickenpox and have not been previously immunized are recommended to have two doses 4–8 weeks apart for effective immunity.

52. **(2)** The live attenuated measles vaccine if given within 72 hours of exposure will provide protection in most cases. The does of IgG would be 0.25 ml/kg given within 6 days of exposure.

53. **(3)** It is not given more often than every 10 years and may be effective for longer periods.

54. **(2)** Influenza outbreaks may affect 60% of those in long-term care and fatality rates are high. All the other groups listed are appropriate for the influenza vaccine but are not as high a priority.

55. **(3)** Prior anaphylaxis and severe hypersensitivity would be considered a contraindication; a mild viral illness would not. The client who is pregnant or lactating may be immunized.

56. **(4)** Pneumococcal and annual influenza immunizations are recommended for those who are 65 years of age and older. Adult Td is offered to those who have not had a booster in the last 10 years.

57. **(1)** Attenuated live-virus vaccines are available for the following communicable diseases: measles, mumps, rubella, poliomyelitis, yellow fever, and smallpox. Rabies vaccine is a killed virus and hepatitis B is a purified viral antigen obtained from the blood of an infected client and then inactivated when manufactured into a vaccination.

58. **(4)** Atopic (allergic) children who have severe food allergy are at an increased risk for the development of an allergic reaction to the measles vaccine. Children with food allergy should be observed for at least 90 minutes in a setting equipped for emergency medical treatment.

59. **(4)** A child who contracts chickenpox for the first time develops antibodies during the period of infection. These antibodies create a naturally acquired, lifelong type of active immunity. Artificially acquired immunity occurs with immunizations. Natural passive immunity occurs with placental transfer. Active acquired immunity occurs with an injection of human or animal serum.

60. **(1)** Standard immunizations are two doses of hepatitis B series, all of the initial DPT series, and two of the polio series. MMR and varicella are not given until 12–15 months.

61. **(2)** Live vaccine can produce serious disseminated disease in a client with an immunocompromised illness such as leukemia, lymphoma, or human immunodeficiency virus (HIV) infection, AIDS, or in clients undergoing cancer chemotherapy. Mild acute illness, concurrent antimicrobial therapy, and a history of nonspecific allergies are not contraindications for use of a live vaccine.

62. **(2)** Adults who enjoy gardening and outdoor activities should have a tetanus vaccine at least every 10 years due to the high-risk activities. A pneumoccocal vaccine is recommended for adults age 65 or older, or for those who have a chronic illness or who are immunosuppressed. Most older adults have had chickenpox as a child and do not require the vaccine.

63. **(4)** The ACP recommends that adults receive a Td booster every 10 years or a single booster at age 50 for clients who have completed full pediatric series, including teenage and young adult boosters.

64. **(1)** Tetanus toxoid induces more persistent antitoxin antibody titers than tetanus toxoid fluid. DPT and DT are for use in children under the age of 7 years; however, they should *not* be used in adults. The recommended dose of DT for an adult is 0.5 ml IM.

65. **(4)** Five to 20% of young adults are susceptible to measles and/or rubella. Influenza and hepatitis B are recommended for students who have exposure to a large number of people. Tetanus is recommended every 10 years, especially in high-risk situations (young adults that participate in outdoor sports). Pneumovax is indicated in a young adult who has a chronic disease, such as diabetes, chronic pulmonary disease, or chronic cardiovascular disease, and is also indicated for young adults who are immunocompromised.

66. **(4)** The most often cause of fever at the 2-month immunization series is the pertussis. This vaccine causes reactions in about 75% of the infants. MMR is not given until 12–15 months of age.

Cardiovascular

4

Physical Examination & Diagnostic Tests

1. The practitioner is performing a physical examination on a healthy male adult. On auscultation, the stethoscope would be placed in what areas to best hear the characteristic heart sounds S_1 and S_2?

   1. S_1 is best heard at the apex and S_2 at the base of the heart.

   2. Both are heard equally well on the right side at the midclavicular line.

   3. On the left side, S_1 is at the area of pulmonic valve and S_2 at the aortic valve.

   4. Both sounds are best heard at Erb's point at the third intercostal space at the sternal margin.

2. On the general assessment of an adult client, the practitioner determines the presence of the apical impulse at the point of maximal impulse (PMI) on the client's chest wall. Where on the chest wall is the PMI normally found?

   1. Second intercostal space at the midclavicular line on the left side.

   2. Right lower sternal border, fifth intercostal space.

   3. Left side at the fifth intercostal space on the midclavicular line.

   4. Left fifth intercostal space, lateral to the midclavicular line.

3. The nurse practitioner is auscultating the carotids for a whooshing sound. The correct procedure is:

   1. Use the diaphragm of the stethoscope.

   2. Use the bell of the stethoscope.

   3. Place the stethoscope 1 inch off the area above the sternocleidomastoid muscle.

   4. Position the client at a 30-degree angle, press firmly with the bell of the stethoscope.

4. When inspecting the precordium, the nurse practitioner is checking for:

   1. Scars and anatomic landmarks.

   2. Pulsations and retractions.

   3. Heaves and cardiac dullness.

   4. Pericardial friction rub and lifts.

47

5. While examining a client in a left lateral decubitus position, the nurse practitioner auscultates a third heart sound (S_3). The nurse practitioner knows:

   1. This sound is normally heard in children and young adults and is considered a physiologic S_3.

   2. This rarely is associated with myocardial failure in the older adult.

   3. This client should be immediately referred to a cardiologist for evaluation.

   4. This is considered a normal splitting of the S_2 during inspiration and is accentuated by positioning.

6. The nurse practitioner knows that the correct auscultatory site for the aortic area is the:

   1. Midclavicular line, fifth interspace, left side.

   2. Left fourth interspace close to the sternum.

   3. Right second interspace close to the sternum.

   4. Midclavicular line, second interspace, left side.

7. The nurse practitioner should include the following in his/her teaching when ordering a lipid profile on a client:

   1. A normal breakfast should be consumed the morning of the exam.

   2. The client should be fasting for 12 hours prior to the exam, with the client's typical diet being ingested for the 7 days prior to the exam.

   3. There are no alcohol or diet restrictions for this test.

   4. The client may take any current medications with a few sips of water before the test.

8. When auscultating the heart sounds of a 72-year-old client with a history of hypertension, the nurse practitioner notes an S_4. This finding could indicate:

   1. A normal variant in people 65 years or older.

   2. The beginning of ventricular failure.

   3. A decreased resistance to ventricular filling.

   4. A severely failing heart.

9. A 55-year-old client has a blood pressure (BP) of 168/100. This is classified as:

   1. Moderate hypertension.

   2. Mild hypertension.

   3. High normal BP.

   4. Severe hypertension.

10. The nurse practitioner is examining a client with a history of rheumatic fever and who is being followed for the development of carditis. During the cardiac auscultation, where on the chest wall is the stethoscope placed to determine the most common murmurs associated with this condition?

    1. At the left sternal border, fourth left intercostal space.

    2. Fifth intercostal space, left side, at the midclavicular line.

    3. Second or third intercostal space at the left of the sternal border.

    4. Second intercostal space on the right of the sternal border.

11. A client presents with unusual coolness in the left hand as compared to the right hand. What is the next step in the examination?

    1. Palpate the radial pulse on both hands for a full minute.

    2. Feel the forehead with the backs of the fingers.

    3. Feel the forearms with the backs of the fingers.

    4. Hold the hand in a dependent position and re-examine in 3 minutes.

12. S_1 and S_2 are identified when the nurse practitioner auscultates for cardiac sounds. The physiology responsible for the production of these heart sounds is:

    1. Contraction of the ventricles and closure of the atrioventricular (AV) valves produces S_1, closure of the semilunar valves forms S_2.

2. Closure of the aortic valve produces S_2, opening of the mitral valve and filling of the left ventricle forms S_1.

3. Opening of the AV valves produces S_1, closure of the semilunar valves produces S_2.

4. Opening of the tricuspid produces S_1, closure of the pulmonic forms S_2.

13. The nurse practitioner is assessing a cardiac client who is experiencing an atrial dysrhythmia. The pulse rate is irregular at 110 bpm and there is concern regarding a pulse deficit. How is a pulse deficit determined in this client?

1. A 12-lead electrocardiogram (ECG) is necessary to determine the presence and length of the P-R intervals.

2. The apical pulse is counted and then the radial pulse is counted; the pulse deficit is determined by the difference in the two rates.

3. The apical pulse is counted and an increase or decrease is correlated with the phases of the respiratory cycle.

4. The apical pulse and radial pulse are determined simultaneously; the pulse deficit is established if the apical rate is higher than the radial rate.

14. The nurse practitioner notes a grade V systolic murmur while examining a client's precordium. Which characteristics describe this type of murmur?

1. Barely audible, faint with the bell of the stethoscope.

2. Heard only with the diaphragm of the stethoscope.

3. Heard with the stethoscope partly off the chest.

4. Heard without the aid of the stethoscope.

15. Normal physiology changes in the geriatric population that affect conductivity and contractility of the myocardium include:

1. Increased automaticity and excitability.

2. Increased contractility and conductivity.

3. Decreased excitability and conductivity.

4. Decreased automaticity and contractility.

16. When assessing temperature of an extremity as part of a peripheral vascular assessment on a client, which part of the hand is the most sensitive?

1. Palm.

2. Fingertips.

3. Back of the wrist.

4. Back of the fingers.

17. A 45-year-old male's lipid profile results are sent to the nurse practitioner. They are as follows: total cholesterol = 287 mM/L; high-density lipoprotein (HDL) = 30 mg/dl; low-density lipoprotein (LDL) = 165 mg/dl; triglycerides = 238 mg/dl. The nurse practitioner interprets these results as:

1. Abnormal; the elevated triglyceride level is of the most concern and should be treated immediately.

2. Borderline; this is considered to be a borderline risk lipid profile.

3. Abnormal; the total cholesterol and LDL levels are elevated, and the HDL is too low.

4. Normal; these results are of no concern; follow up with client in 1 year.

18. Upon examination of a child, the nurse practitioner notes weak femoral pulses. This finding is indicative of:

1. Patent ductus arteriosus.

2. Coarctation of the aorta.

3. Tetralogy of Fallot.

4. Pulmonary stenosis.

19. A client returns to the chest pain clinic 3 weeks post–myocardial infarction (MI) complaining of pericardial pain and elevated temperature. Physical examination reveals a pericardial friction rub. What diagnostic studies are indicated?

1. 24-hour Holter monitoring.

2. Echocardiogram.

3. Complete blood count (CBC) with differential.

4. Cardiac enzymes with myoglobin.

20. In doing a cardiac assessment of a 4-month-old infant, the nurse practitioner notes a machinery-like murmur. This finding is consistent with a diagnosis of:

    1. Coarctation of the aorta.

    2. Patent ductus arteriosus.

    3. Ventricular septal defect.

    4. Aortic stenosis.

21. On assessment of a geriatric client, the nurse practitioner notes bilateral pulsations and distention of the jugular veins when the client's head is elevated 45 degrees. What further assessment needs to be done at this time?

    1. Estimate the level of venous pressure by measuring from the sternal angle to the highest level of venous pulsations.

    3. Place the client in supine position and determine effect of position change on distention and pulsations of jugular vein.

    3. Measure carotid pulses due to the increased left ventricular pressure.

    4. Have the client hold his/her breath to facilitate evaluation for the presence of carotid bruits.

22. The nurse practitioner is examining a woman with a known history of mitral valve disease. What type of murmur heard on auscultation supports a history of mitral stenosis?

    1. Diastolic murmur, heard loudest at the apex with the client on her left side.

    2. Midsystolic ejection murmur heard loudest over the left lower sternal border.

    3. Holosystolic murmur, heard loudest over the apex and left axillary area.

    4. Diastolic murmur, heard loudest with client in sitting position leaning forward.

23. The nurse practitioner is doing an assessment of a client who is 2 weeks post–MI of the left ventricle. The nurse practitioner would pay particular attention to what area of the physical assessment?

    1. The lower extremities and the jugular vein for the presence of systemic venous congestion.

    2. The area on the chest where the PMI is heard most clearly.

    3. The presence of dyspnea and auscultation of crackles in the lungs.

    4. The level of dependent edema and fluid intake over the past 24 hours.

24. Which symptoms would indicate to the nurse practitioner that the client is experiencing intermittent claudication?

    1. Petechiae and itching of the lower part of the leg.

    2. Extensive discoloration and edema of the upper leg.

    3. Profuse rash and discoloration from the trunk down to the feet.

    4. Complaints of pain on walking, relieved by sitting down.

25. Stress testing or the exercise tolerance test is the most widely used diagnostic test in ischemic heart disease. It is most accurate, up to 98%, in the following type client:

    1. Males under the age of 40 with atypical angina pectoris.

    2. Asymptomatic premenopausal females without risk factors.

    3. Males over the age of 50 with typical angina pectoris.

    4. Males on digitalis with typical angina pectoris.

Disorders

26. The diagnosis of hypertension (HTN) should be established on the basis of:

    1. At least three readings with an average systolic BP of 140 mm Hg and a diastolic BP of 90 mm Hg.

    2. At least five readings 1 month apart.

    3. One reading of 140 mm Hg systolic and 90 mm Hg diastolic or above.

    4. One reading taken in three different positions.

27. Two clinical presentations of children with congenital heart disease (CHD) are symptoms of:

    1. CHF and hypoglycemia.

    2. CHF and hypertension.

    3. CHF and peripheral edema.

    4. CHF and cyanosis.

28. A client has a 2-year history of hypertensive heart disease. The nurse practitioner expects the major pathophysiologic change to be:

    1. Right ventricular hypertrophy.

    2. Left atrial dilation.

    3. Left ventricular hypertrophy.

    4. Right atrial dilation.

29. Among the following descriptions, what data most clearly describe atrial tachycardia?

    1. Heart rate of 96, P waves present on each QRS complex, T wave every other beat.

    2. P waves present on every other beat, heart rate of 100, and irregular.

    3. Heart rate of 110, P waves present prior to each QRS complex, and regular.

    4. P waves for every third QRS complex, adequate P-R interval, rate of 90.

30. What clinical manifestation of a myocardial infarction is frequently **not** present in the geriatric cardiac client?

    1. Prolonged severe chest pain.

    2. Diaphoresis, pallor, syncope.

    3. Dyspnea, increasing anxiety.

    4. Gastrointestinal distress, orthopnea.

31. The nurse practitioner is performing an assessment on a client who is having difficulty controlling his left-sided congestive heart failure (CHF). The nurse practitioner understands that the primary symptoms associated with this type of failure are:

    1. Systemic venous congestion.

    2. Dyspnea and pulmonary congestion.

    3. Increased peripheral edema and anorexia.

    4. Atrial fibrillation with a rate around 110.

32. The nurse practitioner is concerned that a post–MI client is developing a problem of constrictive pericarditis. What is one of the characteristic findings and how is it evaluated?

    1. Cardiac tamponade occurs; it is identified by the presence of muffled heart sounds and the presence of a paradoxic pulse.

    2. Pericarditis with a pericardial triphasic friction rub is common; it is best heard at the apical area of the heart.

    3. There is a mitral valve prolapse that is characterized by a late systolic murmur heard at the apex and the left sternal borders.

    4. There are altered waves on the jugular venous pulse; this is determined with a light that is directed tangentially to illuminate the shadows of the pulsations.

33. A geriatric client has a diagnosis of left-sided CHF. The nurse practitioner would identify what common condition frequently associated with CHF?

    1. History of peripheral vascular disease.

    2. History of untreated hypertension.

    3. Current treatment for ventricular dysrhythmias.

    4. History of chronic obstructive pulmonary disease (COPD).

34. In evaluating the effectiveness of cardiopulmonary resuscitation (CPR) on the adult client, the nurse practitioner would note:

    1. Dilated pupils.

    2. Palpable carotid pulse.

    3. Capillary refill within 2 seconds.

    4. Pink and warm skin.

35. The nurse practitioner is evaluating an ECG. The client presented at the clinic with complaints of weakness and fainting. His ECG reveals a cardiac rate of 68, absent P waves, regular QRS complex, T waves are present after each QRS complex. The best interpretation of this information is:

    1. A normal ECG; need to further evaluate client's complaints of weakness.

    2. Third-degree block with junctional rhythm; keep client at rest and transfer to emergency room for cardiology consult.

    3. First-degree block; need to further evaluate possibility of digitalis toxicity and/or levels of cardiac antiarrhythmic medications.

    4. Need to administer sublingual nitroglycerin and refer client for a cardiology consult.

36. The nurse practitioner is conducting a follow-up examination on a client with coronary artery disease (CAD) and a history of pericarditis. What is one of the characteristic physical findings in pericarditis and how is it evaluated?

    1. A paradoxical pulse is common; it is identified by evaluating the changes in the amplitude of arterial pulse pressure associated with the respiratory cycle.

    2. There is a pulse deficit, which is determined by counting the radial pulse and the apical pulse at the same time and evaluating the difference.

    3. A pericardial friction rub is present; it is best heard with the diaphragm of the stethoscope and is loudest to the left of the sternum at the fourth or fifth intercostal spaces.

    4. There is an S_4 present; it is commonly heard at the apex with the bell of the stethoscope and the client in a left lateral position.

37. The typical symptoms of an MI usually experienced by the elderly include:

    1. Dyspnea and diaphoresis.

    2. Back pain and muscle cramping.

    3. Numbness and tingling of the left arm.

    4. Epigastric pain and nausea.

38. Cardiovascular risk factors predisposing females to cardiovascular disease include:

    1. Absence of estrogen adversely affects lipoprotein metabolism.

    2. Fat deposited on the hips mobilizes, raising serum cholesterol.

    3. Coronary arteries are longer and wider in diameter.

    4. Resting ejection fraction is lower.

39. The nurse practitioner is planning the treatment for a geriatric client who has been newly diagnosed with hypertension. What parameters are most important in determining the appropriate pharmacologic therapy?

    1. Determine medications and dosage based on the client's weight, age, and drug availability.

    2. Begin step method utilizing diuretics and β-adrenergic blockers, with the utilization of other medications as necessary.

    3. Initiate lifestyle changes prior to beginning the medications to determine if medication is necessary.

    4. Determine other medical conditions the client is being treated for, side effects, age, and cost of medication.

40. Which statement accurately describes coronary artery disease in geriatric clients?

    1. Cardiovascular disease is increased in the female client who is on estrogen replacement.

    2. A major risk factor for cardiovascular disease in females and males is chronic hypertension.

    3. The majority of geriatric clients with coronary artery disease also have type II diabetes.

    4. Males over 60 years old continue to experience the highest level of coronary artery disease.

41. A client with a history of COPD comes to the clinic for his annual check-up with complaints of increasing difficulty breathing. Assessment findings include S_3 gallop; early

systolic ejection click; and increased P-wave amplitude in leads II, III, and aVF of the ECG. The nurse practitioner would expect to observe which change on the chest x-ray?

1. Hypertrophy of the left ventricle.

2. Hypertrophy of the right ventricle.

3. Hypertrophy of the left atrium and ventricle.

4. Hypertrophy of the right atrium and ventricle.

42. When cardiac output falls in CHF, the body attempts to compensate. What electrolyte imbalances occur as a result of this response?

1. Hypernatremia and hyperkalemia.

2. Hyponatremia and hypokalemia.

3. Hypophosphatemia and hypercalcemia.

4. Hyperphosphatemia and hypocalcemia.

43. When assessing the carotid pulse of a 72-year-old indigent client at a community-based clinic, the nurse practitioner notes a bounding pulse with rapid rise and sudden collapse. The nurse practitioner would include which additional assessment to support this finding?

1. Auscultation for a diastolic murmur.

2. Auscultation for paradoxical pulse.

3. BP in both arms lying, sitting, and standing.

4. BP for an auscultatory gap.

44. Clinical manifestations of CHF in an infant are:

1. Easily fatigued, central cyanosis, tachycardia, tachypnea, splenomegaly.

2. Coughing, diaphoresis, peripheral edema, hepatomegaly.

3. Tachycardia, tachypnea, easily fatigued, paleness, hepatomegaly.

4. Peripheral edema, coughing, splenomegaly, hepatomegaly, tachycardia.

45. The nurse practitioner understands that the pain experienced with angina pectoris or an MI is caused by irritation of the myocardial nerve fibers by the increase in:

1. Blood glucose.

2. Lactic acid.

3. Serum potassium.

4. Serum magnesium.

46. New York Heart Functional Class III for clients with cardiac disease is characterized by:

1. Symptoms are present at rest; any activity leads to increased discomfort.

2. Slight limitation in ordinary physical activity, resulting in fatigue, palpitations, dyspnea, or angina.

3. No physical limitation in activity.

4. Marked limitation in activity; clients are comfortable at rest, but ordinary activity leads to symptoms.

47. The most common causes of chest pain in children are:

1. Ischemic heart disease; congestive heart failure.

2. Gastroesophageal reflux disease; congenital heart disease.

3. Mitral valve prolapse; musculoskeletal.

4. Idiopathic; musculoskeletal.

48. During the history and physical examination of a client with suspected early CHF, which is the most prominent finding?

1. Moist crackles in the lung bases bilaterally.

2. Anorexia with weight loss of 3 lb in 1 week.

3. Increased urinary output, peripheral edema.

4. Facial edema and distended neck veins.

49. Chest pain that is sudden and severe, described as tearing, and accompanied by a decrease in peripheral pulses, may indicate a diagnosis of:

    1. Angina.

    2. Acute myocardial infarction.

    3. Aortic dissection.

    4. Pericarditis.

50. Dietary therapy for hyperlipidemia occurs in two steps, a Step I and Step II diet. A Step I diet includes, as daily intake:

    1. Total fat ≤30% of total calories, <300 mg cholesterol, 8–10% saturated fat.

    2. Total fat ≤30% of total calories, <200 mg cholesterol, <7% saturated fat.

    3. Total fat ≤40% of total calories, <400 mg cholesterol, <15% saturated fat.

    4. Total fat ≤30% of total calories, <2000 total calories, <3 gm sodium.

51. The most frequent life-threatening dysrhythmia experienced by a client with an acute MI is:

    1. Atrial fibrillation.

    2. Ventricular tachycardia.

    3. Third-degree heart block.

    4. Ventricular fibrillation.

52. A young child is scheduled for surgical repair of tetralogy of Fallot. What does the nurse practitioner expect the child's hemoglobin (Hgb) values to show and what kind of lesion does the child have?

    1. Hgb 18 gm/dl, cyanotic.

    2. Hgb, 3 gm/dl, cyanotic.

    3. Hgb, 10 gm/dl, acyanotic.

    4. Hgb 18 gm/dl, acyanotic.

53. In an overweight, older adult female client with an elevated cholesterol level and abnormal lipoprotein profile, the first step in treatment includes:

    1. Prescribing a bile acid sequestrant agent.

    2. Initiation of a diet and exercise program.

    3. Estrogen replacement therapy.

    4. Referral to a cardiologist.

54. Clients with chronic atrial fibrillation are at risk for which condition?

    1. Sudden cardiac death.

    2. Cerebrovascular accident.

    3. Ventricular tachycardia.

    4. Acute myocardial infarction.

55. The nurse practitioner understands that the most common symptom of CHF in adults is:

    1. Anorexia.

    2. Dependent edema.

    3. Dyspnea.

    4. Weakness.

56. The nurse practitioner teaches the cardiac client to avoid foods high in saturated fats, which include:

    1. Nuts, legumes, and seeds.

    2. Fish, shellfish, and mussels.

    3. Palm oil, coconut oil, and butter.

    4. Peanut oil, soybean oil, and olive oil.

57. An elderly male client is complaining of chest pain. A parameter to assist the practitioner to differentiate the chest pain of angina from that of an infarction is:

    1. Myocardial pain with an infarction is more severe.

    2. Anginal pain is more substernal and does not radiate to other areas.

    3. Anginal pain is frequently relieved by nitroglycerin.

    4. Pain from an infarction is always associated with other symptoms.

58. The nurse practitioner is evaluating a client in the office who is complaining of chest pain. The ECG shows some signs of ischemia and the client is to be transferred to the emergency department. What drug

might the nurse practitioner give the client while awaiting transport to the emergency department?

1. Furosemide (Lasix) 40 mg IV.

2. Morphine sulfate 25 mg IV.

3. Streptokinase IV.

4. Acetylsalicyclic acid (aspirin) 81 mg PO.

59. The pathogenesis of superficial thrombophlebitis includes all **except**:

1. Excessive use of oral anticoagulants.

2. Blow to the leg or arm.

3. Recent IV therapy.

4. Secondary to pregnancy.

60. An elderly client is being evaluated for a complaint of dizziness. The symptom that will make the nurse practitioner consider that this is a life-threatening event, as opposed to a disease that is not life threatening, is:

1. The onset of the dizziness occurs in certain positions.

2. It is accompanied by tinnitus.

3. The symptoms worsen when standing and improve when lying down.

4. It is preceded by rapid breathing.

61. A 28-year-old male presents to the nurse practitioner with a history of chest pain that has been increasing over the past several days. The client states that the pain worsens upon lying down. He denies any shortness of breath, cough, or radiation of the pain. He does give a history of a recent infection with coxsackievirus. On exam, it is noted that the client has a cardiac friction rub. One probable diagnosis considered by the nurse practitioner is:

1. Acute myocardial infarction.

2. Pleural effusion.

3. Pericarditis.

4. Esophageal reflux.

62. The nurse practitioner would most likely suspect which differential diagnosis for an elderly client presenting with atrial fibrillation and functional decline?

1. Hyperthyroidism.

2. Hypothyroidism.

3. Sick sinus syndrome.

4. Congestive heart failure.

63. Which assessment made by the nurse practitioner on an older client would be a deviation from the normal aging changes?

1. Decreased exercise tolerance, slightly smaller heart.

2. Grade II/VI systolic ejection murmur.

3. Slight prolongation of the intervals on the ECG.

4. Jugular venous pressure (JVP) of 4 cm.

64. During cardiac auscultation on an older adult, a grade II/VI murmur, heard best at the second right intercostal space, is noted. The murmur is auscultated louder with squatting. There is a small carotid pulse with a delayed upstroke. The client's history is benign, and his activity tolerance is within normal limits for his age. The nurse practitioner would interpret this murmur to be indicative of:

1. Aortic regurgitation.

2. Aortic stenosis.

3. Mitral valve prolapse.

4. Mitral regurgitation.

65. The most frequently diagnosed valvular heart problem in the elderly is:

1. Aortic stenosis.

2. Mitral stenosis.

3. Mitral regurgitation.

4. Aortic regurgitation.

66. A middle-aged male with no known coronary artery risk factors presents with a cholesterol level of 255 mg/dl. The nurse practitioner would:

    1. Start him on an HMG-CoA reductase inhibitor (statins), the most potent lipid-lowering agents.
    2. Start him on a Step I diet, since all clients should be given a trial on a diet.
    3. Repeat cholesterol and obtain HDL and calculated LDL.
    4. Do nothing, since he has no coronary risks other than maleness.

67. The nurse practitioner understands that the most likely cause of hypertension in a young child is:

    1. Glomerulonephritis.
    2. Pheochromocytoma.
    3. Rheumatic fever.
    4. Hyperthyroidism.

68. Which of the following would be pertinent to the past medical history of a child who is being evaluated for cardiovascular disease?

    1. Kawasaki disease.
    2. Hypothyroidism.
    3. Osteogenic sarcoma.
    4. Tourette's syndrome.

69. The nurse practitioner would refer to a pediatric cardiologist for work-up and evaluation within 1–2 weeks a child with:

    1. Signs of exercise intolerance, dyspnea, and elevated pulse.
    2. Poor feeding, increased cyanosis with crying, and dizziness.
    3. Nonfunctional heart murmur, respiratory crackles, and retarded growth and development.
    4. Systolic ejection murmur, grade II, which disappears on sitting.

70. Infective endocarditis prophylaxis may be required for children with congenital heart defects in which of the following conditions?

    1. Dental procedures such as simple adjustment of orthodontic appliances.

    2. Cardiac catheterization.
    3. Tonsillectomy and/or adenoidectomy.
    4. Insertion of tympanostomy tubes.

71. For the congenital heart disease (CHD) child with a permanent pacemaker, electrical safety precautions include avoidance of:

    1. Cellular phones.
    2. Microwave ovens.
    3. Household electrical appliances.
    4. Metal detectors.

72. A child is being worked-up for rheumatic fever. His physical findings are: 103.6°F temperature, migratory joint pain, elected erythrocyte sedimentation rate (ESR). According to the Jones Criteria, what is essential for the diagnosis of rheumatic fever?

    1. History of group A streptococcal throat infection.
    2. Carditis.
    3. Sydenham's chorea.
    4. History of erythema marginatum for past 3 days.

Pharmacology

73. A 75-year-old client presents to the office complaining of "not feeling well." He has a history of chronic lung disease and CHF. His vital signs are pulse 78 and irregular, respirations 26, and BP 158/100. An ECG indicates sinus rhythm and confirms the rate. The P-R interval is 0.28 second, P waves are present, and each is followed by a QRS complex. There are frequent premature atrial beats. The client is on digitalis, potassium, theophylline, hydrochlorothiazide, and a calcium channel blocker. What is the next best action to take?

    1. Obtain serum theophylline, digitalis, and potassium levels.
    2. Increase dosage of calcium blocker and diuretic to obtain better BP control.

3. Order pulmonary function studies to determine progress of pulmonary disease.

4. Refer client to a cardiologist for further evaluation and treatment of CHF.

74. A 49-year-old female was started on a thiazide diuretic for hypertension 1 month ago. She arrives in the clinic complaining of muscle cramps and dizziness. Physical exam findings are:

- BP 132/88 mm Hg (previous 186/112)
- Pulse 112
- Respirations 24
- Tenting positive
- Skin turgor decreased
- Neck veins flat
- STAT serum electrolytes
  - Sodium 114 mEq/L
  - Chloride 92 mEq/L
  - Potassium 3.0 mEq/L
- STAT blood glucose—201 mg/dl

Initial treatment for this client should include fluid replacement:

1. Orally with free water and a potassium supplement.
2. Intravenously with normal saline and regular insulin subcutaneously.
3. Intravenously with 1000 ml of normal saline with 40 mEq KCl at 50 ml/hr.
4. Intravenously with 1000 ml of Ringer's lactate at 250 ml/hr.

75. A client is recovering from an acute episode of thrombophlebitis and is being treated with warfarin (Coumadin) 5 mg PO daily. In reviewing medication information, the nurse practitioner would include what information in her teaching?

1. Decrease the servings of green leafy vegetables and do not take a multivitamin supplement.

2. Limit dairy products, since they tend to decrease medication effectiveness.

3. Do not walk for exercise; aerobic exercises are more effective.

4. Maintain a daily record of intake and output to evaluate renal function.

76. The nurse practitioner is evaluating a client who is complaining of "not feeling good." He has a history of CAD and CHF. Vital signs are pulse 72, respirations 20, BP 130/88, temperature normal. There are no complaints of chest pain or difficulty breathing, and some nausea but no vomiting over the past 2 days, and lower extremities are negative for edema. The client states he has been able to take his medications. His current medications are digoxin (Lanoxin) 0.25 bid, hydrochlorothiazide (Hydrodiuril) 100 mg bid, potassium (Micro-K) 10 mEq daily, and nitroglycerin transdermal patches. What is the priority of care for this client?

1. Obtain a STAT electrocardiogram and WBC.

2. Arterial blood gases and oxygen at 4 L/min.

3. Obtain serum digoxin and potassium levels.

4. Serial cardiac enzymes now and q6h × 2.

77. The nurse practitioner has prescribed losartan (Cozaar) 50 mg PO qd. This medication promotes vasodilation by:

1. Inhibiting conversion of angiotensin I to angiotensin II.

2. Promoting the release of aldosterone.

3. Promoting the synthesis of prostaglandin.

4. Inhibiting calcium influx into smooth muscle cells.

78. A client with a history of hypertension is started on Aldactone 50 mg PO qd. The nurse practitioner instructs the client to call the clinic if which symptoms are experienced?

1. Muscle weakness, fatigue, and paresthesias.

2. Decreased reflex response, nausea, and vomiting.

3. Muscle twitching, numbness of the limbs, and depression.

4. Weight gain, excessive thirst, and fever.

79. A client with a history of unstable angina is seen in the cardiac clinic for a checkup. The assessment reveals increased weight of 10 lb and distended jugular neck veins, and an S_3. What changes in the pharmacologic treatment should be initiated?

    1. Discontinue β-blockers and calcium channel blockers.

    2. Initiate thrombolytic therapy.

    3. Discontinue nitrate and aspirin therapy.

    4. Initiate diruetic and vasoconstrictor therapy.

80. A client arrives at the emergency room of a small rural hospital complaining of "feels like my heart is racing." He is connected to a cardiac monitor that reveals supraventricular tachycardia at a rate of 184, QRS complex <0.10 second, and BP 112/62. Which treatment modality is indicated?

    1. Synchronized cardioversion with 50 joules.

    2. Defibrillation with 100 joules.

    3. Adenosine 6 mg IV push.

    4. Lidocaine 1 mg/kg IV push.

81. An 80-year-old client with a history of glaucoma develops unstable angina and is started on diltiazem (Cardizem) 30 mg PO qid and aspirin 324 mg PO qd in addition to timolol ophthalmic solution (Timoptic) i gtt OD bid. This client would have an increased risk for:

    1. Bleeding episodes.

    2. Fainting episodes and falls.

    3. Rebound supraventricular tachycardia.

    4. Blurred vision.

82. A client with a serum cholesterol of 256 mg/dl, HDL of 38 mg/dl, and LDL of 172 mg/dl is instructed on dietary modifications and niacin (nicotinic acid) 1 gm PO tid. Specific instructions include:

    1. Limiting fluid intake.

    2. Taking measures to minimize orthostatic hypotension.

    3. Administering the drug an hour after eating.

    4. Making slight modifications in diet that are required with drug therapy.

83. When monitoring for the therapeutic effects of verapamil (Calan SR), the nurse practitioner would assess for a(an):

    1. Increase in heart rate.

    2. Decrease in systemic vascular resistance.

    3. Increase in blood pressure.

    4. Decrease in ventricular premature beats.

84. An adult male client with essential hypertension was treated by the nurse practitioner with enalapril (Vasotec) 5 mg daily. After 6 months of therapy, the blood pressure was measured at 150/100 mm Hg. The nurse practitioner recommended sodium restriction and increased the enalapril to 10 mg daily. The client's blood pressure was unchanged after 3 additional months. At this point, the nurse practitioner should:

    1. Double the dose of enalapril.

    2. Add 25 mg of hydrochlorothiazide (Hydrodiuril) daily.

    3. Double the dose of enalapril and add 25 mg of hydrochlorothiazide daily.

    4. Switch to captopril (Capoten) 50 mg tid.

85. When prescribing antihypertensive drug therapy for elderly clients, the nurse practitioner recognizes that elderly clients have decreased receptor sensitivity and a changing baroreceptor response. Which class of antihypertensive agents should be avoided with elderly clients?

    1. Calcium entry antagonists.

    2. Diuretics.

    3. β-Blockers.

    4. Angiotensin converting enzyme (ACE) inhibitors.

86. Medications used in managing ischemic heart disease include:

    1. β-Blockers, sedatives, aspirin.

    2. Nitrates, β-blockers, calcium channel blockers, aspirin.

    3. Vasoconstrictors, aspirin, anxiolytics.

    4. Nitrates, ACE inhibitors, aspirin, lipid-lowering drugs.

87. The nurse practitioner initiates antihypertensive therapy for a middle-aged nonsmoking male. One week later, the client returns for a follow-up visit and complains of a recurrent dry cough since initiating the medications. This is most likely a side effect of a(n):

    1. β-blocker.

    2. Thiazide diuretic.

    3. ACE inhibitor.

    4. Calcium channel blocker.

88. The role of digoxin in the management of CHF is still being defined, but is definitely indicated in CHF:

    1. With atrial fibrillation.

    2. With mitral stenosis.

    3. With normal ejection fraction and sinus rhythm.

    4. Due to acute pericardial disease.

89. The nurse practitioner should monitor the elderly client for which of the most common adverse reactions of digoxin?

    1. Blurred vision.

    2. Confusion.

    3. Diarrhea.

    4. Eating disorder.

90. The nurse practitioner has been successfully treating an older client's hypertension with diet, exercise, and hydrochlorothiazide (Hydrodiuril) 25 mg PO qd for 5 months. During today's clinic visit, the client's blood pressure was 154/90 and temperature was 99.9°F. The physical examination revealed clear breath sounds; S_1 and S_2 with no murmurs, gallops, or rubs; and no JVD. The client denied syncope, headaches, or visual changes, and had a tender and edematous right ankle. Which laboratory values would be most appropriate for evaluation?

    1. Blood urea nitrogen and sodium.

    2. Serum cholesterol and serum calcium.

    3. Serum potassium and blood count.

    4. Serum uric acid and complete blood count.

91. An elderly white male with a long history of COPD has recently developed hypertension. Which class of antihypertensive agents should the nurse practitioner avoid for this client?

    1. ACE inhibitors.

    2. β-Blockers.

    3. Calcium channel blockers.

    4. Diuretics.

92. Which class of pharmacologic agents would the nurse practitioner select for a hypertensive elderly client with a new diagnosis of CHF?

    1. ACE inhibitors.

    2. β-Blockers.

    3. Calcium channel blockers.

    4. Diuretics.

93. A mildly hypertensive male client presents with red, painful swelling of the great toe. In addition to treating the gout, the nurse practitioner also knows he/she must:

    1. Order laboratory studies for diabetes.

    2. Explore for possible alcohol abuse.

    3. Advise him to lose weight.

    4. Change his thiazide antihypertensive.

94. An elderly male with a diagnosis of systolic hypertension for 3 months presents for follow-up care. He is on a no-added-salt diet and has lost 8 lb in 3 months. Weekly BP checks at a senior center average 180s/70s. Health history includes benign prostatic hypertrophy (BPH), diet-controlled type II diabetes, and CAD with an MI 8 years ago. His chief complaint includes periodic angina, occasional heartburn, slowed urinary stream with some dribbling, and decreasing energy level. The BP today is 188/78. Current medications include cimetidine (Tagamet) 200 mg prn, aspirin 325 mg qd, nitroglycerin, and Maalox prn. The client is married and sexually active. Which medication would the nurse practitioner initiate after complete physical, including ECG, and all indicated blood work?

    1. ACE inhibitor.

    2. Diuretic.

    3. α_1-Blocker.

    4. β-Blocker.

95. A geriatric client has been on procainamide (Pronestyl) for 4 years to control his cardiac dysrhythmias. The nurse practitioner would evaluate for what side effect in the chronic use of this medication?

    1. Elevated liver functions.

    2. Appearance of antinuclear antibodies.

    3. Shortened AV interval.

    4. Tachycardia.

96. Secondary prophylaxis for acute rheumatic fever (ARF) in a 25-year-old school teacher includes:

    1. Penicillin V 125–250 mg PO bid indefinitely.

    2. Erythromycin 800 mg PO bid.

    3. One-time dose of 2.0 million units benzathine penicillin G combined with penicillin G procaine (Bicillin C-R) IM.

    4. No medication prophylaxis is needed after client reaches the early 20s.

97. A toddler has ingested some of his grandfather's pills. The toddler is vomiting, feels weak, and has a first-degree AV block pattern on the ECG. The grandfather brings in four medication bottles. Which is the most likely medication the toddler ingested?

    1. Amitriptyline (Elavil).

    2. Digoxin (Lanoxin).

    3. Furosemide (Lasix).

    4. Aspirin.

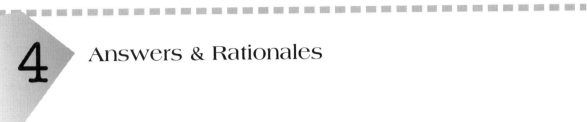

Answers & Rationales

Physical Examination & Diagnostic Tests

1. **(1)** S_1 is heard loudest at the apex, S_2 at the base. Each sound should be carefully assessed as to the intensity of the sound in each area.

2. **(3)** The PMI represents the thrust and contraction of the left ventricle (LV). The LV lies behind the right ventricle (RV) and extends to the left, forming the left border of the heart.

3. **(2)** The correct procedure is to listen for carotid bruits with the bell of the stethoscope, which brings out low-frequency sounds and filters out high-frequency sound. It should be placed very lightly on the neck with just enough pressure to seal the edge.

4. **(2)** The purpose of inspection and palpation of the precordium is to determine the presence and extent of normal and abnormal pulsations. A slight retraction of the chest wall just medial to the midclavicular line in the fifth interspace is a normal finding, whereas marked or active retraction of the rib is abnormal and may indicate pericardial disease. Pericardial friction rubs are heard by auscultation.

5. **(1)** The splitting during inspiration refers to S_1 and S_2. The S_3 is normal in children, young adults, and pregnant women. In the older adult with heart disease, this often signifies myocardial failure.

6. **(3)** The right side of the chest close to the sternal border at the second intercostal space is the correct area to auscultate the aortic valve. The mitral valve is auscultated at the fifth left intercostal space at the midclavicular line. The tricuspid value is auscultated at the fourth left intercostal space at the sternal border. The pulmonic valve is auscultated at the second left intercostal space at the sternal border.

7. **(2)** A 12-hour fast is recommended, due to the influence of intake on cholesterol levels (they may increase). A normal diet for the 7 days prior to the exam is recommended so that an accurate picture of the client's normal life is obtained. Alcohol should not be consumed 48 hours before the test—it may increase cholesterol, HDL, LDL, and triglyceride levels. If possible, all medication should be withheld until the test is over, especially corticosteroids, diuretics, β-blockers, oral contraceptives, and estrogens.

8. **(1)** An S_4 is a normal variant in people 65 years or older and may result from increased resistance to ventricular filling during atrial contraction.

9. **(1)** According to the classification of hypertension, a BP of 168/100 is within the moderate range.

10. **(2)** The fifth intercostal space at the midclavicular line on the left side is the best place to auscultate the closure sounds of the mitral valve. Option #1 describes the area of the tricuspid valve, Option #3 describes the area of the area of the pulmonic valve, and Option #4 describes the aortic valve area.

11. **(3)** It is important to determine if the coolness extends proximally from the hand. Then, palpation of pulses would be appropriate.

12. **(1)** Closure of the AV valves, which allows the filling of both ventricles simultaneously, produces the first heart sound (S_1); closure of the aortic and pulmonic valves produces the second heart sound (S_2).

13. **(4)** The apical and peripheral (radial) pulses must be evaluated simultaneously in order to determine if all of the apical beats are being reflected in the radial pulse. If there is an apical rate of 100 and a radial rate of 90, the client is said to have a pulse deficit of 10 points. This is usually done with two people counting over the same time period.

14. **(3)** A grade V heart murmur is very loud and can be heard with the stethoscope partly off the chest wall. A grade VI murmur is the loudest and is audible with the stethoscope just removed from contact with the chest wall and accompanied by a thrill. A grade I murmur is barely audible or very faint with the bell of the stethoscope.

15. **(4)** The normal aging process impairs automaticity, conductivity, and contractility. Ischemic changes and degeneration decrease sinus node automaticity and conduction velocity resulting in bradycardiac rhythms or atrial fibrillation. The poor myocardial contractility, usually related to hypertension or valvular disease, causes decreased ventricular emptying and increased filling pressures. These changes predispose the elderly to congestive heart failure.

16. **(4)** The most sensitive area on the examiner's hand is the back of the fingers.

17. **(3)** Desired levels for a lipid profile are total cholesterol <200 mg/dl, HDL >35 mg/dl, LDL <130 mg/dl, and triglycerides <250 mg/dl. A high total cholesterol coupled with a low HDL is a positive risk factor for CHD, and is the most concerning for this client. In addition, this client has an elevated LDL level. These parameters, taken as a whole, would mandate intervention in this client.

18. **(2)** Weak or absent pulses are associated with coarctation of the aorta and are not indicative of the other cardiovascular diseases.

19. **(3)** Dressler's syndrome (post-MI syndrome) may develop 1–4 weeks post-MI and is characterized by pericarditis with effusion and fever. Dressler's syndrome is caused by antigen–antibody reactions. Laboratory findings include elevation of WBC and sedimentation rate. Treatment includes corticosteroids.

20. **(2)** A machinery-like murmur is consistent with patent ductus arteriosus (PDA). The turbulent flow of blood from the aorta through the PDA to the pulmonary artery results in a characteristic machinery-like murmur. Coarctation presents with upper extremity hypertension, systolic murmur, and weak or absent femoral pulses. Ventricular septal defect is characterized by a loud, harsh, pansystolic murmur heard best at the lower left sternal border. Aortic stenosis has a systolic murmur.

21. **(1)** Jugular vein distention (JVD) is common in geriatric clients. When it is present with the client's head elevated at a 46-degree angle, then further examination needs to be conducted regarding the venous pressure, which is reflective of pressure in the right heart chambers. Supine position will increase venous pressure and does not provide valid information in this situation. Auscultation for carotid bruits is an important part of assessment but does not have significant value in evaluating JVD.

22. **(1)** Mitral valve stenosis is a diastolic murmur of low intensity heard at the apex of the heart. Option #2 describes characteristics of a murmur with aortic stenosis. Option #3, a holosystolic murmur, is characteristic of mitral regurgitation, which allows for backflow of blood from ventricles into the atrium. Option #4 best describes aortic regurgitation.

23. **(3)** The client had a left ventricular MI. One of the most common complications is left-sided failure resulting in congestive failure. This would be first manifested as pulmonary congestion and difficulty breathing.

24. **(4)** Classically, intermittent claudication is described as pain on activity that is relieved by stopping the activity.

25. **(3)** A positive result on stress testing indicates the likelihood of CAD with 98% accuracy in males over the age of 50. Results are progressively lower in asymptomatic persons, with false-positives increased in asymptomatic men under the age of 40, premenopausal women without risk factors, and clients on digitalis.

Disorders

26. **(1)** A diagnosis of HTN from a single measurement of BP elevation should not be done. A minimum of three readings with an average systolic BP of 140 mm Hg and a diastolic BP of 90 mm Hg establishes the diagnosis. An average of two or more readings taken at each of two or more visits should follow an initial screening. The client should be seated with the arm at heart level. No caffeine or nicotine ingestion should be allowed 30 minutes prior to the reading. The room should be quiet a minimum of 5 minutes, and an appropriate cuff should be used. One high reading should be confirmed within 2 months.

27. **(4)** The majority of cases of CHF in children result from congenital heart disease, and most are during the first year of life. Although the clinical presentation of a child with congenital heart disease will vary with the specific defect, the clinical manifestations usually relate to the degree of CHF or cyanosis.

28. **(3)** In the early stages of hypertensive heart disease, when there is an increased peripheral resistance to blood flow, the most significant change occurring in the heart is left ventricular hypertrophy with an increase in the size of the myocardial cells without a corresponding increase in cell number (i.e., hyperplasia). After a period of time, all of the other options listed occur in the heart.

29. **(3)** Sinus or atrial tachycardia is characterized by a rate at or above 100, P waves are present for each QRS complex, the P-R interval is below 0.20, a T wave occurs after each QRS complex, and the beat is regular.

30. **(1)** The classic chest pain of an infarction may not be present in the geriatric client due to altered pain perception and diminished pain sensation.

31. **(2)** Respiratory symptoms are predominant in clients with left-sided heart failure. Venous congestion and peripheral edema are associated with right-sided failure.

32. **(1)** Cardiac tamponade occurs as a complication of pericarditis. An excessive accumulation of fluids between the pericardium and the myocardium interferes with effective cardiac contraction. The triphasic friction rub is common to pericarditis but is not indicative of a complication of constrictive pericarditis. Jugular venous pressure is utilized to determine levels of venous distention.

33. **(2)** Untreated hypertension causes significant increased work of the left ventricle, eventually causing CHF.

34. **(2)** Palpable carotid pulse with each compression is the best sign of effective CPR. The other answers are appropriate but not the best indicators of effective resuscitation efforts.

35. **(2)** This is a description of complete block with hemodynamic consequences. The client should be seen immediately by a cardiologist for the possibility of pacemaker insertion. First-degree block has characteristic P waves, and a long P-R interval. The client should not just be referred for follow-up; he should be seen by a cardiologist as soon as possible.

36. **(3)** A triphasic friction rub or a pericardial rub occurs in the majority of clients with pericarditis. Paradoxical pulse may occur if constrictive pericarditis and cardiac tamponade are present. Pulse deficits and presence of S$_4$ are not characteristic of problems with pericarditis.

37. **(1)** Elderly individuals experience atypical symptoms of an MI including dyspnea, diaphoresis, vomiting, syncope, confusion, and weakness.

38. **(1)** Cardiovascular risk factors predisposing females to cardiovascular disease include smaller body size, declining estrogen level, heart and thoracic cavity smaller and lighter in size, coronary arteries smaller in diameter, shorter P-R interval, higher resting ejection fraction, increased body fat percentage, and fat distributed in the abdomen that may be mobilized more easily in response to stress and raise serum cholesterol and blood glucose levels.

39. **(4)** The nurse practitioner must consider the geriatric client's other medical problems and treatment prior to prescribing medications for hypertension. Frequently, geriatric clients cannot take the β-blockers due to chronic pulmonary conditions; the client may already be on diuretics for problems of fluid retention. Step therapy is appropriate if there is no other significant medical history. Lifestyle changes should be initiated and medication adjusted as changes are made.

40. **(2)** Hypertension is considered a major factor in the development of CAD in the geriatric client. Female clients have an increased incidence of CAD after menopause; estrogen replacement appears to have cardioprotective effects on the heart, thus decreasing the incidence of CAD. Diabetics have an increased incidence of CAD; however, the majority of CAD clients are not diabetic.

41. **(4)** Cor pulmonale is characterized by hypertrophy of the right ventricle secondary to pulmonary hypertension (resistance). The increased P-wave amplitude (P pulmonale) occurs as the right atrium enlarges.

42. **(2)** Excess secretion of aldosterone predisposes to potassium excretion. Total body sodium content will be above normal, but the excessive secretion of antidiuretic hormone causes greater retention of water, diluting the serum level.

43. **(1)** Waterhammer pulse (bounding with a rapid rise and sudden collapse) is produced by an increase in pulse pressure and may be caused by an increased stroke volume, a decrease in peripheral resistance, or both. Because the nurse practitioner is suspecting either aortic regurgitation or a patent ductus arteriosus (primarily in children), auscultation for a diastolic murmur is indicated.

44. **(3)** The majority of cases of CHF in infants result from congenital heart disease during the first 12 months of life. Symptoms result from the decreased cardiac output and the infant's compensatory mechanisms. Symptoms include tachypnea, dyspnea, tachycardia, paleness, and easy fatigability. Added symptoms include periorbital edema, hepatomegaly, difficult feeding, and persistent cough. Diaphoresis, central cyanosis, and peripheral edema are not necessarily associated with CHF, but may be manifestations of the underlying congenital heart defect of the infant.

45. **(2)** Occlusion of the coronary arteries deprives the myocardial cells of glucose needed for aerobic metabolism. Anaerobic metabolism occurs, which causes the accumulation of lactic acid. Lactic acid irritates the myocardial nerve fibers, sending pain messages to the cardiac nerves and upper thoracic posterior roots located in the left shoulder and arm.

46. **(4)** Option #1 is Functional Class IV. Option #2 is Functional Class II. Option #3 is Class I. Option #4, the correct response, is Functional Class III.

47. **(4)** Common causes of chest pain include cardiac, chest wall, gastrointestinal, neurologic, and psychiatric causes. Ischemic heart disease, CHF, gastroesophageal reflux disease (GERD), and mitral valve prolapse (MVP) are more common in adults than children. Musculoskeletal problems such as costochondritis and idiopathic reasons are more common in children. Idiopathic reasons make up a large percentage of chest pain in children; symptoms appear to be

self-limited and tend to diminish or resolve in 1 year. Cardiovascular causes in children are less common, but are more serious if present and due to congenital heart lesions.

48. **(1)** The moist crackles (rales) heard in the bases of the lung are the most prominent physical examination findings of early CHF. They are caused from transudation of fluid into the alveoli and into the airways. Later findings include distended neck veins, peripheral edema, hepatomegaly, and ascites (rather than weight loss).

49. **(3)** Aortic dissection almost invariably begins with sudden onset of severe chest pain that is tearing or ripping in quality and is accompanied by loss of or decrease in peripheral pulses and neurologic deficits. The pain of angina and acute MI is usually described as a pressure. Pericarditis produces pain that is more gradual in onset.

50. **(1)** A Step I diet involves daily intake of: ≤30% total calorie intake made up of fat, <300 mg/day cholesterol intake, and 8–10% daily saturated fat intake. A decrease to <200 mg/day of cholesterol and 7% saturated fat is a Step II diet, prescribed if Step I is ineffective. The third selection is closer to the current average American's diet. Although watching calorie and sodium intake is important for weight and BP control, it is not part of a Step I diet plan for hyperlipidemia.

51. **(4)** Although the other dysrhythmias may be experienced by the client following an MI, the most life-threatening is ventricular fibrillation. The vast majority of deaths due to ventricular fibrillation happen within the first 24 hours, and, of these deaths, over half occur in the first hour. The majority of out-of-hospital deaths from MI are due to ventricular fibrillation.

52. **(1)** Congenital heart disease is commonly classified as acyanotic or cyanotic. Cyanotic heart defects (right-to-left shunts) include tetralogy of Fallot, severe pulmonary stenosis, pulmonary atresia, tricuspid atresia, and transposition of the great vessels. Children with cyanotic heart disease develop polycythemia to increase the oxygen-carrying capacity of the blood. Additionally, the young child with a cyanotic

heart defect should have a hemoglobin of at least 16 gm/dl.

53. **(2)** Diet and exercise are the mainstay of any treatment program and would be used initially in all cases. A bile acid sequestrant agent or estrogen replacement therapy may eventually be necessary if no improvement is seen with diet/exercise therapy. Referral to a cardiologist is not necessary, unless the client develops symptoms or shows resistance to treatment.

54. **(2)** A cerebrovascular accident is often the outcome of chronic atrial fibrillation due to the blood pooling in the quivering atria. This is the reason why warfarin (Coumadin) is recommended to be maintained at an international normalized ratio (INR) of 2–3. Some trials suggest aspirin may provide adequate anticoagulation in doses of 160–325 mg/day.

55. **(3)** Dyspnea is the most common symptom of CHF. Initially, it is present only with moderate exertion but, as severity of CHF increases, the dyspnea may occur with mild exertion or at rest. Fatigue is another common complaint. Right-sided heart failure is associated with weakness, anorexia, nausea, and dependent edema. Chronic left ventricular failure usually leads to right ventricular failure.

56. **(3)** Palm and coconut oils, along with butter, are very high in saturated fats and should be avoided. The other selections are moderately high in fat content but consist of mostly unsaturated fats.

57. **(3)** Anginal pain is difficult to differentiate from that of an infarction. One of the most characteristic symptoms is the relief of the anginal pain with the administration of sublingual nitroglycerin.

58. **(4)** Aspirin helps prevent the formation of platelet-aggregating substances and may help the occlusion of narrowed coronary arteries. Although Lasix, morphine, and streptokinase all have their place in treating acute MI, it is unlikely that they are available in the average primary care office.

59. **(1)** Superficial inflammation of a vein can be caused by trauma, such as a blow to the arm or leg, recent IV therapy with irritating fluids, or can occur secondary to pregnancy, especially during the postpartum period due to the increase in clotting factors (thromboplastin). Excessive use of oral anticoagulants can lead to bleeding. Deep vein thrombosis (DVT) associated with thrombophlebitis is due to prolonged bed rest, major surgical procedures, injury to the blood vessel wall, and hypercoagulable states (use of oral contraceptives, especially those women who smoke, have cancer, and polycythemia vera).

60. **(3)** Dizziness that improves when lying down and worsens when standing is symptomatic of cardiac involvement and may indicate serious cardiac dysrhythmias. If dizziness occurs in certain positions, it is indicative of benign positional vertigo, which is common in the elderly. Dizziness accompanied by tinnitus is common in acute labyrinthitis and, if preceded by rapid breathing, may be caused by hyperventilation.

61. **(3)** The stated history of a recent coxsackievirus infection, pain that worsens when supine, and a friction rub is classic for viral pericarditis. The client's age makes an acute MI unlikely, and the pain is not typical for pleural effusion or reflux.

62. **(1)** Signs and symptoms of hyperthyroidism in the older adult include progressive functional decline, atrial fibrillation, MI, tachycardia, weakness, fatigue, weight loss, anorexia, diarrhea, nervousness, tremor, pruritus, memory loss, and heat intolerance. Symptoms of hypothyroidism include arthralgia, weakness, decreased mental function, depression, constipation, weight loss, dry coarse skin with yellowish cast, dry sparse hair, and mask-like, puffy face with periorbital edema. Bradycardia would be assessed with both sick sinus syndrome and CHF. Sick sinus syndrome is often associated with the "bradycardia-tachycardia" syndrome.

63. **(4)** A jugular venous pressure of 4 cm is a sign of CHF. Option #1 is a normal sign of aging. Option #2 is a result of sclerosing of the aorta, which occurs with aging. Option #3 is expected with the aging process.

64. **(2)** This assessment is consistent with aortic stenosis. Aortic regurgitation is a diastolic murmur secondary to rheumatic heart disease. There is no history given of rheumatic heart disease. Mitral valve disease is one of the most common valvular disorders. A small percentage of mitral valve prolapse clients do suffer from autonomic dysfunction and complain of palpitations, atypical chest pain, orthostatic dizziness, near-syncope, cold extremities, throbbing headaches, and neurasthenia and manifest tachyarrhythmias. Mitral regurgitation may remain asymptomatic for many years, because the left ventricle dilates and adjusts well to the increase in volume load. Onset of dyspnea and fatigue may not occur for decades.

65. **(1)** Aortic stenosis is most common and caused by calcification. The symptoms would include syncope, angina, and dyspnea on exertion.

66. **(3)** The nurse practitioner needs to repeat the cholesterol and obtain HDL and LDL values before initiating any treatment. The HDL and LDL will help stratify risks and guide aggressiveness of intervention.

67. **(1)** Although all of these conditions can lead to hypertension, the most common in infants and young children is secondary hypertension due to renal disease (i.e., glomerulonephritis, polycystic kidneys, and nephrosis). Endocrine-induced hypertension is the second most common cause.

68. **(1)** The top two conditions known to play a causative role in the development of cardiovascular disease in children are untreated streptococcal infections involving group A β-hemolytic streptococcus (leads to cardiac valve problems) and Kawasaki disease (leads to coronary artery aneurysm).

69. **(4)** Options #1, #2, and #3 are considered unstable and acute and these clients should be immediately referred to a pediatric cardiologist. Children with a murmur need to be further evaluated, but it is not considered emergency as long as they are asymptomatic, have normal activity and exercise, and are growing normally.

70. **(3)** Procedures for which endocarditis prophylaxis is recommended include dental

procedures known to induce gingival bleeding, such as cleaning; tonsillectomy and/or adenoidectomy; and surgical procedures that involve respiratory mucosa. Endocarditis prophylaxis is not recommended for insertion of tympanostomy tubes, cardiac catheterization, simple dental procedures, or endotracheal intubation.

71. **(4)** For the child with a pacemaker, an electric shock may irreparably damage the pacemaker and thus immediate surgical replacement would be necessary. There is no risk of electromagnetic interference between the permanent pacemaker and household items such as electrical appliances, radios, electronic equipment, cellular phones, or microwave ovens. Ovens and pacemakers have filtering systems that prevent interference with the pacemaker's function. Metal detectors have an electromagnetic field that could alter the pacemaker's function temporarily. In addition, the alarm will be set off as a result of the metal in the pacemaker.

72. **(1)** According to the Jones Criteria, a diagnosis of rheumatic fever is highly likely if, in addition to two major manifestations (carditis, polyarthritis, Sydenham's chorea, erythema marginaturm, and subcutaneous nodules), or one major and two minor manifestations (arthralgia, fever, elevated ESR, C-reactive protein, and prolonged P-R interval), there is evidence of a preceding group A streptococcus infection.

Pharmacology

73. **(1)** This client is presenting with symptoms of digitalis toxicity—first-degree block and increasing cardiac irritability. If the potassium level is low, it may be precipitating the toxicity. Also, it is important to determine that serum theophylline levels remain within the therapeutic range. There is no evidence presented to indicate that the pulmonary disease is progressing. The blood pressure may be adequately controlled for this client; further information should be obtained prior to adjusting the medications. Based on the information presented, referral to a cardiologist is not appropriate at this time.

74. **(3)** Thiazide diuretics inhibit sodium reabsorption, promoting the excretion of sodium, chloride, and water. As the extracellular fluid volume decreases, plasma renin activity and aldosterone levels increase, resulting in potassium loss. Treatment is to restore the volume with normal saline and correct the potassium depletion. If the sodium is increased too rapidly, irreversible neurologic damage can occur.

75. **(1)** Vitamin K is an antidote for Coumadin. Increased intake of green leafy vegetables could cause an increase in vitamin K levels and decrease the effectiveness of the medication. Also, multivitamin supplements may contain additional vitamin K.

76. **(3)** The client presents with the classic profile of digitalis toxicity, which is frequently related to hypokalemia, especially since the potassium replacement is rather low for an adult and there is history of poor eating and nausea. The actions listed in the other options may be taken; however, it is important to determine the presence of hypokalemia and digitalis toxicity, so it may be addressed immediately.

77. **(1)** ACE inhibitors such as losartan (Cozaar) decrease the conversion of angiotensin I to angiotensin II, a potent vasoconstrictor, and inhibit the release of aldosterone.

78. **(1)** Aldactone is a potassium-sparing diuretic. Clients should be instructed on signs of hyperkalemia.

79. **(1)** β-Blockers are myocardial depressants that suppress heart rate and contraction (negative inotropic). Calcium channel blockers decrease AV conduction, which suppresses heart rate. Both drugs are contraindicated with the onset of left ventricular dysfunction.

80. **(3)** The American Heart Association's Advanced Cardiac Life Support (ACLS) guidelines recommend adenosine as the drug of choice for emergent treatment of supraventricular tachycardia, when a client is hemodynamically stable.

81. **(2)** The combination of calcium channel blockers and β-adrenergic blocking agents, systemic or ophthalmic, may result in excessive hypotension.

82. **(2)** Niacin can cause vasodilatation, leading to orthostatic hypotension. Antihyperlipidemic drugs may cause constipation. Antihyperlipidemic effectiveness is enhanced when taken before or with meals.

83. **(2)** Calcium channel blockers depress the rate of discharge from the sinoatrial node and conduction velocity through the AV node, causing a decrease in heart rate; relax the coronary and systemic arteries, producing vasodilation (decrease in afterload and blood pressure); and decrease myocardial contractility (negative inotropic effect).

84. **(2)** The dose of the client's medication had been doubled by the nurse practitioner according to the recommended protocols. The aim of therapy is to use the drugs alone or in combination to return arterial pressure to normal levels with minimal side effects. Since the therapy had been continued, doubled, the next step is to add a low-dose thiazide diuretic. Therefore, the hydrochlorothiazide addition is the correct choice. Because of reduced side effects, the ACE inhibitors are used alone first, with a slight preference for certain ACE inhibitors (enalapril over captopril and losartan [Cozaar] over both of them).

85. **(3)** Blood pressure should be lowered cautiously using smaller doses of calcium entry antagonists, ACE inhibitors, or diuretics in the elderly. β-Blockers are not appropriate in normal doses for the elderly because of decreased β-receptor sensitivity in these clients. Larger doses also result in depression, impotence, fatigue, and declining mental function. Elderly clients are especially likely to experience CHF and peripheral vascular insufficiency from β-adrenergic blocker toxicity.

86. **(2)** Nitrates are venous and arterial dilators that decrease myocardial oxygen demand. β-Blockers have an antianginal effect and reduce myocardial oxygen demand. Calcium channel blockers relieve myocardial ischemia by reducing myocardial oxygen demand and dilating coronary arteries. Aspirin is effective for primary and secondary prevention of myocardial infarction. Unless contraindicated, small doses of ASA (162–325 mg daily) should be prescribed for clients with angina. Clients remaining symptomatic when treated with nitrates, β-blockers, or calcium channel blocking drugs should be treated with a β-blocker plus a combination of another agent. Appropriate combinations are a nitrate or a β-blocker plus a calcium channel blocker other than verapamil. Combination therapy does not include sedatives, vasoconstrictors, ACE inhibitors, or lipid-lowering drugs.

87. **(3)** Adverse side effects of ACE inhibitors include cough (1–30%), headache, and dizziness. Adverse effects of calcium channel blockers include peripheral edema, dizziness, headache, nausea, and tachycardia. Adverse effects of thiazide diuretics include nausea, vomiting, diarrhea, dizziness, and headache. Side effects of β-blockers include fatigue, impotence, depression, and shortness of breath.

88. **(1)** Digoxin, once a first-line drug for all clients with CHF, is now used in clients with atrial fibrillation, other tachycardias, and left ventricular dysfunction. By controlling the ventricular rate in the client with atrial fibrillation or tachycardias, cardiac output increases. In cases of diastolic dysfunction with a sinus rhythm, digitalis is of no benefit. Digoxin is of relatively little value in most forms of cardiomyopathy, myocarditis, mitral stenosis, and chronic constrictive pericarditis.

89. **(2)** Noncardiac adverse reactions include a change in the mental status. Although visual disturbances; diarrhea; and anorexia, nausea, or vomiting are also adverse reactions, they are not the most common in the elderly.

90. **(4)** The assessments point to gout. A side effect of a thiazide diuretic is hyperuricemia. Blood for a CBC should be drawn prior to therapy. The other distractors are not addressing the assessment of a tender and edematous right ankle. The cardiac assessments were benign. There are no indications of a

concern for hypo- or hypernatremia or hypo- or hyperkalemia.

91. **(2)** β-Blockers increase peripheral vascular resistance, a phenomenon that already occurs with normal aging, so these drugs can precipitate or worsen symptoms of asthma, COPD, peripheral vascular disease, sexual dysfunction, or CHF. The other classes have no effect or decrease the effect on peripheral resistance.

92. **(1)** ACE inhibitors have been shown to prolong life in clients with CHF by improving overall cardiac function. Options #2 and #3 should be contraindicated in CHF. Although Option #4 may be correct, it is not a priority to Option #1.

93. **(4)** The most likely precipitating cause of his gout is the thiazide diuretic used to control his hypertension, since it blocks the excretion of uric acid. Although gout may be more common in obese clients, alcoholics, and diabetics, these conditions are not indicated here.

94. **(1)** The ACE inhibitor will preserve renal function and have less impact on sexual functioning. The nurse practitioner must monitor potassium and carefully follow renal status for change. The ACE inhibitor has fewer negative side effects or interactions with the other medical conditions of this client.

95. **(2)** Eighty per cent of the clients who chronically use procainamide develop antinuclear antibodies. Twenty per cent of these clients develop a lupus-like syndrome.

96. **(1)** Secondary prevention or preventing the recurrent attacks of acute rheumatic fever is controversial. Some authorities identify reaching the early 20s and 5 years since the last ARF attack as the criteria to stop the use of prophylactic penicillin, unless the client is at increased risk of exposure to streptococcal infections, as are school teachers or health professionals. Other authorities recommend lifelong prophylactic drug therapy. Although erythromycin is an alternative medication for penicillin-sensitive individuals, the dose in Option #2 is for a client having a dental or surgical procedure. The secondary prophylaxis dose for erythromycin is 250 mg PO bid.

97. **(2)** Nausea, vomiting, and anorexia are common side-effect symptoms for many medications. The first-degree AV block is what confirms the ingestion of digoxin in this situation. Tricyclic antidepressant medication toxicity is characterized by agitation and anticholingeric symptoms. Lasix symptoms include hypokalemia, weakness, and cardiac arrhythmias. Aspirin toxicity symptoms includes tinnitus, mental confusion, gastrointestinal symptoms, and rapid, deep respirations.

5

Respiratory

Physical Examination & Diagnostic Tests

1. The nurse practitioner knows that normal breath sounds that have a low pitch and soft intensity and are heard better on inspiration are called:

   1. Bronchial.

   2. Vesicular.

   3. Bronchovesicular.

   4. Rhonchi

2. When auscultating for vocal resonance in a client with possible consolidation of lung tissue, the nurse practitioner hears "a-a-a" when the client says "e-e-e." This is called:

   1. Tactile fremitus.

   2. Bronchophony.

   3. Whispered pectoriloquy.

   4. Egophony.

3. The nurse practitioner understands the following about hyperresonance in percussion of the lungs:

   1. It is a normal finding in the adult client.

2. It occurs commonly in pediatric clients.

3. It is characterized by soft intensity, high pitch, short duration, and extreme dullness quality.

4. It is characterized by loud intensity, high pitch, medium duration, and dull quality.

4. What is the correct procedure when percussing the chest?

   1. Start at the right upper side of the anterior chest and move to the left side.

   2. Begin at the upper left side of the posterior chest and compare to the respective anterior side, moving from front to back.

   3. Percuss systematically and symmetrically the anterior chest, moving from left to right side, then do the posterior chest.

   4. Percuss the posterior chest and then measure for diaphragmatic excursion on the anterior chest.

5. The nurse practitioner understands that pleural friction rubs are:

   1. Auscultated in the lower anterolateral chest.

   2. Heard best at the end of expiration.

   3. Characterized by a continuous, low-pitched, snoring sound heard early in inspiration.

   4. Noted when the client says "e-e-e" and the examiner hears through the stethoscope "a-a-a."

6. Normal physiologic changes in the respiratory system of the geriatric client include:

   1. Increased rigidity of the rib cage and an increase in the anteroposterior (AP) diameter of the chest.

   2. Increased ciliary action resulting in a more forceful and recurrent cough.

   3. Increase in number of smaller alveoli with a decrease in residual capacity.

   4. Decrease in AP diameter of rib cage with decrease in lung expansion.

7. When assessing for tactile fremitus, the nurse practitioner would place her hands over what area of the client's chest?

   1. On the anterior chest at the level of the sixth intercostal space.

   2. At the level of bifurcation of the bronchi on the posterior chest wall.

   3. At the apex on the anterior chest wall.

   4. At the level of the diaphragm on the posterior chest wall.

8. On assessment of the client's respiratory status, crepitation is felt over the third rib at the midaxillary line on the left side. The interpretation of this finding is:

   1. There is consolidation of fluid in the left lower lobe of the lung.

   2. Severe inflammation is present on the visceral pleural surfaces of the left lung.

   3. An increase in pressure has occurred in the pleural cavity on the right lung.

   4. Air is present in the subcutaneous tissue from an air leak in the respiratory system.

9. An important anatomic landmark on the anterior thoracic wall is the angle of Louis. Where on the thorax is this landmark present?

   1. The mid-nipple line on either side of the manubrium.

   2. Bilaterally at the manubriosternal junction.

   3. Midline at the base of the suprasternal notch.

   4. Just below the clavicle but above the manubrium.

10. During the assessment of a geriatric client's respiratory status, the nurse practitioner determines the presence of coarse tactile fremitus posteriorly at the second intercostal space. The best interpretation of this finding is:

    1. Increased air trapping in the alveoli on the affected side.

    2. Presence of fluid or solid mass within the lungs.

    3. Increased pressure in the bronchial tree.

    4. Presence of hyperactive airway disease.

11. When the lateral diameter of the chest is the same size as the AP diameter, the nurse practitioner correctly documents this finding as a:

    1. Biot deviated chest.

    2. Pigeon chest.

    3. Funnel chest.

    4. Barrel chest.

12. Cystic fibrosis is the preliminary diagnosis for a young girl who was brought to the clinic for evaluation. The test that will be used to rule out cystic fibrosis is:

    1. Hemoccult test.

    2. Sweat chloride test.

    3. Sputum culture and sensitivity.

    4. Glucose tolerance test.

13. The nurse practitioner is planning a community screening program for lung cancer in geriatric clients. Which examination is best to use for this program?

    1. Bronchoscopy with biopsy for cytology.

    2. Arterial blood-gas studies.

    3. Pulmonary function test.

    4. Chest x-ray and comparison with previous x-ray.

14. An adult male client comes to the clinic with the chief complaint of "coughing up blood." He has no history of respiratory or cardiac problems. His vital signs are pulse 96, respirations 28, blood pressure 140/92, temperature of 99°F orally. The initial diagnostic evaluation of this client includes:

    1. Electrocardiogram, pulmonary function studies, sputum cytology.

    2. PPD skin test, chest x-ray, sputum smear for acid-fast bacillus.

    3. Arterial blood-gas studies, CBC, chest x-ray.

    4. Direct bronchoscopy with biopsy and complement fixation antibody titer.

15. A client comes to the clinic complaining of difficulty breathing, lethargy, and coughing up blood in his sputum. He has no history of chronic illness or major health problems. The nurse practitioner orders diagnostic tests to determine the problem. What diagnostic test results would require immediate treatment of this client?

    1. Positive sputum smear for acid-fast bacillus.

    2. Sputum culture positive for *Pneumocystis carinii*.

    3. Presence of hemolysis on complement fixation test.

    4. Oxygen saturation 94%, leukocyte count >5000 white blood cells (WBC)/mm^3.

16. When assessing the pulmonary function studies of a client, which assessment finding is seen in chronic air flow limitation such as emphysema?

    1. Decrease in forced vital capacity (FVC) and forced expiratory volume timed (FEV$_1$).

    2. Increase functional residual capacity (FRC) and residual volumes (RV).

    3. Decrease residual volume (RV) and increase in total lung capacity (TLC).

    4. Increase in forced expiratory volume timed (FEV$_1$) and total lung capacity (TLC).

17. When interpreting purified protein derivative (PPD) skin tests in clients at a long-term care facility, the nurse practitioner identifies positive results in individuals with:

    1. Redness or erythema at the site.

    2. An induration reaction of $\geq$5 mm.

    3. An induration reaction of $\geq$10 mm.

    4. An induration reaction extending to 15 mm.

Disorders

18. A client has received a blunt trauma injury to his chest. An assessment finding that would be most indicative of further respiratory complications would be:

    1. Complaints of increased pain over the affected area.

    2. Oximetry readings consistently around 90%.

    3. Decreased breath sounds on the affected side.

    4. Fever of 102°F and increased sputum production.

19. The nurse understands that the following characteristic is more likely to occur when the adult client has pneumonia (due to *Streptococcus pneumoniae*) rather than bronchitis:

    1. Rusty sputum.

    2. Cough.

    3. Dyspnea.

    4. Wheezing

20. A child is recovering from tuberculosis. What information should be included in a teaching plan for her home care?

    1. It is critical for the child to take medications at the prescribed time; do not skip doses or allow the supply to run out.

    2. Respiratory isolation procedures need to be carried out at home; the child should avoid contact with immediate family members.

    3. It will be necessary for the parent to return to the clinic every week to have the child's sputum checked for viable bacteria.

    4. The child may experience a rash along with nausea and vomiting from the medications and the parent should decrease the dosage if this occurs.

21. What would be a priority intervention for a client experiencing a respiratory arrest?

    1. Start chest compressions at 15 compressions and two breaths.

    2. Open the airway with a head tilt and chin lift.

    3. Give oxygen via a rebreathing mask at 10 L/min.

    4. Pinch the nose and give two breaths.

22. A client comes to the emergency room complaining of difficulty breathing. What is most important to establish initially in this client?

    1. What type of activity produces the dyspnea.

    2. The presence of consolidation via a chest x-ray.

    3. Arterial blood-gas levels with respect to oxygen pressures.

    4. Presence of bilateral breath sounds over the lower lobes.

23. A client is severely dyspneic and the history strongly suggests the possibility of a foreign body in the bronchi. What observation would contribute to the documentation of this problem?

    1. Unilateral retraction of the right chest wall.

    2. Presence of crepitation on the anterior chest wall.

    3. Retraction of the lower chest wall.

    4. A friction rub heard over the area of the bronchi.

24. The nurse practitioner is assessing a client who is complaining of shortness of breath and chest discomfort. His respirations are shallow and at a rate of 26. When evaluating the diaphragmatic excursion, it is determined that the diaphragm on the right is slightly higher than on the left side. The best interpretation of these findings is:

    1. This is normal due to the liver on the right side.

    2. There may be atelectasis in the right lower lobe.

    3. Consolidation is present in the right lower lobe.

    4. This indicates the presence of early stages of chronic obstructive lung disease.

25. A 22-year-old male comes to the office complaining of chest pain and shortness of breath. He states the problems started suddenly after running sprints in basketball practice. He states he has no past history of pulmonary problems. He is about 72 inches tall and weighs approximately 145 lbs, his pulse rate is 118, his respiratory rate is 30, there are decreased breath sounds, and there is hyperresonance over the left lung. The best diagnosis for this client is:

    1. Spontaneous pneumothorax.

    2. Exercise-induced asthma.

    3. Pulmonary edema.

    4. Acute bronchiectasis.

26. A young woman presents at the clinic with complaints of tingling in her face and hands, sudden shortness of breath, and vague chest discomfort. She appears very anxious and denies any history of respiratory problems. On examination her hands are cool to touch; her vital signs are respirations 34, pulse regular at a rate of

100, blood pressure 110/76, and normal temperature. Respiratory examination reveals bilateral breath sounds with tachypnea, no adventitious sounds, and normal percussion and visual examination of the chest. The best immediate treatment is:

1. Rebreathing into a paper bag and encouraging controlled diaphragmatic breathing.

2. Albuterol (Proventil) two puffs with a metered-dose inhaler.

3. Oxygen at 4 L and arterial blood gases after 30 minutes.

4. Establish an IV, infuse 500 ml normal saline for volume depletion.

27. An 18-month-old infant is brought into the emergency room He is awake, lethargic, and in severe respiratory distress. His mother states that he has not been sick and was playing on the floor when he suddenly began coughing, choking, and gagging. He has expiratory wheezes and there are decreased breath sounds over the right lower lobes. His respirations are 36, pulse is 130, and temperature is normal. A portable chest x-ray shows hyperinflation on expiratory views. The best treatment for this infant is:

1. Bronchoscopy as soon as possible.

2. Cool mist therapy with racemic epinephrine.

3. Antibiotics with chest physiotherapy.

4. Immediate endotracheal intubation and ventilation.

28. A 4-month-old client presents to the office with a history of several days of rhinorrhea, cough, low-grade fever, and increased respiratory rate. The most likely diagnosis is:

1. Croup.

2. Epiglottitis.

3. Tracheitis.

4. Bronchiolitis.

29. A newly diagnosed COPD client is being discharged from the hospital. The nurse practitioner is discussing home care with the client. What information is important for the practitioner to include in the home care teaching?

1. Use the bronchodilator prior to exercising.

2. Maintain bed rest for the first few days at home.

3. Decrease amount of fluid intake to prevent fluid overload.

4. Maintain flow rate on oxygen around 5–7 L.

30. A client is admitted to a rural emergency department by ambulance. Primary assessment reveals:

- Respirations: 38/min with of accessory muscles, prolonged expiration and wheezes

- ECG: Sinus tachycardia rate 140

- Blood pressure: 192/98

- Lethargic: Responds to name only by opening eyes

- Cyanosis of lips

Therapeutic interventions initiated by emergency medical technicians include:

- Intravenous therapy of D_5W at 30 ml/hr

- Oxygen therapy at 48% by venturi mask

STAT arterial blood gases (ABGs) indicate:

- pH = 7.24

- $PaCO_2$ = 82 mm Hg

- HCO_3 = 36

- PaO_2 = 76 mm Hg

Prior to obtaining a second set of ABGs, the nurse practitioner would:

1. Assist respirations with bag-valve mask with 100% oxygen.

2. Administer 1 ampule of sodium bicarbonate.

3. Change oxygen delivery to nasal cannula at 2 L.

4. Disconnect the supplemental oxygen.

31. Instructions to the elderly client with COPD concerning nutritional therapy would include foods that are:

    1. High caloric, high protein, low carbohydrate.

    2. High caloric, low protein, high carbohydrate.

    3. Low caloric, high protein, low carbohydrate.

    4. Low caloric, low protein, high carbohydrate.

32. Age-associated changes that increase the risk for pneumonia in the elderly client include an increase in:

    1. Compliance of the chest wall.

    2. Diameter of the trachea and bronchi.

    3. Lung parenchyma.

    4. Cough forcefulness.

33. An adult client arrives at the clinic complaining of difficulty breathing, a cough, and chest pain. History indicates the client was discharged from the hospital 2 days ago after a cesarean section and has a 15-pack-year smoking history. Diagnostic studies should include:

    1. Sputum for culture and sensitivity.

    2. Cardiac troponin proteins.

    3. Pulse oximetry.

    4. Arterial blood gases.

34. The nurse practitioner is aware that the flu or influenza:

    1. Can be caused by receiving a flu vaccine when one's resistance is low.

    2. Is characterized by a slow, insidious onset of chills, fever, and muscle aches.

    3. In older adults may persist for several weeks with symptoms of lack of energy and extreme tiredness.

    4. Is primarily contagious in the early autumn and spring.

35. During a physical exam of a 2-year-old diagnosed with possible cystic fibrosis, the child passes a stool. The nurse practitioner would expect the stool's appearance to be:

    1. Yellow and loose.

    2. Small and constipated.

    3. Green and odorous.

    4. Large and bulky.

36. An adult client with a history of asthma calls to tell the nurse practitioner that she is "blowing 55%" on the peak flowmeter. What advice would the nurse practitioner give this client?

    1. Call an ambulance immediately.

    2. Use a bronchodilator now and come in for evaluation in the office today.

    3. Come in for office evaluation this week.

    4. Refer to a pulmonary physician.

37. An elderly client is evaluated by the nurse practitioner for a complaint of cough, fever, chest pain, and sputum production. In gathering a history on this client, it is important to know if the client has:

    1. Received the pneumococcal vaccine.

    2. Traveled out of the country.

    3. Pets in the household.

    4. Recently started new medications.

38. An elderly client presents with signs and symptoms that make the nurse practitioner suspect the diagnosis of pneumonia. Which assessment would the nurse practitioner most likely evaluate during the examination?

    1. Chest pain with inspiration.

    2. Confusion with a low-grade temperature.

    3. Congested, productive cough.

    4. Fever with leukocytosis.

39. In developing a plan for an older client with pneumonia, the nurse practitioner understands that 30–40% of community-acquired pneumonia is caused by which organism?

    1. *Haemophilus influenzae.*

    2. *Klebsiella pneumoniae.*

3. *Mycobacterium tuberculosis.*

4. *Streptococcus pneumoniae.*

40. Which plan would be most appropriate to include in the health promotion plan for an older client who is at risk for developing pneumonia?

    1. Administer the pneumococcal vaccination annually.

    2. Administer the pneumococcal vaccination and yearly influenza immunization.

    3. Sputum culture annually along with a chest x-ray.

    4. PPD done every 3–5 years.

41. The nurse practitioner evaluates an older client with a current history of alcoholism. The client presents with an elevated temperature, congested cough producing rusty sputum, and occasional chills. The suspected diagnosis is bacterial pneumonia. The Gram-stained sputum smear would most likely reveal which organism?

    1. *Haemophilus influenzae.*

    2. *Klebsiella pneumoniae.*

    3. *Staphylococcus aureus.*

    4. *Streptococcus pneumoniae.*

42. An elderly client residing in a nursing home has recently been exposed to tuberculosis (TB). The nurse practitioner interprets the initial PPD test to be negative. Which plan would be most appropriate at this time?

    1. Evaluate client in another year.

    2. Repeat PPD test in 1 week.

    3. Ignore results and immediately begin ethambutol.

    4. Evaluate client in 6 months, since he is asymptomatic at this time.

43. The nurse practitioner knows that Horner's syndrome is commonly associated with:

    1. Chronic bronchitis.

    2. Pulmonary tuberculosis.

    3. Pancoast's syndrome of lung cancer.

    4. Pulmonary embolism.

44. An adult client who smokes presents with complaints of breathlessness. The nurse practitioner notes on examination dilated blood vessels on the chest and mild edema of the head and supraclavicular area. She recognizes this condition as:

    1. Thyroid abnormality.

    2. Chronic bronchitis with mild congestive failure.

    3. Asthma with fluid retention.

    4. Superior vena cava obstruction.

45. A 3-year-old client with a history of asthma presents to the office for evaluation by the nurse practitioner. The child has never used a peak flowmeter. What quick tool can the nurse practitioner use to assess the severity of this child's distress?

    1. An arterial blood gas study.

    2. The child's inability to complete a sentence.

    3. A chest x-ray.

    4. The presence of a runny nose.

46. An elderly client presents with postural hypotension, and laboratory studies reveal hyponatremia. The most likely cause of this is:

    1. Diabetic ketoacidosis.

    2. Severe trauma.

    3. Bronchogenic carcinoma.

    4. Antacid overuse.

47. The nurse practitioner knows the following about asthma in the elderly:

    1. Subcutaneous epinephrine is standard therapy.

    2. It is usually of the allergic-type.

    3. Attacks are usually preceded by viral infections.

    4. Clinical presentation is usually dyspnea, costal retraction, and fever.

48. Clinical signs and symptoms of late-phase asthma include:

    1. Bronchoconstriction refractory to bronchodilator therapy.

    2. Sneezing, watery eyes, and cough.

    3. Wheezing and increased sputum production.

    4. Bronchodilation secondary to release of histamine.

49. The nurse practitioner is assessing a client for asthma. What is a common clinical manifestation of asthma?

    1. Pruritis.

    2. Diffuse crackles.

    3. Nocturnal exacerbation.

    4. Chronic hypoxemia.

50. During a routine follow-up visit for a client with asthma, she states that she has been doing fine except that, when she goes out for dinner, she notices she has increased bronchospasm and wheezing. Which would be an appropriate response?

    1. "Have you been taking your medication?"

    2. "Do you usually have wine with dinner?"

    3. "I recommend you do not go out for dinner."

    4. "Does going out to dinner make you stressed?"

51. A mother tells the nurse practitioner that her child has nocturnal asthma attacks. The nurse practitioner would expect the mother to explain that the attacks are the worst:

    1. At midnight.

    2. 2 hours after going to bed.

    3. Immediately after falling asleep.

    4. At 4 AM.

52. The nurse practitioner understands the following concerning tuberculosis:

    1. Infants are more likely than children to present with wheezing and rales.

    2. Older children develop disseminated disease and meningitis more often than infants.

    3. Affected infants and young children are more likely to have a PPD skin test of 15 mm or more.

    4. Adults are rarely the source of the disease when a child develops tuberculosis.

53. During a 4-month visit to the clinic for routine care, the mother reports that her infant who was diagnosed with bronchopulmonary dysplasia (BPD) has been vomiting after each gastrostomy feeding. The nurse practitioner notes that the infant's weight gain is adequate and would recommend:

    1. Referral to the pediatrician for follow-up.

    2. Reduction in the amount of formula for the gastrostomy feeding.

    3. Addition of 3 oz of Pedialyte for the next two feedings.

    4. Positioning of the infant in a prone position after feedings with the head and trunk elevated.

54. A 3-year-old male who is up-to-date on his immunizations is brought to the office by his mother with a fairly rapid onset of stridor and a high-pitched wheeze. In view of this information, the differential diagnosis that could be considered less likely than the other is:

    1. Croup.

    2. Foreign body aspiration.

    3. Epiglottitis.

    4. Bacterial tracheitis.

Pharmacology

55. The nurse practitioner is following up on a client who is experiencing acute asthmatic problems. Albuterol (Proventil) by metered-dose inhaler has been ordered as treatment. Which client response would indicate to the nurse practitioner that the client understands how to take his medication?

1. "I will take one puff of the medication and then wait a minute before taking the second puff."

2. "I will take two puffs of the medication every 4 hours, even if I am not short of breath."

3. "It is important for me to take this medication on a regular cycle to prevent future attacks."

4. "I will take two puffs, one right after the other, whenever I begin to get short of breath."

56. A client who was recently diagnosed with tuberculosis calls the clinic because her urine is reddish orange. She is taking isoniazid (INH; Laniazid), rifampin (Rifadin), and pyrazinamide. An appropriate response for the nurse practitioner to make would be:

    1. "This is a urinary tract infection symptom; drink plenty of fluids."

    2. "This is a normal response to the rifampin."

    3. "Often this is an indication of liver toxicity. Stop the medications."

    4. "This is probably bleeding and you should see a physician immediately."

57. A 15-year-old female comes into the emergency room with complaints of extreme shortness of breath. She is confused and her past medical history is not available. Her vital signs are pulse 124, respirations 32, blood pressure 124/80, and temperature normal. Physical examination reveals diffuse expiratory wheezes, hyperresonance on percussion, and a prolonged expiratory phase. The best treatment for this client includes:

    1. Aminophylline by mouth.

    2. Beclomethasone (Beclovent) inhaler.

    3. Epinephrine by injection.

    4. Albuterol (Proventil) metered-dose inhaler (MDI).

58. A client with a history of bronchial asthma is seen in the clinic for increased episodes of difficult breathing. The client has been taking theophylline 100 mg PO tid. The client is a 40-year-old obese male with an 18-pack-year history of cigarette smoking and an excessive intake of coffee daily, and who eats a low-carbohydrate, high-protein diet. Which identified factors decrease the therapeutic effects of the theophylline?

    1. Age and gender.

    2. Coffee intake and weight.

    3. Age and weight.

    4. Smoking history and diet.

59. A 70-year-old man comes to the clinic with complaints that he is experiencing increased difficulty breathing over the past few days. He has a history of chronic obstructive lung disease and coronary artery disease. He was recently diagnosed with hypertension. Examination reveals no jugular vein distention, slight increase in the AP diameter of the chest, and no productive cough; breath sounds are present but expiratory wheezes are noted bilaterally, and he denies complaints of chest pain. His vital signs are pulse 72, respirations 34, and blood pressure 170/100. His current medications are ipratropium bromide (Atrovent) inhaler two puffs q6h, nitroglycerin transdermal patches, and propranolol (Inderal) 60 mg PO bid. The best treatment for this client is:

    1. Discontinue the propranolol (Inderal) and begin verapamil (Calan) 80 mg PO tid qd.

    2. Begin theophylline (Theo-Dur) 200 mg q12h PO.

    3. Discontinue the propranolol (Inderal) and begin on atenolol (Tenormin) 50 mg PO qd.

    4. Start beclomethasone (Beclovent) inhaler two puffs 3–4 times daily.

60. The recommended range for maintaining serum theophylline levels is:

    1. 0.05–2 µg/ml.

    2. 5–15 µg/ml.

    3. 20–25 µg/ml.

    4. 30–40 µg/ml.

61. A client in a long-term facility whose roommate has been diagnosed as having active tuberculosis should be started on chemoprophylaxis:

    1. As soon as possible and initiated at the time of screening skin testing.

    2. In 72 hours after PPD skin test results are obtained.

    3. Only if PPD skin test results are positive.

    4. In 3 months if the repeated skin test is positive.

62. In adults with asthma, the most common reason outpatient treatment fails, resulting in hospitalization, is:

    1. Exposure to allergens.

    2. Increased use of steroids.

    3. Improper inhaler technique.

    4. Use of cromolyn inhalers.

63. Which can elevate theophylline levels?

    1. Concomitant treatment with cimetidine (Tagamet).

    2. Intravenous ampicillin.

    3. Heavy smoking.

    4. History of seizure disorder.

64. A client with a long history of chronic airflow limitation has noticed a change in sputum over the past few days (increased amount of thick, yellow-green mucus, congestion). Appropriate therapy is:

    1. Hismanal 10 mg PO qd.

    2. Augmentin 500 mg PO tid × 10 days.

    3. Tylenol with codeine.

    4. Vancenase MDI 2 puffs prn.

65. Which medication is most effective in promoting a decrease in airway inflammation as well as providing long-term medication coverage in a client with asthma?

    1. Isoetharine (Bronkometer).

    2. Beclomethasone diproprionate (Vanceril, Beclovent).

    3. Albuterol (Proventil, Ventolin).

    4. Pirbuterol (Maxair).

66. The nurse practitioner is planning prophylactic treatment for a client with asthma. What is the best medication to use for the asthmatic client who is not currently experiencing an exacerbation?

    1. Antibiotics.

    2. Inhaled glucocorticoids.

    3. β_1-Agonist.

    4. Methacholine challenge.

67. Clients with asthma need to be instructed to:

    1. Begin their inhaled steroids as soon as symptoms appear.

    2. Using the metered-dose inhaler, take two puffs on the β-agonist prn.

    3. Use their inhaled steroids when they experience bronchospasm.

    4. Start their antibiotic regimen when they experience bronchospasm.

68. The nurse practitioner understands that an appropriate medication regimen for a child with tuberculosis is:

    1. Singular drug therapy with rifampin (Rifadin).

    2. Combination therapy with streptomycin, pyrazinamide, and rimantadine (Flumadine).

    3. Combination therapy with isoniazid, pyrazinamide, and rifampin.

    4. Singular therapy with pyrimethamine (Fansidar).

69. During a routine well-child exam of a 4-year-old, the nurse practitioner learns that the paternal grandmother has just been diagnosed with active tuberculosis. The mother states that the grandmother had stayed in their home for a week during the summer. The child has no signs of tuberculosis and has a negative PPD. The nurse practitioner should:

    1. Prescribe no medications, but schedule a repeat PPD in 2 months.

2. Administer 1 ml gamma globulin IM.

3. Start the child on a combination of isoniazid and rifampin therapy for 15 months.

4. Start the child on isoniazid therapy for 3 months and then re-evaluate.

70. A client presents in the clinic with a dry hacking, nonproductive cough that is interfering with her sleep. The nurse practitioner would encourage the client to purchase an over-the-counter preparation that contains:

1. Pseudoephedrine.

2. Phenylpropanolamine.

3. Guaifenesin.

4. Dextromethorphan.

71. Indications for antibiotic use in a child with asthmatic bronchitis would include:

1. History of two episodes in 4 months.

2. Rhinitis and a productive cough.

3. High fever and rales.

4. Low-grade fever and sibilant wheezes.

72. A 10-year-old on INH prophylactically for exposure to tuberculosis complains of headache, palpitations, a rash, and diarrhea. Management would be based on:

1. Avoidance of tyramine- and histamine-containing foods.

2. Addition of pyridoxine to the diet.

3. Changing the INH to rifampin (Rifadin).

4. Evaluate for hepatic impairment.

73. What is the initial treatment of choice for children diagnosed with bronchiolitis?

1. Increase fluids, albuterol (Ventolin) in saline inhalation every 4–6 hours.

2. Prednisolone (Pediapred) immediately and continue over 3–5 days.

3. Diphenhydramine HCL (Benadryl) every 4–6 hours as long as symptoms persist.

4. Amoxicillin over 10–14 days and aerosol humidification.

74. A 10-year-old boy is experiencing problems with wheezing, coughing, and shortness of breath about 4 hours after basketball practice. He has normal respirations and only experiences the problems after exercise. He is experiencing no other respiratory problems and the physical exam is within normal limits. What is the treatment of choice for this child?

1. Albuterol (Ventolin) 20–30 minutes prior to exercise.

2. Cromolyn sodium (Intal) two puffs each morning.

3. Theophylline (Theo-Dur) PO, bid.

4. Beclomethasone (Beclovent) two puffs 3–4 times daily.

75. A client with chronic asthma is seen in the clinic complaining of vomiting and stomach cramps. He is confused and is unsure what medications he is currently taking. His vital signs are blood pressure 158/92, pulse 152 and irregular, and respirations 28 and shallow. What stat diagnostic study should be obtained?

1. Serum electrolytes.

2. Digoxin level.

3. Theophylline level.

4. Arterial blood gases.

76. A client is seen in the clinic complaining of increased difficulty breathing and an intermittent productive cough that worsens in the evening. The history revels that the client has a 20-pack-year history of smoking. Breath sounds are clear to auscultation, there is no evidence of fever, and chest radiography is within normal limits. The nurse practitioner instructs the client concerning the importance of smoking cessation and fluid therapy and prescribes:

1. Erythromycin 500 mg PO qid × 14 days.

2. Albuterol 2 mg PO tid.

3. Mucomyst inhalation 10 ml of 10% solution q4h prn.

4. Tetracycline 100 mg q12h × 14 days.

77. When initiating preventive care to decrease the incidence of pneumonia in clients in an extended-care facility, the nurse practitioner would identify clients receiving immunosuppressive therapy, repeated antibiotic use, sedation, and:

    1. β_1-Adrenergic blocking agents.

    2. Calcium channel blockers.

    3. Diuretics.

    4. Histamine$_2$ antagonists.

78. An older adult client presents with complaints of dyspnea, cough, fatigue, and dependent edema that has been worsening over the past few days. In planning the treatment for this client, the nurse practitioner considers:

    1. Streptokinase therapy.

    2. Hospitalization for evaluation of heart function.

    3. Prescription for furosemide (Lasix) 40 mg PO qd.

    4. Addition of a calcium channel blocker to the client's medications.

79. A client with a history of Parkinson's disease has a positive TB skin test and INH is ordered as a prophylactic medication. Prior to beginning INH, it is important for the nurse practitioner to determine:

    1. Is the client's Parkinson's condition being treated with levodopa (Larodopa).

    2. How long the client has been diagnosed with Parkinson's disease.

    3. How much respiratory compromise the client is currently experiencing.

    4. The adequacy of urinary output and renal function.

80. A geriatric client is seen for an upper respiratory infection and the nurse practitioner decides to prescribe erythromycin. On review of the client's history, what current medication would be a contraindication to the administration of erythromycin?

    1. Cisapride (Propulsid).

    2. Lisinopril (Zestril).

    3. Moexipril (Univasc).

    4. Atenolol (Tenormin).

Answers & Rationales

Physical Examination & Diagnostic Tests

1. **(2)** The sounds heard over normal lung tissue are called vesicular breath sounds. The inspiratory phase of the vesicular breath sound is heard better than the expiratory phase and is about 2.5 times longer for these low-pitched, soft sounds. Bronchial breath sounds are normally heard over the trachea and usually indicate pathology. Bronchial breath sounds are high-pitched, loud sounds with a shortened inspiratory and lengthened expiratory phase. Bronchovesicular breath sounds have an intermediate pitch and intensity with equal duration of expiratory and inspiratory sounds heard mainly over the second interspace anteriorly and between the scapulae posteriorly. Rhonchi are abnormal breath sounds that are low pitched with a snoring quality.

2. **(4)** Tactile fremitus is a palpable vibration of the thoracic wall that is produced when the client speaks. Bronchophony is the increase in loudness and clarity of vocal resonance. Whispered pectoriloquy is exaggerated bronchophony and is heard through a stethoscope when the client whispers a series of words (e.g., "ninety-nine"). In egophony, the spoken voice has a nasal or bleating quality when heard through a stethoscope and the spoken "e-e-e" sounds like "a-a-a."

3. **(2)** Hyperresonance is an abnormal percussion tone in adults but occurs normally in a child's lung. It is characterized by very loud intensity, very low pitch, long duration, and a booming quality.

4. **(3)** Both the anterior and posterior chest are to be percussed systematically and symmetrically, moving from left to right. Diaphragmatic excursion is usually only measured on the posterior chest.

5. **(1)** Pleural friction rubs are loud, dry, creaking or grating sounds produced by the rubbing together of inflamed and roughened pleural surfaces that are heard best during the latter part of inspiration and the beginning of expiration and in the lower anterolateral chest. Option #3 is characteristic of sonorous rhonchi.

6. **(1)** With aging, there is a decrease in the number of alveoli, and the alveoli become rigid and lose the ability to recoil. The loss of alveolar elasticity affects the ability of the client to exhale effectively, and there is an increase in the residual volume. There is also a decrease in basilar inflation and a decrease in the ability to expel foreign matter. The AP diameter of the chest increases, as seen in clients with kyphosis.

7. **(2)** The bifurcation of the trachea or bronchi on the posterior chest wall is the best area for assessment of tactile fremitus. Care should be taken to avoid the area over the scapula.

8. **(4)** Crepitation or crepitus (also called subcutaneous emphysema) results from air bubbles under the skin from a rupture somewhere in the respiratory system, or less commonly from an infection by a gas-producing organism. Crepitation always requires attention.

9. **(2)** This landmark can be used to determine the position of the second rib and intercostal space and corresponding spaces below that level. It is a visible and palpable angle of the sternum at the point where the second rib attaches to the sternum.

10. **(2)** Fluid or solid mass transmits the vibrations so that tactile fremitus may be felt on the exterior chest wall. Increased air trapping will cause a decreased or absent fremitus. A reactive airway results in wheezing due to edematous airway.

11. **(4)** The adult chest is somewhat asymmetric and the AP diameter is often one half the transverse diameter.

12. **(2)** Sweat chloride test is positive for cystic fibrosis due to the abnormal amount of sodium chloride in the sweat. Hemoccult is a test for blood in the stool. Sputum culture and sensitivity is performed to determine what medication is effective against an organism. Glucose tolerance test is performed to diagnose diabetes.

13. **(4)** For preliminary screening, the chest x-ray is the best, since it is less expensive and less invasive. It is even more beneficial if it can be compared to previous chest x-rays. All of the other options are beneficial in diagnosing malignancy, but the x-ray is best for a screening program.

14. **(2)** The client should be initially evaluated for tuberculosis. Pulmonary function studies, ABG studies, and bronchoscopy are not indicated at this time. Complement fixation studies are done to diagnose atypical pneumonia.

15. **(1)** The positive sputum for acid-fast bacillus is indicative of active tuberculosis. The *P. carinii* is a common organism in healthy respiratory tracts; it becomes a problem if the client is immuno-compromised. Hemolysis on a complement fixation test is a negative finding. When

oxygen saturation is low and the leukocyte count is within normal ranges, treatment is not as important as for tuberculosis.

16. **(2)** Hyperinflation due to air trapping causes an increase in FRC, RV, and TLC (which may be twice normal). A corresponding decrease in FVC and FEV_1 occurs. This causes a flattening of the diaphragm, decreased inspiratory efficiency, and increased work of breathing.

17. **(3)** Positive interpretation of PPD skin test results are as follows:

Induration	Positive in:
≥5 mm	Individuals with human immunodeficiency virus (HIV) infection
	Recent close contact with individuals with active TB
	Individuals with chest x-ray indicating healed TB
≥10 mm	Medically underserved individuals
	IV drug users
	Clients in long-term care facilities
≥15 mm	All individuals

Disorders

18. **(3)** The most common respiratory complication after a traumatic injury to the chest is pneumothorax caused from a fractured rib. Oximetry readings at 90% and increased pain are expected at this point and may not be indicative of a problem.

19. **(1)** Pneumococcal pneumonia due to *S. pneumoniae* often presents abruptly with high fever, shaking chills (rigor), cough productive of purulent or rusty sputum, headache, and pleuritic chest pain. In acute bronchitis, cough is the primary symptom and initially is dry and nonproductive. Fever, dyspnea, wheezing, and possible mucoid sputum production are also characteristic of acute bronchitis.

20. **(1)** On discharge, a client must understand the importance of taking medications as prescribed. If doses are missed, it will increase the mutation of the tubercule bacillus and decrease the effectiveness of the medication. Respiratory isolation at

home is not necessary and if she experiences problems of rash, nausea, and vomiting, she should contact her health care provider. Weekly sputum checks are not necessary.

21. **(2)** According to the American Heart Association, the protocol for cardiopulmonary resuscitation (CPR) (rescue breathing) due to respiratory arrest would be to open the airway by tilting the head and lifting the chin.

22. **(1)** It is most important to determine what precipitates the dyspnea. Is it present during rest or does it occur with activity? What level of activity precipitates the problem? This is important information necessary in order to determine the severity of the client's complaint.

23. **(1)** The most common area for a foreign body obstruction is the right bronchi; this will produce a unilateral retraction of the right chest wall. Retraction of the lower chest occurs with lower respiratory problems such as asthma. A pleural friction rub is heard when there is inflammation between the visceral and parietal pleura. Crepitation is present when air is leaking into the subcutaneous tissue.

24. **(1)** This is a normal finding due to the bulk of the liver. Atelectasis and consolidation will present with normal diaphragmatic movement but with dullness to percussion over the affected area. Obstructive lung disease will result in hyperresonance and limited diaphragmatic excursion, but it will be bilateral.

25. **(1)** Spontaneous pneumothorax occurs in healthy, thin young adults, especially after strenuous exercise; predominant symptoms include sudden pain and dyspnea. The clinical hallmark of asthma is wheezing; with pulmonary edema there is frequently coughing, frothy sputum, and crackles heard on auscultation. Bronchiectasis is most often chronic and is characterized by moist crackles and wheezing on ausculation; cough is usually present.

26. **(1)** The situation described is hyperventilation; by slowing the breathing, and breathing into a paper bag the carbon dioxide levels will be restored and the acid-base problem resolved. Albuterol, oxygen, ABGs, and IV fluids are not appropriate initial treatment.

27. **(1)** The child has the symptoms and history that are consistent with a partial airway obstruction from aspiration of a foreign body. Direct laryngoscopy or bronchoscopy are necessary to remove the foreign body. Chest physiotherapy may dislodge the object and force it farther into the airway. Antibiotics and epinephrine are not going to be effective. There is no need to intubate the infant if the foreign body can be removed.

28. **(4)** Croup, epiglottitis, and tracheitis are all middle respiratory tract infections with a rapid onset. Bronchiolitis is a lower respiratory tract infection that has a more gradual onset and no "barking" sound to the cough.

29. **(1)** In order to prevent dyspnea on activity, the bronchodilator should be used prior to walking or increased physical activity. The client should not stay in bed but should be encouraged to gradually increase activity. Fluid intake of 2–3 L/day should be encouraged, unless there are cardiac problems. The oxygen level should not exceed 3- to 4-L flow.

30. **(3)** Elevated bicarbonate levels of blood are expected in clients with chronic hypercapnia. Hypoventilation and acidemia can result when too much oxygen is delivered. Supplemental oxygen should not be discontinued because the PaO_2 levels decrease faster than the stimulus to breathe returns to eliminate the accumulated store of carbon dioxide. Discontinuing supplemental oxygen, even for a short period of time, could cause serious complications.

31. **(1)** Nutritional needs are meet by high-caloric, high-protein foods. High-carbohydrate foods need to be avoided in clients who retain CO_2 because carbohydrates metabolize into CO_2 as a waste product.

32. **(2)** Age-associated physiologic changes include:

- A decreased compliance of the chest wall, making deep inspiration difficult.
- The trachea and bronchi increase in diameter, increasing dead space and resulting in a decrease of volume of air reaching the alveoli.
- The lung parenchyma become less elastic, which decreases the function of the alveoli.
- Breathing becomes more shallow and cough forcefulness decreases due to respiratory muscles weakening.

33. **(4)** The client is at risk for a pulmonary embolism as a result of hypercoagulation related to giving birth, smoking, and vascular injury (recent surgery). Assessment reveals common symptoms of pulmonary embolism: dyspnea, cough, and pleuritic pain. Diagnostic tests include ABGs, 12-lead electrocardiogram (ECG), chest x-ray, and echocardiogram.

34. **(3)** The flu or influenza is a highly contagious respiratory infection that occurs epidemically during the winter cold months. It is characterized by a sudden onset of chills, elevated temperature (101°–104°F), headache, fatigue, muscle pain, dry cough, laryngitis, rhinorrhea, and red eyes following a waiting period of 24–48 hours from time of exposure via respiratory droplets from an infected person or indirectly by drinking from a contaminated glass. Flu vaccines do not cause the flu; they are made with a killed virus.

35. **(4)** In cystic fibrosis the stools are large, bulky, and foul smelling (steatorrhea). Yellow stools are indicative of liver or gallbladder problems. Green stools often indicate a rapid transit time and may be associated with an infection.

36. **(2)** This client is considered to be in the "yellow" zone of personal best peak flow but is close to the "red" zone (50% or less of personal best). The client should use her bronchodilator immediately and if not improved may need emergency intervention by the nurse practitioner.

37. **(1)** The pneumococcal vaccine is recommended for elderly clients, since their immune system is less efficient. The symptoms of fever, chest pain, and sputum production are suggestive of pneumonia.

38. **(2)** Confusion may be the first sign that the elderly client is septic. The client may not have a temperature or leukocytosis. The client may not experience any discomfort or a cough.

39. **(4)** *Streptococcus pneumoniae* is the most common cause of community- and nursing home–acquired pneumonia. *Haemophilus influenzae* is common in elderly clients with underlying chronic diseases (e.g., COPD, diabetes). *Klebsiella pneumoniae* and other gram-negative bacteria are pathogens in alcoholics, immunocompromised hosts, and hospitalized clients. *Mycobacterium tuberculosis* is an infrequent cause of pneumonia.

40. **(2)** Pneumococcal vaccination and yearly influenza immunization will decrease complications and hospitalizations for the older client. The pneumococcal vaccination is not administered annually. Options #3 and #4 are not recommended. The PPD should be done annually for high-risk clients.

41. **(2)** *Klebsiella pneumoniae* and other gram-negative bacteria are important pathogens in alcoholics, immunocompromised hosts, and hospitalized clients. *Haemophilus influenzae* is common in elderly clients with underlying chronic diseases (e.g., COPD, diabetes mellitus). *Staphylococcus aureus* generally affects elderly clients recovering from influenza; it is also frequent in hospitalized clients and diabetics. *Streptococcus pneumoniae* is the most common bacterial pathogen (30–40% of pneumonia cases), and the most common cause of community- and nursing home–acquired pneumonia.

42. **(2)** Up to 25% of elderly clients with newly diagnosed TB have a negative tuberculin skin test due to waning cellular immunity with senescence. If the initial PPD test is negative, a repeat PPD test 1 week later is recommended in elderly clients. The repeat test is useful to stimulate a booster phenomenon in clients whose initial infection occurred many years in the past.

The other options contain incorrect information.

43. **(3)** Horner's syndrome, which is paralysis of the cervical sympathetic nerves resulting in ptosis, loss of sweating, constriction of the pupil, and sinking of the eyeball on one side, is very commonly associated with malignant tumors in the upper lung leading to nerve compression.

44. **(4)** Superior vena cava obstruction is a complication of malignancy involving the mediastinum and rapidly progresses into an oncologic emergency.

45. **(2)** In children too young to properly use a peak flowmeter, the inability to cry or complete a sentence may indicate an acute asthma attack. An ABG study is usually not performed in office settings and a chest x-ray will most likely agitate the child and take too long to process.

46. **(3)** Hyponatremia results from an overproduction of antidiuretic hormone caused by an ectopic production from the bronchogenic tumor. Ketoacidosis and trauma result in fluid loss causing hypernatremia, as does overuse of sodium-containing antacids.

47. **(3)** In older individuals the asthma is usually accompanied by infection. It is rarely allergic, and costal retraction and fever are not usually seen. Subcutaneous epinephrine is not standard treatment but is sometimes indicated in emergent situations.

48. **(1)** Late-phase asthma occurs at 6–12 hours after the initial or acute bronchoconstrictive phase. The inflammatory response is the result of mast cell degranulation and release of histamine. Histamine acts on the lung by causing bronchoconstriction, vascular permeability, and vasodilatation. In late-phase asthma, bronchoconstriction is refractory to most bronchodilator therapy.

49. **(3)** Nocturnal exacerbation of asthma is a common clinical sign. It is linked to the variation in circulating catecholamines and vagal tone. Chronic hypoxemia and diffuse crackles are seen in the client with chronic bronchitis. Pruritus is often seen in contact allergic reactions.

50. **(2)** Asking the client about the consumption of wine with dinner is the most appropriate response. Many wines, especially white wines, contain sulfites that can trigger a mild allergic response.

51. **(4)** Nocturnal asthma attacks are generally the worse at 4 AM, when bronchial constriction occurs due to changes in the circadian rhythm that affect bronchial reactivity.

52. **(1)** In addition to more symptoms of wheezing and rales, infants are more likely to develop disseminated disease such as meningitis and to have a negative PPD skin test. Usually, the transmission of the disease can be traced to an affected adult living in the household.

53. **(4)** Maintaining a high caloric intake is important in the care of infants with BPD to promote growth and nourishment of developing lung tissue. Sometimes, infants have gastroesophageal reflux (GER) after feedings. Initially, positioning should be tried, then feedings may be thickened or given in smaller amounts more frequently. If the problem persists or if the weight gain is not adequate, then referral to a pediatrican is indicated.

54. **(3)** If this child is up-to-date on his immunizations, he should have had his *Haemophilus influenzae* type b vaccine (HIB), the most common cause of epiglottitis. A dramatic decline in the incidence of epiglottis and *Haemophilus influenzae* type b infections is associated closely with the history of the HIB vaccines. Considering the age of this child and the suddenness of the onset, the most likely diagnosis is foreign body aspiration.

Pharmacology

55. **(1)** In order for the medication to be most effective, there needs to be a 1-minute lapse time between the two puffs of medication. The first puff will open the upper airways. This will allow more effective penetration of the lower tract with the second puff of medication.

56. **(2)** The client would not stop taking the medications, as this is a common side effect of rifampin. Also, soft contact lenses may become discolored.

57. **(4)** β-Agonist (albuterol) MDI is the first line of treatment to decrease airflow obstruction. Aminophylline by mouth would take too long to be effective. Epinephrine is used predominantly for anaphylactic reaction. Beclovent is a steroid inhaler that is most effective when used prophylactically rather than in acute episodes.

58. **(4)** The use of tobacco increases the metabolism of theophylline, causing a need for greater dosage than required in nonsmokers. A high-protein, low-carbohydrate diet increases the metabolism of theophylline and decreases serum concentrations. Coffee (and other xanthine-containing beverages) may increase the central nervous system effects of xanthine derivatives.

59. **(1)** β-Blockers (Inderal and Tenormin) are known to cause exacerbation of chronic respiratory problems. Another antihypertensive, such as a calcium channel blocker, should be considered. The client's pulse is 74 and his blood pressure remains elevated, which indicates the β-blocker is probably not effective in decreasing the blood pressure in this client. Theophylline derivatives are not indicated unless other medications are not effective. Drug interactions and increased levels of toxicity present problems in the elderly client.

60. **(2)** Therapeutic plasma levels range from 5–15 μg/ml. Drug levels of 20 μg/ml or greater are associated with toxicity.

61. **(1)** Chemoprophylaxis is initiated at the time of the screening skin testing. Skin testing should be repeated in 3 months if initial test results are negative. If the second skin testing is negative, chemoprophylaxis can be stopped.

62. **(3)** One of the most common causes of outpatient treatment failure is improper inhaler technique. While exposure to allergens may trigger an asthma attack, the proper use of inhalers will control those attacks. Use of both steroids and cromolyn inhalers has decreased the severity of asthma attacks.

63. **(1)** Theophylline is used in the treatment of chronic lung disease and can accumulate in toxic levels. Cimetidine decreases the hepatic clearance of theophylline. Nicotine and some antiseizure drugs may actually increase clearance, and ampicillin does not change the clearance.

64. **(2)** Antibiotic therapy is indicated when there is a change in color, consistency, or amount of sputum. Cough suppressants and antihistamines should be avoided.

65. **(2)** Beclomethasone diproprionate is a long-acting corticosteroid that stabilizes mast cells and greatly reduces mast cell degranulation when exposed to allergens. All of the other medications are bronchodilators used for rapid reversal of bronchospasm.

66. **(2)** Treatment of the client with asthma includes inhaled glucocorticoids for their anti-inflammatory effects. Antibiotics are indicated if there is a concurrent infection such as acute bronchitis. β₂-Agonists are used for their bronchodilator effects and rapid onset of action. Methacholine challenge is used in the diagnosis of asthma.

67. **(2)** Clients with asthma should be instructed to keep their inhaled β₂-agonist with them at all times in case of bronchospasm and use them prn. The β₂-agonists are effective in reversing bronchospasm. Inhaled steroids are long acting and will not give immediate relief; therefore, the client should be instructed to use them regularly as prescribed and use their inhaled β₂-agonist prn. Beginning antibiotics is not indicated for acute bronchospasm.

68. **(3)** These are the common drugs used for combination therapy for the treatment of tuberculosis in children. Rimantadine is an antiviral; Fansidar is an antimalarial. Singular therapy is not indicated due to the virulence of the tubercle bacillus.

69. **(4)** Close contacts of clients with an active case of tuberculosis should be placed on isoniazid single-drug therapy, even if the

tuberculin skin test is negative. This early treatment will destroy the tubercle bacilli before hypersensitivity develops. The isoniazid should be continued for 3 months for those people whose skin test remains negative and there is no evidence of disease. If there is a positive skin test conversion, isoniazid (10–20 mg/kg) should be continued for 1 year. If the child develops symptoms of tuberculosis, he should be given isoniazid and rifampin (10 mg/kg) for 1 year.

70. **(4)** Dextromethorphan is specific for control of coughing. Guaifenesin is an expectorant, and Options #1 and #2 are decongestants to decrease nasal and upper respiratory congestion.

71. **(3)** Rhinitis and a productive cough are common and not cause for concern unless the mucus begins to change color and is accompanied by a high fever. The wheezes are also common, if the mucus is loose. A high fever and rales indicate further deterioration and possible bacterial infection.

72. **(2)** Pyridoxine (vitamin B$_6$) is added to prevent peripheral neuropathy. Tyramine- and histamine-containing foods such as tuna, aged cheese, and yeast vitamin supplements cause interaction with monoamine oxidase (MOA) inhibitors. Anorexia, jaundice, malaise, and fatigue would be signs of hepatic involvement.

Bronchiolitis

73. **(1)** Bronchodilators are frequently effective for acute episodes. Antibiotics and antihistamines are not effective and should not be used. The condition is usually treated symptomatically. If the child does not improve, consult a physician.

74. **(1)** Medications should be taken only when the child is going to exercise and anticipates respiratory difficulty. Intal and Beclovent are steroids and do not provide immediate relief, and theophylline should be avoided unless symptoms get progressively worse

and cannot be controlled with inhalation therapy.

75. **(3)** The drug therapy regimen for chronic asthma usually includes theophylline. Symptoms of toxicity include anorexia, nausea, vomiting, confusion, restlessness, tachycardia, dysrrhythmias, and seizures.

76. **(2)** The hallmark clinical presentation of acute bronchitis is a productive cough. The nurse practitioner should rule out pneumonia. This was accomplished with this client through the normal chest x-ray and breath sounds. Bronchodilators (Albuterol) have been found to eliminate the cough of acute bronchitis. Antibiotic therapy (erythromycin and tetracycline) is not recommended. Research has demonstrated that antibiotic-susceptible organisms rarely cause acute bronchitis.

77. **(4)** Histamine H$_2$ antagonists neutralize the normal gastric acid barrier, allowing for an increased colonization of gram-negative bacilli and *Staphylococcus aureus*.

78. **(2)** Worsening dyspnea and fatigue with increasing cough may be indicative of early pulmonary edema. Clients with pulmonary edema require hospitalization with oxygen therapy, IV furosemide (Lasix), and morphine. Clients who are suspected to have pulmonary edema ***should not*** be treated on an outpatient basis. Calcium channel blockers are of little benefit in heart failure.

Parkinson/Tb

79. **(1)** INH requires concurrent administration of vitamin B$_6$ to prevent problems of optic neuritis. Vitamin B$_6$ will decrease the effectiveness of levodopa. If the client is to receive INH, his antiparkinson medication needs to be re-evaluated.

80. **(1)** Combination of cisapride (Propulsid) and erythromycin-based antibiotics can precipitate fatal dysrhythmias. Another antibiotic should be considered. (*Testing tip: three of the distractors are antihypertensive medications; only one is different and it is the correct answer.*)

Immune & Allergy

Physical Examination & Diagnostic Tests

1. When taking the history of a client with known allergies, what is the most important information to determine?

   1. Reaction associated with each allergen.

   2. Drug allergies.

   3. Food allergies.

   4. Environmental exposure.

2. Which test is used to determine the concentration of gamma globulins that contain most of the immunoglobulins?

   1. Immunofixation electrophoresis.

   2. Complement fixation.

   3. Protein electrophoresis.

   4. Antinuclear antibodies (ANA).

3. Diagnostic studies used in the differential diagnosis of systemic lupus erythematosus (SLE) include:

   1. CBC, SMA-12, and ESR.

   2. Chest radiograph and coagulation profile.

   3. ANA, ESR, and C-reactive protein.

   4. CBC, urinalysis, and chest radiograph.

4. Which tests are appropriate for the nurse practitioner to order in an initial work-up for asymptomatic clients at risk for human immunodeficiency virus (HIV) infection?

   1. CD4 count and HIV ELISA.

   2. Serology for cytomegalovirus, herpes simplex virus, and Epstein-Barr virus.

   3. HIV ELISA and Western blot.

   4. Hepatitis screen and Western blot.

5. The nurse practitioner would anticipate which laboratory finding in a client with joint pain, "butterfly rash," photosensitivity, weight loss, and fever?

   1. Presence of antinuclear antibodies.

   2. Negative serum complement level.

   3. Increased red blood cell (RBC) and white blood cell (WBC) count.

   4. Glycosuria.

6. When assessing a client for angioedema, the nurse practitioner would examine the:

   1. Neck and ears.

   2. Heart sounds.

   3. Abdomen.

   4. Eyes and mouth.

7. Clients who believe they have been exposed to HIV should have an HIV antibody test how soon after the exposure?

   1. The next day and 2 months later.

   2. 6 months after exposure and again at 12 months.

   3. 6–12 weeks after exposure and again at 6 months.

   4. 4 weeks and 12 weeks.

8. The most reliable test for the presence of specific immunoglobulin E (IgE) antibody is:

   1. Skin testing.

   2. Radioallergosorbent testing (RAST).

   3. Smears for eosinophils.

   4. Complete blood count.

9. To diagnose allergic rhinitis in the primary care office setting, the nurse practitioner would consider performing:

   1. A nasal smear for eosinophils.

   2. A total serum IgE.

   3. Skin testing.

   4. Radioallergosorbent tests (RAST).

10. The nurse practitioner is evaluating the TB skin test on an immunocompetent child who has no risk factors for tuberculosis. The purified protein derivative (PPD) is considered positive when it measures:

    1. 5 mm.

    2. 10 mm.

    3. 15 mm.

    4. 20 mm.

Disorders

11. A new mother tells the clinic nurse that her infant was born HIV-positive. She asks the nurse how long her baby has to live. The nurse's response would be based on the knowledge that:

    1. The antibodies present in the baby's blood may reflect the antibodies received from the mother at the time of birth.

    2. If antibodies are present at birth, the baby has the acquired immunodeficiency syndrome (AIDS) in an active form.

    3. Since the baby is HIV-positive, the child will develop full-blown AIDS within 3 years.

    4. The antibodies detected at birth indicate presence of the HIV; the test does not indicate when the child will develop AIDS.

12. Client education regarding common antigens of anaphylaxis includes:

    1. Extreme weather.

    2. Egg albumin.

    3. Pungent odors.

    4. Animal dandruff.

13. The nurse practitioner understands that an HIV infection results in a reduction of:

    1. Helper T cells.

    2. Suppressor T cells.

    3. Killer T cells.

    4. Suppressor B cells.

14. Which assessment finding is commonly associated with a diagnosis of SLE?

    1. Excitability, diarrhea, vomiting.

    2. High fever, measle-like rash on limbs, weight gain.

    3. Joint pain, malar rash, photosensitivity.

    4. Weight loss, diarrhea, epigastric pain.

15. After a repeat HIV antibody test, a client continues to test positive but is asymptomatic. The nurse understands

which of the following about possible transmission of the virus by the client?

1. The client is infectious when symptoms are active.

2. The client is infectious for life.

3. The dormant virus is not infectious while the client is asymptomatic and the T-cell count is high.

4. Laboratory tests should be done monthly to identify the infectious periods of the disease process.

16. A young woman has just received news of a positive HIV test. She does not want her sexual partner to be informed. What is the most appropriate response to her decision?

1. Respect for her decision, since she is the client.

2. Letting her know that you have a legal responsibility to inform her partner.

3. Counseling her about your ethical responsibility to inform all sexual partners.

4. Noting her decision in the record for future reference.

17. The nurse practitioner has been assigned a new client. The problem list indicates this client has CREST syndrome. The nurse practitioner will be following this client for:

1. Scleroderma.

2. Dental caries.

3. Systemic lupus erythematosus.

4. Rheumatoid arthritis.

18. A client presenting with complaints of fatigue, malaise, arthralgias, oral ulcers, malar rash, and a positive ANA would most likely be diagnosed as having:

1. Rheumatoid arthritis.

2. Fibromyalgia.

3. Scleroderma.

4. Systemic lupus erythematosus.

19. The most common clinical manifestations of Sjögren's syndrome are:

1. Corneal dryness and lack of saliva.

2. Increased urination and hunger.

3. Abdominal discomfort and headaches.

4. Joint destruction and alopecia.

20. An elderly female client presents to the nurse practitioner with a low-grade temperature and a unilateral throbbing headache. She also reports scalp sensitivity and some visual disturbances. Lab results show a markedly elevated ESR and anemia. She has been relatively healthy except for a recent history of polymyalgia rheumatica (PMR). Symptoms indicate a clinical presentation of:

1. Bacterial menigitis.

2. Acute migraine headache.

3. Temporal (giant cell) arteritis.

4. Subdural hematoma.

21. A middle-aged female client presents with weight loss, heartburn, dysphagia, dry cough, pain, stiffness of the fingers and knees, and Raynaud's phenomenon. The nurse practitioner recognizes these as the symptoms of:

1. Rheumatoid arthritis.

2. Lupus erythematosus.

3. Graft-versus-host disease (GVHD).

4. Scleroderma.

22. The erythematous confluent macular eruption of the face known as the butterfly rash is characteristic of:

1. Allergic drug eruption.

2. Systemic lupus erythematosus.

3. Rosacea.

4. Seborrheic dermatitis.

23. The nurse practitioner is discussing general health care with a female client with SLE who is in remission. Important points to include are:

    1. Avoid getting pregnant.

    2. Decrease physical and psychological stress.

    3. Avoid isometric and aerobic exercise.

    4. Maintain diet low in fat and carbohydrates.

24. A 50-year-old male client presents with complaints of frequent sinus infections, a decrease in the ability to hear, and arthralgias. Laboratory findings are RBC—mild normochromic and normocytic anemia; elevated ESR; mild hypergammaglobinemia (elevated immunglobulin A); proteinuria; and hematuria with granular or cellular casts. Physical examination findings include mild conjunctivitis, vasculitic dermatitis, chronic cough, chest pain, dyspnea, paranasal sinus pain, occasional epistaxis, and imbalance of intake and output. A tentative diagnosis is:

    1. Connective tissue disease.

    2. Wegener's granulomatosis.

    3. Pulmonary neoplasm.

    4. Infectious granulomatous disease.

25. A client presents with sneezing, watery eyes, postnasal drip, full head, and sore throat. The best diagnosis for this client is:

    1. Acute bronchitis.

    2. Allergic rhinitis.

    3. Asthma exacerbation.

    4. Influenza.

26. A 70-year-old woman presents with complaints of morning headache, malaise, and anorexia. The nurse practitioner suspects:

    1. Pneumonia.

    2. Temporal arteritis.

    3. Herpes zoster.

    4. Postmenopausal symptoms.

27. When teaching a client about risk factors and prevention of transmission of HIV, which statement is most appropriate?

    1. HIV can be transmitted by casual kissing.

    2. Unprotected oral sex with an infected partner is not advised.

    3. Sharing an office with an HIV-positive person increases the risk of exposure to the HIV.

    4. Using the same bathroom as an infected family member puts you at risk of exposure to HIV.

28. Signs and symptoms that alert the nurse practitioner to identify a client who is at an increased risk for HIV infection include:

    1. Night sweats.

    2. Malaise and fatigue.

    3. Frequent sexually transmitted diseases.

    4. Swollen glands and diarrhea.

29. HIV is classified as a:

    1. Cytomegalovirus.

    2. Herpetic virus.

    3. Papillomavirus.

    4. Retrovirus.

30. The most frequently occurring symptoms of SLE are:

    1. Splenomegaly and Raynaud's syndrome.

    2. Pulmonary effusions and hepatomegaly.

    3. Butterfly rash on the face and lymphadenopathy.

    4. Fever, arthritis, arthralgia, and weight loss.

31. A systemic IgE-mediated antigen–antibody response resulting in a life-threatening massive release of mediators is:

    1. Generalized seizures.

    2. Allergic rhinitis.

    3. Anaphylaxis.

    4. Status asthmaticus.

32. The release of histamine results in:

    1. Bronchospasm, vasodilatation, and vascular permeability.

    2. Bronchodilatation, vasodilatation, and vascular permeability.

    3. Smooth muscle contraction, decreased vascular permeability, and vasoconstriction.

    4. Pain, increased vascular permeability, and bronchodilatation.

33. Following a bone marrow transplant (BMT), the nurse practitioner can expect the peak onset of an acute graft versus host disease (GVHD) to occur:

    1. Between 10 and 15 days posttransplant.

    2. Between 30 and 50 days posttransplant.

    3. Between 1 and 5 days posttransplant.

    4. At 100 days posttransplant.

34. A client has a history of recent BMT. The nurse practitioner identifies signs and symptoms of GVHD to include:

    1. Fever, headache, and mental status changes.

    2. Chills, fever, and urticaria over flank area.

    3. Increased serum bilirubin, maculopapular rash, and green, watery diarrhea.

    4. Decreased RBC, hematocrit, and hemoglobin; petechiae; and increased bleeding tendencies.

35. The pathogenesis of SLE is characterized by autoantibody development. This results in:

    1. Increased T suppressor cell.

    2. B-cell decrease.

    3. Polyclonal hypogammaglobinlinemia.

    4. Decreased T suppressor cells and inhibited cell activity.

36. The cell responsible for the activation of the immune response is:

    1. Band neutrophil.

    2. T4 lymphocyte.

    3. Segmented neutrophil.

    5. B lymphocytes.

37. A 22-year-old male presents with breathlessness, weight loss, nonproductive cough, temperature of 38°C (100.4°F), pulse 124, respirations 36, blood pressure 120/78, and a history of a positive HIV serum test. Based on this information, what is the most accurate diagnosis?

    1. *Klebsiella pneumoniae.*

    2. Kaposi's sarcoma.

    3. *Pneumocystis carinii* pneumonia.

    4. Lymphoma.

38. An adult is brought into the clinic and the family states he has a history of anaphylactic reactions. What signs and symptoms indicate to the nurse practitioner the client is experiencing another reaction?

    1. Cough, wheezing, and hives.

    2. Severe malaise, pallor, stridor, and dyspnea.

    3. Anxiety, nasal congestion, and tachycardia.

    4. Rhinorrhea, nausea, and gastrointestinal cramping.

39. A nurse at the clinic experiences a needle stick from a client with known hepatitis. What immunoglobulin (Ig) should be administered to provide passive immunity?

    1. IgE.

    2. IgA.

    3. IgG.

    4. IgC.

40. Which sign and/or symptom is indicative of a type I hypersensitivity reaction?

    1. Contact dermatitis.

    2. Immediate wheal-and-flare reaction.

    3. Hematuria.

    4. High fever.

41. Which clients are at risk for developing HIV/AIDS?

    1. Immunocompromised clients.

    2. Sexually active teenagers.

    3. Elderly adults.

    4. Marijuana users.

42. Cardiovascular effects of anaphylaxis include:

    1. ST-segment and T-wave changes.

    2. Hypertension.

    3. Prolonged P-R intervals with elevated Q-T segment.

    4. Elevated serum enzymes.

43. When assessing a client for SLE, what ophthalmologic findings would the nurse practitioner determine to be consistent with this condition?

    1. Retinal hemorrhages.

    2. Conjunctivitis.

    3. Cotton-wool spots.

    4. Arteriovenous (AV) nicking.

44. What information does the nurse practitioner include in the education for the client with allergic rhinitis?

    1. Monitor air quality and the allergy index.

    2. Use a surgical-type mask when going outdoors.

    3. Remain inside during allergy season.

    4. Avoid working in the garden or yard.

45. A nurse from the operating room comes into the clinic with complaints of shortness of breath, itching, reddened hands, and wheezing. He indicates that, when he is not working, he does not seem to have the symptoms. Based on the history and symptoms the nurse practitioner would further evaluate for:

    1. Sick building syndrome.

    2. Bronchitis.

    3. Latex allergy.

    4. Contact dermatitis.

46. Which statement is true regarding latex allergy?

    1. It usually only produces symptoms of contact dermatitis and allergic rhinorrhea.

    2. It is a progressive disease that worsens with continued exposure.

    3. It affects <5% of the health care population.

    4. It is an autoimmune response.

47. Children who have chronic allergic rhinitis often present with clinical symptoms that include:

    1. Mouth breathing and nasal polyps.

    2. Allergic shiners and Dennie's lines.

    3. Thick nasal discharge and sneezing.

    4. Flushed face and fever.

48. Common sites for adolescent atopic dermatitis are:

    1. Cheeks, forehead, and scalp.

    2. Wrists, ankles, and antecubital fossae.

    3. Antecubital fossae, face, neck, and back.

    4. Palmar creases and extensor surface of legs.

Pharmacology

49. Drugs that have been associated with a lupus-like syndrome include:

    1. Sulfonamides (Septra DS), penicillin (Pen-Vee K, Penicillin G).

    2. Progestin/estrogen combination of oral contraceptives.

    3. Nonsteroidal anti-inflammatory drugs (NSAIDs; Motrin).

    4. Procainamide (Pronestyl), hydralazine (Apresoline).

50. Clients newly presenting with signs and symptoms of SLE would have their medication profile reviewed to determine if they are on any medication that may have caused a drug-induced lupus. Which drug would be most suspect?

    1. Digoxin (Lanoxin).

    2. Procainamide (Pronestyl).

    3. Trimethoprim-sulfamethoxazole (Bactrim).

    4. Cimetidine (Tagamet).

51. A client is diagnosed with temporal (giant cell) arteritis. The medication of choice is:

    1. Prednisone (Deltasone).

    2. Ibuprofen (Motrin).

    3. Indomethacin (Indocin).

    4. Azathioprine (Imuran).

52. The clinic is notified that a child is being brought in with a bee sting and that the child is having difficulty breathing. Which medication should the nurse practitioner have available for the child's initial care?

    1. Lidocaine topical ointment.

    2. Epinephrine.

    3. Prednisone.

    4. Benadryl elixir.

53. The standard drug used for malaria prophylaxis is:

    1. Ampicillin (Polycillin, Omnipen).

    2. Doxycycline (Vibramycin).

    3. Ceftriaxone (Rocephin).

    4. Chloroquine phosphate (Aralen).

54. Treatment for allergic rhinitis includes:

    1. Antihistamines, corticosteroids, and environmental control.

    2. Antibiotics, antihistamines, analgesics, and allergen control.

    3. Cholinergic agents, antibiotics, and analgesics.

    4. Nasal saline, corticosteroids, and antibiotics.

55. Development of an adverse drug reaction is dependent on which factors?

    1. Client age, prior drug reactions, genetic factors, and degree of exposure.

    2. Client gender, oral route of administration, and history of atrophic disease.

    3. Client age, gender, and genetic factors.

    4. Genetic factors, prior drug reactions, and client gender.

56. A medication frequently used for the prophylaxis as well as initial treatment of *Pneumocystis carinii* pneumonia (PCP) is

    1. Fluconazole (Diflucan).

    2. Amphotericin B (Fungizone).

    3. Trimethoprim-sulfamethoxazole (Septra, Bactrim).

    4. Acyclovir (Zovirax).

57. When instructing clients with allergic rhinitis about the use of nasal decongestants, it is important for them to understand:

    1. The condition is self-limiting and will resolve in a matter of weeks whether or not the client is re-exposed to the allergen.

    2. A nasal decongestant used continuous for greater than 3 days can result in a worsening of the symptoms.

    3. It is not necessary to avoid exposure to the allergen once therapy has been initiated.

    4. Allergic rhinitis is only seen in the spring and fall; the condition requires treatment during these seasons only.

58. The major advantage to use of second-generation antihistamines such as astemizole (Hismanal) and loratadine (Claritin) is:

    1. Decreased cost.

    2. Increased anticholinergic activity.

    3. Delayed absorption.

    4. Do not cross the blood-brain barrier.

59. What is the desired action of sympathomimetics (adrenergics) when used in the treatment of allergic rhinitis?

    1. Promote vasoconstriction in nasal mucosa.

    2. Block mast cell degranulation.

    3. Decrease the effect of histamines.

    4. Increase degranulation and end-organ response.

60. The nurse practitioner is prescribing astemizole (Hismanal) for a geriatric client's allergy problems. When considering the client's current medications, which medication would be a contraindication to the administration of astemizole?

    1. Erythromycin ethylsuccinate (E.E.S.).

    2. Verapamil (Calan).

    3. Propranolol (Propranolol).

    4. Captopril (Capoten).

61. Cromolyn sodium is used to:

    1. Reduce the histamine load.

    2. Antagonize the effects of histamine.

    3. Stabilize the mast cell membrane.

    4. Reduce antiemetic activity.

62. In the elderly client, histamine$_1$ (H$_1$) blockers may cause which side effects?

    1. Ataxia.

    2. Nausea.

    3. Diarrhea.

    4. Gastrointestinal upset.

63. What information is important for the nurse practitioner to include when teaching a client about the use of antihistamines?

    1. Use of topical antihistamines is safe and has relatively few side effects.

    2. Do not use over-the-counter (OTC) medications without consulting the health care provider.

    3. Constipation and urinary retention are expected side effects and do not need to be reported.

    4. Once the antihistamine therapy has been taken for 3 days, avoidance of allergens is not necessary.

64. A primary advantage of using loratadine (Claritin) in treating a client with seasonal allergies is that it:

    1. Is supplied as an enteric-coated pill.

    2. May be prescribed on a once-a-day dosing.

    3. Costs considerably less than other medications.

    4. Effectively decreases nasal secretions.

65. What medications are the choice of treatment in secondary therapy for the client with an anaphylactic reaction?

    1. Antibiotics and anticholinergics.

    2. NSAIDs.

    3. Decongestants and expectorants.

    4. Antihistamines and corticosteroids.

66. An appropriate antihistamine to recommend for a child with allergic rhinitis is:

    1. Diphenhydramine (Benadryl).

    2. Dextromethorphan (Benylin).

    3. Guaifenesin (Robitussin).

    4. Brompheniramine (Dimetane).

67. A child who weighs 30 lb (13.6 kg) arrives in the office with a complaint of an allergic reaction to peanuts. The child has hives on most of her body and is beginning to wheeze; she is in acute distress. The nurse practitioner administers:

    1. Diphenhydramine (Benadryl) 50 mg PO.

    2. Diphenhydramine (Benadryl) 25 mg PO.

    3. Epinephrine (Adrenalin) 0.14 ml of a 1:1000 solution.

    4. Epinephrine (Adrenalin) 0.3 ml of a 1:1000 solution.

68. During a well-child visit, it is noted that the patient, an 8-year-old male, is taking 50 mg grapeseed extract three times a day for allergies. The practitioner bases teaching on the knowledge that:

    1. Grapeseed extract is not safe in children under age 12.

    2. The client may need loratadine (Claritin) for breakthrough episodes.

    3. Grapeseed extract can be toxic for children.

    4. The client will need to be monitored for seizures.

69. Children on antihistamines chronically will need supplements due to decreased absorption of:

    1. Calcium.

    2. Iron.

    3. Magnesium.

    4. Niacin.

6 Answers & Rationales

Physical Examination & Diagnostic Tests

1. **(1)** The reaction to each allergen is important to know. Often clients will indicate they have an allergy to a particular food or medication, such as nausea, stomach pain, or diarrhea, and consider it an allergy. The signs and symptoms of the reaction, speed of onset, how long it lasts, and what successful treatment has been used in the past are important information. Both drug and food allergies should be explored.

2. **(3)** In protein electrophoresis, proteins are electrically separated on a strip. It is a screening test to measure various proteins in body fluids, usually serum or urine. It assists in screening for diseases that are characterized by an increase or decrease in immunoglobulins. Complement fixation and ANA are diagnostic studies for rheumatoid problems.

3. **(3)** Although all of the tests included in the answer may be included in a complete physical examination, laboratory tests, specific to the diagnosis of SLE include the ANA, ESR, and C-reactive protein. During flares the ESR and C-reactive protein are elevated. The ANA titer in a client with SLE is positive at a 1:80 ratio.

4. **(3)** The initial screening test for HIV is the ELISA. If the test is positive, confirmation of antibodies is done with a Western blot. Although serology and hepatitis screening along with a CBC and tuberculosis skin test are routinely performed, the initial work-up starts with an ELISA test. The CD4 count is performed during the active disease process.

5. **(1)** The majority of clients with SLE have the presence of ANA in their blood. There is leukopenia, thrombocytopenia, lymphopenia, and a positive LE cell prep. Proteinuria with cellular casts is often noted.

6. **(4)** Angioedema is most easily seen in the eyes and mouth. It is edema of the mucous membrane tissue. It can also be observed on the tongue, feet, hands, and genitalia. Diffuse erythema may be seen in the upper body parts. Gastrointestinal symptoms such as vomiting, cramping, and diarrhea may also be seen.

7. **(3)** The HIV antibody develops between 6 and 12 weeks after exposure. Because of the variability of antibody development, it is recommended that the test be repeated in 6 months to confirm the findings.

8. **(1)** The most reliable test for the presence of the specific IgE antibody is the skin test. RAST is less sensitive than skin testing and is difficult to standardize and reproduce results. The smear for eosinophils and the CBC are not specific for IgE antibody.

9. **(1)** A nasal smear for eosinophils is a simple office procedure. Many clients who have uncomplicated allergic rhinitis have a normal serum IgE. Skin testing should be performed by allergy-trained providers only. RAST testing is higher in cost and lower in sensitivity.

10. **(3)** A positive PPD for an immunocompetent child is 15 mm. A child who is HIV-positive, immunocompromised, or exposed to an active case of TB is considered positive at 5 mm. The child (<4 years of age) that has a chronic disease or has been exposed to HIV-positive people or people born in a foreign country is considered positive at 10 mm.

Disorders

11. **(4)** It is important to give the mother as much hope as possible but still be realistic about the condition. There is no way to tell when or if the child will convert to active AIDS. Many infants seroconvert to HIV-negative status.

12. **(2)** Egg albumin is just one of many identified common antigens that may result in anaphylactic reaction. Others include vaccines, allergen extracts, sulfonamides, penicillins, hormones, legumes (especially peanuts), berries, nuts, seafoods, and venom bites (bee, wasp, yellow jacket bites). Changes in weather, and strong scents and odors, are triggers that may precipitate an asthma attack resulting in bronchospasm and wheezing.

13. **(1)** There is a severe, life-threatening reduction of helper T cells, along with an increase in suppressor T cells. The helper T cells help amplify or increase the production of antibody-forming cells from the B lymphocytes after an encounter with an antigen. Killer T cells are produced after mature helper T cells interact with an antigen. Suppressor T cells suppress the formation of antibody-forming cells from the B lymphocytes, which, when their numbers are increased, have a detrimental effect on the immunity and ability of the HIV client to make antibody-forming cells.

14. **(3)** The symptoms most commonly experienced are joint pain, fatigue, Raynaud's phenomenon, chronic or low-grade or recurrent fever, sun sensitivity, hair loss, weakness, butterfly (malar) facial rash, and weight loss. Typically, the pulmonary, cardiac, renal, and central nervous systems are involved.

15. **(2)** HIV infection creates a chronic infectious state in the body that is transmitted via blood or body fluids and transplacentally.

16. **(3)** Ethical response includes notification of all persons at risk.

17. **(1)** CREST (**C**alcinosis, **R**aynaud's phenomenon, **E**sophageal dysfunction, **S**clerodactyly, **T**elangiectasia) is associated with a slow progressive form of scleroderma. *Malaise fatigue*

18. **(4)** This client is presenting with 4 of the 11 criteria necessary for diagnosing SLE. There is no singular test for SLE, but the presence of these characteristics plus lab results can differentiate the diagnosis. *oral ulcers malar rash ⊕ ANA arthralgias*

19. **(1)** Corneal dryness and lack of saliva are the most common clinical manifestations of Sjögren's syndrome. Clients may also have joint inflammation, but this rarely leads to joint destruction.

20. **(3)** About 40% of temporal (giant cell) arteritis clients have a history of PMR. The other diagnoses may have some of these symptoms, but only arteritis has all the symptoms listed in the situation. It is especially critical to note visual disturbances, as these clients can develop sudden blindness.

21. **(4)** The symptom of Raynaud's phenomenon differentiates this as scleroderma. The esophageal dysfunction is often an initial complaint in this disease, which is four times more common in females.

22. **(2)** The butterfly rash is one of the characteristic symptoms of SLE.

23. **(2)** Psychological and physical stress can exacerbate SLE. A balanced diet helps to limit the side effects of some of the medications, while regular exercise helps to reduce arthralgia and myalgia. Barrier contraception is recommended for the female with SLE. Pregnancy is usually allowed during periods of remission.

24. **(2)** Wegener's granulomatosis is a multisystem disorder that occurs equally in both sexes. Peak occurrence is between 40 and 60 years of age. The disease usually targets the upper respiratory tract and the kidney. Connective tissue disease, pulmonary neoplasm, and infectious granulomatous disease would be considered in the differential.

[handwritten margin note: nn. Chrome mild +IgA proteinuria hematuria]

25. **(2)** The signs and symptoms presented are classic for allergic rhinitis. Acute bronchitis would present with cough and yellow or green sputum production. An asthma exacerbation would present with wheezing, chest tightness, decreased forced vital capacity, and history of exposure to an allergen. Influenza presents with fever, chills, and general malaise.

26. **(2)** The nurse practitioner should rule out temporal arteritis, an inflammatory disorder of unknown etiology affecting large- and medium-sized arteries. It occurs two times more frequently in women, most frequently in the elderly, and rarely in the African-American population.

[handwritten margin note: 11A malaise anorexia]

27. **(2)** Unprotected oral sex with an HIV-positive person puts one at risk for exposure to the virus. Contact such as casual kissing, or sharing an office or bathroom, does not transmit the virus. The virus is transmitted in bodily fluids and secretions.

28. **(3)** Frequent sexually transmitted diseases would alert the nurse practitioner to the client's lack of protected sex and the possibility of multiple partners. Night sweats, malaise, fatigue, swollen glands, and diarrhea can be associated with many other illnesses.

29. **(4)** The HIV virus is a retrovirus. It contains an enzyme, reverse transcriptase, that copies RNA into DNA. When the virus binds to a CD4 receptor, it inserts its RNA and enzymes into the cell, where a copy of the virus's RNA is made and enters the nucleus of the cell. As the infected host cell reproduces, the HIV DNA is duplicated and passed on.

30. **(4)** Although any of the above-mentioned clinical symptoms can be present in clients with SLE, fever, weight loss, and arthritis and arthralgias occur most often. Butterfly rash of the face and lymphadenopathy occur <50% of the time. Pulmonary effusion, hepatomegaly, splenomegaly, and Raynaud's syndrome occur in less than a third of the cases.

31. **(3)** The massive release of mediators triggers a series of events in target organs. Prior sensitization to the antigen must have occurred to trigger an anaphylactic reaction. Anaphylaxis may result from injection of an antigen, ingested food or drugs, or inhaled antigens.

32. **(1)** The release of histamine results in bronchospasm, vasodilatation, and vascular permeability leading to wheezing, increased mucous production in the lung, and edema of the airway.

33. **(2)** The onset of acute GVHD occurs between 30 and 50 days post-BMT. It results from immunocompetent donor T lymphocytes attacking the host tissues.

34. **(3)** The signs and symptoms of GVHD include maculopapular rash, generalized erythroderma with desquamation, increased bilirubin, increased serum glutamic-oxaloacetic transaminase (SGOT) and/or increased alkaline phosphatase, abdominal cramping, and diarrhea. Infection is characterized by fever, mental status changes, and headaches. Decreased RBC, hematocrit, and hemoglobin and petechiae are signs of anemia. Fever, chills, and urticaria are indications of a reaction to white cells in the marrow.

35. **(4)** T lymphocytes are the white cells responsible for control of the immune response. In SLE, T suppressor cells are decreased and cell activity is inhibited. This results in hypergammaglobulinemia and B-cell proliferation.

36. **(2)** The T4 lymphocyte is known as the T *[handwritten: Helper Cells]* helper cell. These cells are responsible for the proliferation of lymphocytes and macrophages causing activation of the cells in response to an antigen. The B lymphocytes are effector cells that mediate humoral responses by production of antibodies. The band neutrophil and segmented neutrophil are slightly mature and fully mature neutrophils, respectively. Neutrophils are the most abundant cells in the bone marrow and blood.

37. **(3)** Based on the history of an HIV-positive test and the symptoms presented, the client is at risk for development of *Pneumocystis carinii* pneumonia. Further examination would include obtaining a chest radiograph, and pulse oximetry to determine oxygen saturation. The lack of purplish lesions is considered in ruling out Kaposi's sarcoma. *Klebsiella pneumoniae* is a nosocomial infection, not community acquired. Lymphoma in HIV usually occurs as non-Hodgkin's lymphoma as a primary site in the brain.

38. **(2)** Severe malaise, pallor, stridor, and dyspnea are signs and symptoms associated with a severe anaphylactic reaction. Symptoms may occur immediately or up to 2 hours after exposure. Severe reactions require immediate intervention.

39. **(3)** IgG is the major antibody against viruses and bacterias and is the principal mediator of the secondary immune response, which requires repeated response to the same antigen. There is no IgC antibody. IgA is the secretory immunoglobulin found in tears, saliva, and mucous secretions of the lung and gastrointestinal tract. IgE mediates allergic reactions.

40. **(2)** A type I hypersensitivity reaction causes an immediate wheal-and-flare reaction. Contact dermatitis is seen in a type IV (delayed) reaction. Hematuria is seen in a type II reaction caused by the presence of preformed circulating cytoxic antibodies, such as in a blood transfusion reaction or autoimmune hemolytic anemia. High fever can be seen in the type III hypersensitivity reaction when large quantities of antigen—antibody complexes are released in the body.

41. **(2)** Sexually active teenagers are the fastest growing group of HIV-positive clients because of unprotected sexual activity. Immunocompromised clients and elderly adults are at no greater risk for developing HIV than is any other group. Risk factors for the development of HIV include unprotected sexual contact with someone of unknown HIV status, multiple sexual partners, intravenous drug use, hemophilia, and blood transfusions received prior to 1985.

42. **(1)** Changes in the electrocardiogram (ECG) are associated with coronary ischemia and myocardial ischemia. Although the electrocardiographic changes suggest myocardial injury, there is no change in the serum enzymes. Other signs and symptoms include hypotension and tachycardia.

43. **(3)** Cotton-wool spots are the most common ophthalmologic problem associated with SLE. Retinal hemorrhages and AV nicking can be seen in the client with hypertension. Conjunctivitis is an infection of the conjunctiva.

44. **(1)** Clients with allergic rhinitis should monitor the air quality and allergy index in their area. A surgical-type mask will not filter out small allergens. Remaining inside during allergy season is an unrealistic expectation and can lead to depression and isolation for the client. Clients can enjoy a summer garden if they are careful about the types of plants and flowers they plant. For example, the client with an allergy to ragweed should avoid daisies, dahlias, and chrysanthemums.

45. **(3)** The incidence of latex allergies has increased dramatically since the onset of BSI precautions and increased use of latex gloves. Because of a change in the manufacturing of the gloves, in an effort to keep up with the increased demand, there is a higher protein count in the gloves. The increased exposure has led to a proliferation of health care workers being diagnosed with the illness.

46. **(2)** Latex allergy is a progressive disease that worsens with continual exposure. The symptoms range from contact dermatitis to anaphylaxis. Currently, latex allergy affects 17% of health care workers and 39% of dental professionals. Latex allergy is an acquired immune response to the latex protein allergen. There is no vaccine, and the only defense is to avoid contact with latex.

47. **(2)** The typical allergic facies consists of allergic shiners, Dennie's lines (extra wrinkles below the lower eyelids), and mouth breathing. Nasal polyps are uncommon in childhood allergic rhinitis. The nasal discharge with allergies is usually clear.

48. **(3)** Adolescent through adulthood atopic dermatitis common sites are the popliteal and anticubital fossae, face, neck, upper arms and back, dorsa of the hand, feet, fingers, and toes.

Pharmacology

49. **(4)** Procainamide (Pronestyl), hydralazine (Apresoline), and isoniazid have been shown to induce a lupus-like syndrome. Discontinuation of the medication results in disappearance of the clinical signs and symptoms. Antibiotics such as sulfonamides (Septra DS) and penicillin (Pen-Vee K, Penicillin G) have been associated with anaphylactic reactions in some clients. Oral contraceptives may cause increased blood pressure and increase the risk for development of thromboemboli. NSAIDs such as Motrin have been associated with gastrointestinal upset and gastric pain, especially when taken on an empty stomach.

50. **(2)** Procainamide (Pronestyl) is one of the most common offenders. Twenty per cent of clients receiving this drug develop clinical drug-induced SLE. The other drugs listed have not been associated with SLE.

51. **(1)** Temporal arthritis, seen primarily in the elderly, can lead to blindness if not treated immediately with corticosteroids. The usual daily dose of prednisone is 60 mg, divided dose initially, then single morning dose (never use every-other-day steroids). Begin a *slow taper* after 4 weeks if asymptomatic and the ESR is decreased. Tapering of the dose is very individualized, and the client may be on medications for several months to years. Average time for disease remission is 3–4 years (range 1–10 years).

52. **(2)** Epinephrine would be the first-line drug to be injected for the treatment of the respiratory distress associated with an anaphylactic reaction. The dosage for epinephrine (1:1000, SC) is 0.01 ml/kg for a child and 0.3–0.5 ml/kg for an adult. Benadryl's onset of action is not fast enough. Lidocaine would only topically treat the pain and not the respiratory problem. Anti-inflammatory medications would not be given initially, but possibly later if needed.

53. **(4)** Chloroquine phosphate is the standard drug used for malaria prophylaxis. The dosage is 5 mg/kg body weight up to 300 mg for an adult. Doxycycline (Vibramycin) is often used to treat diarrhea associated with traveling to areas where diarrhea is common from drinking the water; it is also used to treat chlamydia and pelvic inflammatory disease. Ceftriaxone (Rocephin) is used in bacterial septicemia or problems of the respiratory and urinary tracts. Ampicillin (Polycillin, Omnipen) is used to treat a variety of organisms and as prophylaxis for bacterial endocarditis.

54. **(1)** Unless there is a secondary bacterial infection, antibiotics are not indicated. Antihistamines and reduction of exposure to the allergen will help to reduce the symptoms. For continued control and stabilization of the mast cell, corticosteroids are indicated.

55. **(1)** Adults are at greater risk for development of adverse drug reactions, probably due to the increased number of medications used and the amount of exposures. Clients with prior drug reactions are more likely to develop reactions to new drugs. The risk of an adverse drug reaction occurs in the first 2–3 weeks of therapy. Prolonged course of drug use, high dosage, and intermittent therapy increase the risk of an adverse reaction. Genetic factors may contribute to increased mediators and influencing metabolic pathways. Gender has no effect except in muscle relaxants and chymopapain, where women are at greater risk of developing an adverse drug reaction. Route of drug administration contributes to the risk with IV, IM SC, PO, and topical in the order of greatest to least risk.

56. **(3)** Trimethoprim-sulfamethoxazole (Septra, Bactrim) is used to treat as well as prevent *Pneumocystis carinii* pneumonia. Usually a 21-day course of the drug is indicated. It may take 7–10 days to see a clinical response. Fluconazole (Diflucan) and amphotericin B are antifungal drugs, and acyclovir (Zovirax) is an antiviral used primarily to treat herpes simplex virus types 1 and 2 and herpes zoster (shingles).

57. **(2)** The chronic use of nasal decongestants for greater than 3 days can result in a rebound effect when discontinued. This will

lead to an increased nasal congestion as a result of reflex vasodilatation. The condition may take as long as 2–3 weeks to resolve. Allergic rhinitis is not a self-limiting illness associated only with the spring and fall. Even though therapy is initiated, the client should be instructed to avoid exposure to the allergen as much as possible.

58. **(4)** The second-generation antihistamines do not cross the blood-brain barrier; therefore, they do not cause sedation and/or psychomotor dysfunction. There is little anticholinergic activity and less dry mouth and constipation. The cost of these antihistamines is 15–30 times greater than the first-generation antihistamines. The medications are rapidly absorbed within 1–2 hours of oral administration on an empty stomach.

59. **(1)** Sympathomimetics (adrenergics) cause vasoconstriction, reducing edema and secretions. Inhaled corticosteroids stabilize mast cells and block degranulation.

60. **(1)** Macrolides (erythromycin) and Hismanal should not be administered concurrently. Fatal dysrhythmias may be precipitated by this combination.

61. **(3)** Chromolyn sodium is used to stabilize the mast cell membrane to prevent release of histamine when the cell comes in contact with an antigen. It does not affect the amount of histamine released from the cell, antagonize the effects of histamine, or reduce antiemetic activity.

62. **(1)** The use of H_1 blockers can cause paradoxical central nervous system stimulation resulting in ataxia in the elderly. Antihistamines can cause many simultaneous side effects in the elderly that can interfere with their daily living: dry mouth, constipation, as well as impaired vision, gait, and thinking.

63. **(2)** The client should be instructed not to use over-the-counter medications without consulting the nurse practitioner or pharmacist. The client should be cautioned on the extended use of topical antihistamines. Antihistamines do not affect circulating histamine; therefore, it is important for the client to avoid exposure to a known allergen. Constipation and urinary retention are adverse effects that should be reported to the nurse practitioner.

64. **(2)** An advantage of using loratadine (Claritin) is the once-a-day dosing, which helps with client compliance. The cost is greater than some of the other first-generation antihistamines. Loratadine/pseudoephedrine (Claritin D) is available in an antihistamine/decongestant with twice-a-day dosing or loratadine/pseudoephedrine extended release (Claritin D 24 Hour) is available for once-a-day dosing.

65. **(4)** Medications such as antihistamines and corticosteroids are used to counter mediator release and block release of additional mediators. NSAID, antibiotics, and decongestants are not indicated in the treatment of anaphylaxis.

66. **(4)** Both Benadryl and Dimetane are antihistamines and could be prescribed. The Dimetane would have less central nervous system sedating effects than the Benadryl. Benylin is an antitussive and Robitussin is an expectorant.

67. **(3)** While Benadryl will help with the itching and can certainly be administered after the child's distress is relieved, the immediate concern is to prevent respiratory arrest from swelling of the mucosa of the throat. The usual dose for children is 0.01 ml/kg of the 1:1000 solution.

68. **(2)** Grapeseed extract is a common alternative therapy for allergies with few side effects. It is often not as effective during peak allergy seasons and an antihistamine is needed for breakthrough allergy symptoms.

69. **(2)** Antihistamines block the absorption of iron, folate, and vitamin B_{12}.

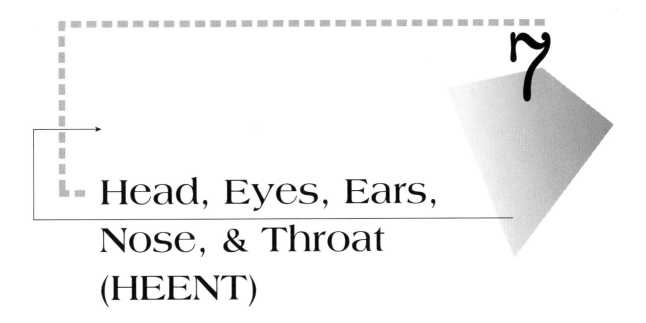

Head, Eyes, Ears, Nose, & Throat (HEENT)

Physical Examination & Diagnostic Tests

Head

1. In examining the mouth of a school-age child, the nurse practitioner notes that the central and lateral permanent incisors have surface pitting and are stained brown. This condition is most suggestive of:

   1. The mother taking tetracycline during pregnancy.

   2. Poor dental hygiene.

   3. Dental fluorosis.

   4. Going to bed with a bottle during infancy.

2. The nurse practitioner is examining lymph nodes in the neck. What is palpated in the anterior triangle of the neck?

   1. Posterior cervical chain.

   2. Anterior superficial chain.

   3. Periauricular lymph nodes.

   4. Supraclavicular lymph nodes.

Eyes

3. When using an ophthalmoscope, the nurse practitioner:

   1. Holds the ophthalmoscope in the right hand (uses right eye) while examining the client's left eye.

   2. Starts the examination with the lens set at zero.

   3. Begins in a position 1 inch from the eye to check the red light reflex.

   4. Examines the anterior chamber in a well-lighted room and asks the client to focus on an object.

4. The visual screening for a 4-year-old child is recorded as 20/40 in both eyes. The nurse practitioner should now:

   1. Have the child return in 1 month to have his vision rechecked.

   2. Refer the child to an ophthalmologist.

   3. Recheck his vision to make sure that it is accurate.

   4. Record the findings as normal for age.

5. The nurse practitioner checking for strabimus would use which test?

   1. Cover-uncover test.

   2. Bruchner's test.

   3. Ishihara's test.

   4. Snellen's test.

6. The nurse practitioner observes lid lag in a client with:

   1. Myasthenia gravis.

   2. Hyperthyroidism.

   3. Hordeolum.

   4. Chalazion.

7. The nurse practitioner is examining an elderly woman. There is a glossy white circle around the pupils of her eyes, and the pupil has a decreased reaction to the direct light reflex. There is a history of presbyopia. Correct interpretation of these findings is:

   1. Beginning development of cataracts with a significant decrease in visual acuity.

   2. Normal changes in the eyes as a result of the aging process.

   3. A decrease in depth perception and the early eye changes associated with glaucoma.

   4. Visual changes secondary to long-term treatment with digitoxin and corticosteroids.

8. The nurse practitioner is preparing to examine the eyes of an adult client. In order to examine the optic disc and retinal vessels, the practitioner uses what aperture on the ophthalmoscope?

   1. Small aperture.

   2. Red-free filter.

   3. Slit.

   4. Grid.

9. When testing the eyes for the presence of a normal consensual response, the nurse practitioner will:

   1. Shine the light into the client's pupil and observe the rate of pupillary constriction.

   2. Direct the light into one pupil and observe for the constriction or response of the other pupil.

   3. Hold a card in front of one eye and have the client focus on a fixed object, remove the card, and observe movement of the newly uncovered eye.

   4. Ask the client to focus on an object, then direct a light source to the bridge of the nose while observing for symmetrical reflection in both eyes.

10. On ophthalmic examination, there appears to be a narrowing or blocking of the vein at the point where an arteriole crosses over it. The significance of this finding is:

   1. The client needs to be evaluated for chronic hypertension.

   2. This may be indicative of increased ocular pressure associated with glaucoma.

   3. The finding is associated with papilledema causing decreased venous drainage.

   4. This may represent a small embolus in the retinal vessels.

11. When examining the eyes, the nurse practitioner determines that the pupils change in size when the client focuses from a close object to a distant object. This is interpreted as:

    1. Normal visual accommodation.

    2. Intact extraocular motor nerves.

    3. Appropriate consensual response.

    4. Visual acuity within normal limits.

12. During a preschool screening for visual acuity, the nurse practitioner would also assess for:

    1. Pupils that are equal and reactive.

    2. Intraocular pressure by tonometry.

    3. Diplopia.

    4. Strabismus.

Ears

13. When examining the ears of an adult client, the nurse practitioner determines the tympanic membrane is gray and translucent. This is interpreted as:

    1. Scarring from previous infections.

    2. Decreased circulation to the membrane.

    3. Presence of serous fluid behind the membrane.

    4. Normal characteristics of the adult ear.

14. The purpose of conducting the Rinne test is to determine conduction of sound through the bone and through the auditory canal. A normal Rinne test is described as:

    1. Equal conduction through the mastoid bone and the ear canal.

    2. Air conduction twice as long as bone conduction.

    3. Bone conduction twice as long as air conduction.

    4. Sound is clearer with bone conduction than air conduction.

15. When assessing the tympanic membrane, specific landmarks are determined and described according to the face of a clock. Where are the normal landmarks for the right tympanic membrane located?

    1. Direct light reflex at 5- to 6-o'clock position, malleus at 1- to 2-o'clock position with umbo in center.

    2. Manubrium slanted to the left with malleus at 10-o'clock position.

    3. Direct light reflex in center of membrane with malleus at 9-o'clock position.

    4. Umbo to the left with anterior malleolar folds at 10-o'clock position.

16. A 4-year-old's pure tone audiometry reveals 25 dB in the left ear and 43 dB in the right ear. The nurse practitioner would interpret these findings as:

    1. Inconclusive because a pure tone audiometry is not accurate under age 5.

    2. Within normal limits for age.

    3. Normal hearing in the left ear and moderate hearing loss in the right ear.

    4. Mild hearing loss in the left ear and normal hearing in the right ear.

17. The nurse practitioner knows that if an infant has low or obliquely set ears there is also an increased incidence of:

    1. Cataracts.

    2. Hyaline membrane disease.

    3. Genitourinary defects.

    4. Cardiovascular anomalies.

Nose

18. The nurse practitioner understands that nasal mucosa:

    1. Is redder than oral mucosa.

    2. Is pale and translucent in appearance.

    3. Appears pink and boggy, without exudate.

    4. Appears dark pink with watery secretion.

Throat

19. Throat cultures are indicated for the following suspected causes of pharyngitis:
    1. Rhinovirus and coronavirus infection.
    2. Group A β-hemolytic streptococci.
    3. Mononucleosis.
    4. *Candida albicans*.

20. The following statement is true regarding tonsils:
    1. Large tonsils in children are more prone to tonsillitis than small tonsils.
    2. Tonsils enlarge as the child grows older.
    3. Most hypertrophied tonsils in children are normal.
    4. The majority of tonsillitis is due to a β-hemolytic streptococcus infection.

21. An adolescent arrives at the nurse practitioner's clinic with a complaint of low-grade fever, sore throat, a slight headache, and fatigue. On physical examination, the nurse practitioner found exudative tonsils bilaterally, red pharynx with white patches, and enlarged posterior cervical neck nodes. The nurse practitioner would expect to find:
    1. Positive rapid strep test.
    2. Positive monospot test.
    3. Decreased white blood cell (WBC) count.
    4. Positive viral throat cultures.

Disorders

Head

22. An adult client presents to the nurse practitioner's office with a white plaque near the base of the tongue. The nurse practitioner notes that the plaque does not wipe off and assesses it as:
    1. Hemangioma.
    2. Leukoplakia.
    3. Papilloma.
    4. Erythroplasia.

23. Which of the following are predominant risk factors for oral carcinoma?
    1. History of dental infections, age <40.
    2. Tobacco use, alcohol use.
    3. Herpes simplex virus type 1, tobacco use.
    4. Alcohol use, history of dental abscess.

24. The hallmark of early oral cancer is:
    1. Tissue retraction.
    2. Thickening oral tissues.
    3. Persistent (>14 days) local inflammation.
    4. Halitosis and cough.

25. A adult male client is being evaluated for a complaint of a sore throat. He states that he has difficulty swallowing and has some mouth pain. On exam, the nurse practitioner finds that the client's mouth, tongue, and pharynx are coated with white curd-like plaques that are difficult to remove with a tongue blade. The course of treatment for this client should include:
    1. Referral to an ear, nose, and throat specialist for evaluation.
    2. Amoxicillin 500 mg PO tid × 10 days.
    3. Encourage the client to have human immunodeficiency virus (HIV) screening.
    4. Clear liquids only for the next few days.

26. The nurse practitioner knows that the most common site for head and neck cancer to occur is the:
    1. Sinuses.
    2. Oral cavity.
    3. Larynx.
    4. Nasal cavity.

27. The nurse practitioner taking a history on a preschooler learns that the family does not have fluoridated drinking water. Taking into consideration the concerns about fluorosis, the most appropriate nursing intervention would be to:
    1. Prescribe 5 ml of 0.02% fluoride solution (Fluorinse) once daily.

2. Instruct patients to use a pea-size fluoridated dentrifice and to supervise toothbrushing.

3. Instruct parents to use bottled drinking water.

4. Refer to dentist for topical application of fluoride.

Eyes

28. A client who is a sheet metal worker complains of something in his right eye since this morning. Before beginning treatment, the nurse practitioner should:

    1. Instill local anesthetic.

    2. Check the visual acuity.

    3. Flush the eye with tap water for 30 minutes.

    4. Stain the eye with fluorescein.

29. A mother reports that her toddler awoke this morning with eye redness and a swollen eyelid. The nurse practitioner notes that the child is afebrile and the eyelid is nontender and uniformly swollen. The most likely diagnosis is:

    1. Blepharitis.

    2. Hordeolum.

    3. Insect bite.

    4. Dacryocystitis.

30. Upon examination of a 2-week-old infant, the nurse practitioner notes that the infant's left eye is watering and there is crusted material on the eyelids. No edema or erythema is noted. The nurse practitioner would make the diagnosis of:

    1. Nasolacrimal duct obstruction.

    2. Conjunctivitis.

    3. Congenital dacrocystocele.

    4. Corneal abrasion.

31. A client is being prepared for cataract surgery. What information is important for the nurse practitioner to explain to the client?

    1. The procedure is short and the client usually goes home the morning after the surgery.

    2. Both eyes will be patched for the first 24 hours and it is important for the client to stay in bed.

    3. There may be problems with headache and eye pain for the first 24 hours; take the pain medication provided.

    4. Client usually go home in 2–3 hours after the surgery; there will be increased tearing, but it should not be painful.

32. A client works as a welder. He finished work about 8 hours ago and discovered the protective glass on his welding hood was cracked. He is complaining of agonizing pain and photophobia. The correct diagnosis and action are:

    1. Chemical keratitis; dilate with atropine twice daily.

    2. Viral conjunctivitis; sulfonamide drops four times daily.

    3. Corneal abrasion; binocular patching with polymyxin ointment.

    4. Ultraviolet keratitis; binocular patching and 1% cyclopentolate (Cyclogyl) drops.

33. A geriatric client presents at the clinic with complaints of blurred vision that has been getting increasingly worse over the past 2 years. There is also a problem with glare, but no problems with pain. The nurse practitioner would first evaluate for the presence of:

    1. Glaucoma.

    2. Retinal detachment.

    3. Degeneration of macula.

    4. Cataracts.

34. An adult client presents to the nurse practitioner for evaluation of a red, itchy eye for 1 day. The client states that when he awoke the eye was matted shut. The client can recall no trauma to the eye. The pupils are equal and reactive and the client denies any pain to the eye. The nurse practitioner treats this client for:

    1. Conjunctivitis.

    2. Corneal abrasion.

    3. Glaucoma.

    4. Iritis.

35. Which assessment of the eye is a deviation from the commonly occurring age-related changes?

    1. Arcus senilis.

    2. Presbyopia.

    3. Sensitivity to glare.

    4. Sustained nystagmus.

36. During a routine physical examination on a 30-year-old client, the nurse practitioner identifies arcus cornealis. The significance of this disorder is:

    1. High potential for future blindness.

    2. None, normal variant of aging process.

    3. Abnormal lipid metabolism requiring medical management.

    4. Hereditary variant of no consequence.

37. A 70-year-old client comes to the clinic complaining of an increased sensitivity to glare, difficulty adapting to darkness, and altered depth perception. The nurse practitioner should suspect:

    1. Cataract.

    2. Macular degeneration.

    3. Glaucoma.

    4. Normal age-related changes.

38. A 6-week-old infant is brought to the clinic by her mother. The mother is very concerned that the child's eyes are crossed. The best action for the nurse practitioner is:

    1. Explain to the mother this is not abnormal, the child should be re-evaluated at 3 months of age.

    2. Refer the infant to an ophthalmologist.

    3. Provide the mother with normal saline eye drops for the infant.

    4. Have the mother alternate patching one eye then the other every 6 hours.

39. In assessing a child with bacterial conjunctivitis, the nurse practitioner finds:

    1. Minimal tearing, moderate itching, and profuse exudate.

    2. Severe itching, moderate tearing, and minimal discharge.

    3. Minimal itching, moderate tearing, and mucoid exudate.

    4. Minimal itching, moderate tearing, and profuse exudate.

40. The nurse practitioner makes the diagnosis of nasolacrimal obstruction in a 1-week-old infant who presents with "laking" of the right eye and a yellow discharge in the inner canthus of both eyes. Which of the following interventions would be contraindicated?

    1. Neosporin ophthalmic gtts.

    2. Massaging the lacrimal duct for 1 minute qid.

    3. Cleansing the eye with warm water qid.

    4. Dexamethasone (Decadron) ophthalmic gtts.

Ears

41. A child is diagnosed by the nurse practitioner with acute otitis media. During pneumatic otoscopy, the nurse practitioner expects the tympanic membrane (TM) to be:

    1. Immobile, painful, with absent or decreased landmarks.

    2. Mobile, painful, with absent or decreased landmarks.

3. Immobile, not painful with landmarks visualized.

4. Mobile, not painful, full, bulging.

42. In teaching clients how to avoid acoustic trauma due to noise in the very loud range, the nurse practitioner knows that noise is loudest from a:

1. Vacuum cleaner.

2. Power mower.

3. Clothes washer.

4. Food blender.

43. A geriatric client is complaining of difficulty hearing. He relates that the problem seems to be getting worse over the past few years. What finding would support a diagnosis of presbycusis?

1. Unable to hear a watch tick at 1–2 inches from the ear.

2. Rinne test indicates air conduction greater than bone conduction.

3. History of long-term tetracycline antibiotics for chronic infections.

4. Long-term family history of chronic hearing loss.

44. A 6-year-old child is seen by the nurse practitioner for ear pain. The child is afebrile. The left ear canal is markedly edematous and moderately inflamed with thick, yellowish drainage at the external meatus. The child denies putting anything in the ear canal, but the nurse practitioner finds that the child swims frequently. The most likely diagnosis is:

1. Acute otitis media.

2. Serous otitis media.

3. Sinusitis.

4. Otitis externa.

45. Which of the following organisms is least likely to cause otitis media?

1. *Moraxella catarrhalis.*

2. *Streptococcus pneumoniae.*

3. *Chlamydia trachomatis.*

4. *Haemophilus influenzae.*

46. Risk factors for acute otitis media include:

1. Second-hand smoke, attending day care, American Indians and Eskimos.

2. Chinese race, previous otitis media, many siblings.

3. Higher socioeconomic level, full-time day care, allergies.

4. Summer season, full-time day care, premature at birth.

47. Which assessment of the ear would indicate a deviation from the normal aging process?

1. Dull, retracted, white tympanic membrane.

2. An elongated lobule.

3. A sensorineural hearing loss.

4. Bulging tympanic membrane with a distorted cone of light.

48. The nurse practitioner indicates an ~~refer to AC~~ understanding of conductive hearing loss in the older client with which statement?

1. "This has occurred due to damage of the eighth cranial nerve from gentamycin."

2. "This is a result of an inner ear infection."

3. "This is a normal part of aging and is referred to as presbycusis."

4. "This may be reversible after the cerumen is removed from the ear canal."

49. A 6-year-old child is examined by the nurse practitioner because of fluctuating hearing problems. The child is afebrile and denies otalgia. The mobility of the tympanic membrane is decreased when the nurse practitioner performs pneumatic otoscopy. The tympanic membrane is opaque with no visible landmarks. The child denies putting anything in the ear, and the mother states the child does not swim frequently. The most likely diagnosis is:

1. Acute otitis media (AOM).

2. A foreign body.

3. Otitis media with effusion (OME).

4. Otitis externa.

50. Sensory hearing loss is common in industrial settings and preventable with the use of adequate hearing protection. This type of hearing loss is usually first noted with changes at what level?

    1. 500 Hz.

    2. 200 Hz.

    3. 3000–4000 Hz.

    4. Above 4000 Hz.

Nose

51. An adult client presents to the nurse practitioner's office with fever and complaints of right facial pain, copious yellow nasal discharge, and acute pain and headache when bending over for 5 days. There is no transillumination of the right maxillary sinus and that area is very tender to palpation. The client's diagnosis is:

    1. Chronic sinusitis.

    2. Acute sinusitis.

    3. Dental abscess.

    4. Temporal arteritis.

52. The nurse practitioner teaches the mother of a school-age child the following as the most effective preventive measure against the common cold:

    1. Judicious use of vitamin C during cold season.

    2. Ensuring adequate sleep and fluids.

    3. Meticulous handwashing, preferably with an antibacterial soap.

    4. Avoiding contact with children and adults who have a runny nose, cough, and sore throat.

Throat

53. A 20-year-old client presents to the nurse practitioner's office with a chief complaint of "severe sore throat" for 3 days. The client states he also ran a fever, but does not know how high it got, and he has been very tired with the sore throat. The physical exam revealed enlarged tonsils with large patchy exudate, inflamed pharynx, and nontender posterior cervical lymphadenopathy. The rest of the physical exam was nonremarkable. The nurse practitioner would make the diagnosis of:

    1. Infectious mononucleosis.

    2. Leukemia.

    3. Scarlet fever.

    4. Oral candidiasis.

54. Which of the following clinical findings are associated with bacterial streptococcal pharyngitis?

    1. Rhinorrhea.

    2. Cough.

    3. Enlarged tonsils with exudate.

    4. Small oral vesicles.

Pharmacology

55. The antibiotic(s) of choice for acute sinusitis in the adult is (are):

    1. Amoxicillin (Amoxil) 500 mg PO tid × 14 days; trimethoprim-sulfamethoxazole (Bactrim) DS PO 1 q12h × 14 days; penicillin V potassium (Pen-Vee K) 500 mg bid PO × 14 days.

    2. Trimethoprim-sulfamethoxazole DS PO 1 q12h × 14 days; penicillin V potassium (Pen-Vee K) 500 mg PO bid × 14 days.

    3. Penicillin G 150,000 U IM × 1; Amoxicillin 500 mg PO tid × 14 days.

    4. Amoxicillin 500 mg PO tid × 14 days; trimethoprim-sulfamethoxazole DS 1 q12h PO × 14 days.

56. A geriatric client is diagnosed with chronic open-angle glaucoma. She has a past history of bradycardia and first-degree atrioventricular block. In consideration of her treatment, what medication is to be avoided?

    1. Pilocarpine (Isopto Carpine).

    2. Timolol (Timoptic).

    3. Hydrochlorothiazide (Diuril).

    4. Acetazolamide (Diamox).

57. Which antibiotic would be appropriate for the nurse practitioner to prescribe for β-lactamase production by strains of *Haemophilus influenzae* and *Moraxella catarrhalis* in a child with acute otitis media?

    1. Amoxicillin (Amoxil).

    2. Erythromycin-sulfisoxazole (Pediazole).

    3. Penicillin V potassium (Pen-Vee K).

    4. Metronidazole (Flagyl).

58. Prophylactic antibiotics are indicated for which of the following clients?

    1. A 3-year-old with two episodes of AOM in the previous winter.

    2. A 2-year-old with three episodes of AOM within the last 6 months.

    4. A 4-year-old with history of prophylactic antibiotics in last 2 years but without evidence of AOM this year.

    4. A 2-year-old with three episodes of AOM over last 9 months.

59. The treatment plan for a client diagnosed with infectious mononucleosis includes which of the following?

    1. Rest during acute phase.

    2. Avoid exercise during acute phase.

    3. Corticosteroids during acute phase.

    4. Ampicillin orally for 10 days.

60. An adolescent client has had yellowish green nasal discharge and frontal headache for a week. The adolescent's temperature has gone up to 101.2°F on most afternoons and she has a cough that worsens when she lies down. The physical exam is within normal limits except for the drainage and a slightly erythematous pharynx. She does not have any drug allergies and has not been on any medications in the last few months. Which medication would be best to prescribe for her?

    1. Diphenhydramine hydrochloride (Benadryl).

    2. Erythromycin (E-Mycin).

    3. Pseudoephedrine hydrochloride (Sudafed).

    4. Amoxicillin (Amoxil).

61. A toddler (weight 18 kg) is diagnosed as having bilateral otitis media. His last ear infection was 6 months ago and he has no known drug allergies. An appropriate medication to prescribe would be:

    1. Ampicillin, 125 mg/kg, 1 tsp PO tid × 7 days.

    2. Corticosteroid otic solution, 3 gtts both ears × 10 days.

    3. Amoxicillin, 250 mg/kg, 1 tsp PO tid × 10 days.

    4. Doxycycline, 250 mg, 1 tsp PO tid × 10 days.

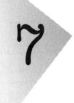

Answers & Rationales

Physical Examination & Diagnostic Tests

Head

1. **(3)** Dental fluorosis causes surface pitting and staining, especially to the central and lateral permanent incisors. Tetracycline would have caused staining of all the teeth. Dental caries would be more indicative of poor dental hygiene. "Baby teeth," not the permanent teeth, would be affected by going to bed with a bottle.

2. **(2)** The conceptualization of triangles is useful in determining the location of palpable lymph nodes in the neck. The sternocleidomastoid muscle is the division between the anterior (containing the anterior superficial cervical chain) and the posterior (containing the posterior cervical chain) triangles. The trapezius muscle marks the posterior border of the posterior triangle. The supraclavicular or scale nodes are palpated in the angle formed by the clavical and the sternocleidomastoid muscle.

Eyes

3. **(2)** The correct use of the ophthalmoscope involves using the right hand and right eye to examine the client's right eye. The room should be semidarkened for best visualization. The examiner initially inspects the lens and vitreous body from a distance of about 12 inches (at zero setting) and moves closer to the eye, usually rotating the lenses to the positive numbers (+15 to +20), which assists in focusing on near objects.

4. **(4)** A 4-year-old's normal acuity is 20/40; therefore, none of the other answers is appropriate.

5. **(1)** Cover-uncover tests for strabismus; Bruchner's tests the red reflex; Ishihara's tests color perception; and Snellen's tests far vision.

6. **(2)** If the lid margin falls above the limbus (junction line where the sclera and cornea meet) so that some sclera is visible, hyperthyroidism may be present. The lid may lag behind the limbus as the gaze moves from an upward to a downward position. Ptosis is a drooping lid margin that falls at the pupil or below and may indicate an oculomotor lesion or myasthenia gravis. A chalazion is an inflammation or cyst of the meibomian glands that lie within the posterior portion of the eyelid. A localized infection of the small glands around the eyelashes in the hair follicle at the lid margin is called a hordeolum.

7. **(2)** With cataracts there is a clouding of the lens, not a circle around the pupil. The circle around the pupil is arcus senilis, which is normal in the geriatric client. The visual acuity of the client cannot be determined from the information provided. There are no observable pupillary changes in the beginning stages of glaucoma, which is identified by checking the intraocular pressure.

8. **(2)** The red-free filter is used to examine the optic disc for pallor and vascular changes as well as to assess for retinal hemorrhages. The small aperture is used for small pupils, the slit is for the anterior eye, and the grid is for estimating the size of lesions found in the fundal area.

9. **(2)** Consensual response is pupillary constriction of one eye when there is a direct light stimulus to the pupil of the other eye.

10. **(1)** Arteriovenous nicking is associated with longstanding hypertension. Intraocular pressure cannot be determined from an ophthalmic examination. Papilledema is associated with swelling around the optic disc, and small emboli are represented by an abrupt impediment or severe narrowing of an arteriole not associated with where the retinal veins and arteries cross.

11. **(1)** Changes in pupil size when focusing from near to distant objects is normal accommodation. Extraocular eye movements refer to the ability to move the eye. Consensual response is constriction of the eye in response to light being shined in the opposite eye. The Snellen eye chart is used to determine the visual acuity.

12. **(4)** Strabismus (malaligned eyes) can be a precursor for amblyopia (decreased visual acuity). It is important to detect strabismus as early as possible in preschool children. Options #1 and #3 are components of a neurologic assessment. Tonometry exams are performed to assess for glaucoma.

Ears

13. **(4)** This describes the normal characteristics of the tympanic membrane. There is no evidence of scarring or fluid.

14. **(2)** The normal Rinne test is air conduction is twice as long as bone conduction (AC > BC).

15. **(1)** This describes the correct position for these landmarks on the right ear. In Option #2, the manubrium slants to the right with the malleus at the 1- to 2-o'clock position for the right ear. Option #3 describes the correct position for the left ear. In Option #4, the umbo is in the center with anterior folds at the 1- to 2-o'clock position for the right ear.

16. **(3)** Pure tone audiometry is appropriate after age 3. 0–25 dB = normal; 26–40 dB = mild hearing loss; and 41–55 dB = moderate hearing loss.

17. **(3)** Low-set or obliquely set ears occur more frequently in children who also have genitourinary defects. None of the other defects are associated with low-set ears.

Nose

18. **(1)** Nasal mucosa is redder than oral mucosa. Increased redness of the nasal mucosa usually indicates infection. Pale, boggy turbinates along with watery secretion often occur with allergic rhinitis. The normal secretion is mucoid. Purulent, crusty, or bloody secretions are abnormal.

Throat

19. **(2)** Rapid screening for strep can be done from a throat swab with antigen agglutination kits, but there is a 5–10% false-negative rate; therefore, it is suggested that culture should be performed. The heterophile antibody test (monospot test), which rapidly detects heterophile antibodies, compares with the sensitivity and specificity (95% specific and 90% sensitive) of older heterophile antibody tests to diagnose mononucleosis. *Candida albicans* and rhinovirus are not diagnosed by bacterial cultures. Oral candidiasis can be diagnosed with a potassium hydroxide smear.

20. **(3)** Enlarged tonsils are common in young children. As the child grows older, the tonsils recede in size. Only about 25–30% of tonsillitis is caused by the β-hemolytic streptococcus. Option #1 is a false statement.

21. **(2)** The client in this situation had risk factors (age) and symptoms of mononucleosis, therefore the monospot or heterophile antibody test should be conducted. The classical triad of mononucleosis symptoms include sore throat, fever, and posterior cervical lymphadenopathy with or without mild tenderness. Rapid screening for strep can be done from throat swab with antigen agglutination kits and would be obtained first, however would probably be negative. A WBC count would be ordered for bacterial pharyngitis, in that WBC elevation is found with bacterial infection and a decrease is associated with viral agents.

Disorders

22. **(2)** Leukoplakia is a white patch present on the oral mucosa that cannot be rubbed off. Hemangiomas are benign blood vessel proliferations of the lips, tongue, or buccal mucosa. Erythroplasia is an asymptomatic, red, velvety lesion of the mouth. Papillomas are benign verrucous lesions that are manifestations of human papillomavirus infection.

23. **(2)** The high risk factors for oral cancer are tobacco and alcohol use. The risk increases with the number of cigarettes smoked per day. The disease is age related, occurring in those over 40 years of age and increasing with age. The male/female ratio is 3:1. Other risk factors are use of cigars, pipes, and smokeless tobacco. Human papillomavirus has been considered in the etiology for squamous cell carcinoma in the upper head and neck.

24. **(3)** Erythroplasia is accompanied by an inflammatory reaction in a client with suspected oral cancer. If the erythematous lesion persists over 14 days, a high suspicion of early oral cancer exists. Tissue retraction and thickening of the oral tissues are later signs of oral cancer. Halitosis (odor) may be associated with dysfunction within the oral cavity, nasal cavity, sinuses, or esophageal disorders. Cough is the primary symptom of respiratory disorders such as acute bronchitis or pneumonia.

25. **(3)** Adults who present with thrush (oral candidiasis) may be immunologically impaired. It is important to make the diagnosis of HIV early to start treatment modalities. Treatment with amoxicillin may actually worsen the condition.

26. **(2)** The nurse practitioner knows the risk factors for head and neck cancer include tobacco and alcohol use; poor oral hygiene; and occupational exposure to asbestos, coke, nickel, wood, or leather. The most common site is in the oral cavity, accounting for 48% of the head and neck cancer diagnoses.

27. **(2)** A fluoridated dentifrice should be used in a small amount (pea-size) and children under 6 should be supervised so that they do not swallow too much toothpaste, which would put them at risk for fluorosis. The dose of fluoride rinse is too high plus it is inappropriate to prescribe to a preschooler. Bottled water does not contain fluoride. Topical application, though appropriate, is not the best answer.

Eyes

28. **(2)** Check the visual acuity before treatment as a basis for comparison in the event of complications. Local anesthetic will be helpful for the exam. Flushing at this point is unlikely to be helpful, and staining the eye should come later when preparing to examine for abrasion under ultraviolet light.

29. **(3)** Generalized, diffuse swelling and erythema of the eyelid is associated with an insect bite. Blepharitis is a chronic inflammatory condition characterized by erythema and scaling of the lid margins. Hordeolum, or stye, is an acute, purulent inflammation of the sebaceous glands (usually the meibomian or zeisian) of the eyelids and usually does not involve the entire eyelid. It may be painful, especially over the gland. Dacryocystitis is an inflammation of the lacrimal sac characterized by erythema and swelling over the lacrimal duct.

30. **(1)** Nasolacrimal obstruction occurs in up to 6% of infants. Signs and symptoms include a wet eye with mucoid discharge. There may also be irritated skin and conjunctivitis associated with this condition. There is no redness that would be indicative of

conjunctivitis. Congenital dacrocystocele presents at birth as a bluish subcutaneous mass. There would be more signs of irritation and pain with a corneal abrasion.

31. **(4)** Clients go home almost immediately after the procedure. Eye patches may be worn for the first 24 hours. Care should be taken to protect the operative eye from injury. There is some discomfort, but pain should not be a problem. The client can be up and around as tolerated.

32. **(4)** Ultraviolet burns of the cornea caused by a welding arc are treated with binocular patching.

33. **(4)** Cataracts are characterized by painless loss of visual acuity over a period of time. Retinal detachment most often occurs suddenly, with partial loss of the field of vision. Glaucoma results in the loss of peripheral vision, and macular degeneration primarily involves the central vision field.

34. **(1)** In corneal abrasion, glaucoma, and iritis the chief complaint is pain. Conjunctivitis presents with no pain and with a history of purulent discharge.

35. **(4)** Sustained nystagmus is indicative of a neurologic complication. The other options include normal age-related changes.

36. **(3)** Arcus cornealis is the deposit of lipids at the junction of the cornea and sclera that is present in many people over age 50. When identified in younger individuals, it points to a disorder of lipid metabolism.

37. **(4)** These assessments are normal age-related changes. Signs and symptoms of cataracts include reduced visual acuity; painless, progressive loss of vision; and sensitivity to light, especially during night driving. Reduced color discrimination and double vision may also be seen. Macular degeneration will present with a loss of the central vision. Primary open-angle glaucoma will present with occasional headaches and occasionally halos around lights, and may be asymptomatic in early stages. Primary angle-closure glaucoma will present with episodes of blurred vision, halos around lights at night, and redness with congestion.

38. **(1)** Strabismus is not an uncommon or abnormal occurrence in infants up until 3 months of age.

39. **(4)** Classic signs of bacterial conjunctivitis include those symptoms listed along with complaints of eyelids being "glued shut" upon arising in the morning. Option #2 is indicative of allergic conjunctivitis. Option #3 is indicative of viral conjunctivitis.

40. **(4)** Steroid (dexamethasone) medications are not used to treat nasolacrimal obstruction in infancy. Due to the yellow discharge in the eye, it would be appropriate to prescribe an antibiotic to prevent and/or treat conjunctivitis. Cleansing the eye with warm water and massaging the lacrimal duct are both appropriate interventions.

Ears

41. **(1)** The diagnosis of otitis media is clinical, made by otoscopy based on the appearance of the tympanic membrane. The bony landmarks are absent or decreased. The tympanic membrane may be full, bulging, or retracted with pus, and the light reflex is distorted. Pneumatic otoscopy reveals decreased or absent mobility of the tympanic membrane. Erythema is an inconclusive finding, especially in children, because the redness may be due to crying rather than infection.

42. **(2)** Although all of these household appliances are noisy, the client should wear ear plugs or muffs when using a power lawn mower regularly for long periods of time.

43. **(1)** Inability to hear a watch tick at 1–2 inches from the ear is a classic sign of hearing loss characteristic of advancing age. The Rinne test will indicate bone conduction is two times greater than air conduction. Tetracyclines are not ototoxic and the family history may or may not contribute to the problem.

44. **(4)** The client has the clinical findings of otitis externa, an inflammation and/or infection of the external ear canal predisposed by excessive wetness, such as swimming. Common organisms responsible for otitis externa include *Pseudomonas aeruginosa*, *Proteus mirabilis*, and *Enterobacter aerogenes*. Sinusitis clinical findings focus on sinus tenderness and a purulent nasal discharge. Clinical findings of otitis media include ear pain, full or bulging tympanic membrane, decreased or negative mobility, and possible erythema. Findings associated with serous otitis media include opaque or translucent tympanic membrane with presence of air bubbles; landmarks may be absent and the light reflex may be diffuse or absent.

45. **(3)** The key factor that contributes to acute otitis media (AOM) is a dysfunctional eustachian tube that may allow bacteria from the nasopharynx to the middle ear. The most frequent bacterial organisms that infect the middle ear, especially in children, are similar to those of the nasopharynx: *S. pneumoniae*, *H. influenzae*, and *M. catarrhalis*. *Escherichia coli* and *Klebsiella* cause about 15% of AOM cases in babies under 6 weeks old. Viruses may also cause AOM. *Chlamydia trachomatis* is not a frequent causative agent.

46. **(1)** AOM occurs more during the fall, winter, and spring than summer. American Indians and Eskimos have more repetitive and severe otitis media than members of other races. Children who attend day-care centers have more frequent infections than those that do not. Members of lower socioeconomic levels are more at risk than those at higher levels. Other risk factors are children who live with many siblings or homes with smokers, children who have developmental abnormalities, or male gender.

47. **(4)** This would be indicative of an inflammation of the middle ear (acute otitis media). The other options include normal changes that occur with aging.

48. **(4)** Conductive hearing loss may result from acute otitis media, perforation of the eardrum, and obstruction of the ear canal, as by cerumen. The other distractors result in sensorineural hearing loss.

49. **(3)** The client with otitis externa, "swimmer's ear," or inflammation of the external auditory canal presents with ear pain. The most common clinical findings include redness and swelling of the external ear canal, pain with manipulation of movement of auricle, no swelling or pain over mastoid, and the tympanic membrane is not usually involved. The TM is involved in acute otitis media. There was no evidence in the case of the child placing a foreign body in the ear. The most significant distinction between otitis media with effusion and acute otitis media is that clinical findings of acute infection, such as fever and otalgia are lacking in OME. OME is the most common cause of hearing loss in children. OME clinical findings include: relatively asymptomatic, decreased mobility, bulging opaque TM with no visible landmarks.

50. **(4)** This type of hearing loss presents with high-frequency loss, above the 4000-Hz level, and then progresses into voice frequencies at 2000–3000 Hz.

Nose

51. **(2)** The client is experiencing the classic characteristics of acute sinusitis. Chronic sinusitis has nasal discharge, congestion, headache, or cough for over 30 days. A dental abscess has a constant, severe tooth-associated pain, and jaw tenderness. Temporal arteritis causes pain in the jaw, tongue, and face but no nasal discharge.

52. **(3)** Tranmission of cold viruses is indirect (e.g., self-inncoulation from virus on surfaces of inanimate objects to mucous membranes of the nose and mouth). It is less likely to be spread by the aerosol route. Thus the client should avoid touching the nose and mouth unless the hands have been thoroughly washed. It is impractical to avoid contact, as cold viruses are found everywhere. Although may individuals believe vitamin C prevents colds, there is little research to support the claim.

Throat

53. **(1)** Mononucleosis is commonly seen in adolescents and young adults. It often presents with fever, exudate on the tonsils, generalized lymphadenopathy, malaise,

posterior cervical adenopathy, and palatine petechiae. Leukemia presents with anorexia, irritability, lethargy, and bone pain. The peak incidence is 3- to 5-year-olds. Scarlet fever presents in children 2–10 years old with fever, abdominal pain, headache, sore throat, and strawberry tongue. Oral candidiasis presents with white curd-like plaques on an erythematous mucosa. The tongue is red with a white coat.

54. **(3)** Characteristics of bacterial pharyngitis include headache, mild to severe erythema of tonsils with white or yellow exudate, dysphagia, positive anterior cervical nodes, sore throat with dysphagia, fever >101°–102.5°F, and nausea. Viral organisms that cause herpangina present with small oral vesicles. Cough is the primary symptom of acute bronchitis. Rhinorrhea is associated with allergic rhinitis.

Pharmacology

55. **(4)** Amoxicillin (Amoxil) is the first-line antibiotic for acute uncomplicated sinusitis in the adult because of cost-effectiveness, efficacy, and cure rates ranging from 67–100%. Even though 35% of *H. influenzae* and 75% of *M. catarrhalis* produce β-lactamase, cure rates when using amoxicillin have not been significantly different. Therefore, several other drugs may be utilized with similar clinical response to amoxicillin. These include ampicillin, trimethoprim-sulfamethoxazole (Bactrim), cefaclor (Ceclor), cefuroxime axetil (Ceftin), loracarbef (Lorabid); and amoxicillin–clavulanate potassium (Augmentin).

56. **(2)** β-Adrenergic blockers cause problems with bradycardia; the timolol (Timoptic) can be absorbed systemically from the eye and should not be used.

57. **(2)** Amoxicillin is ineffective against β-lactamase production. Erythromycin-sulfisoxazole, trimethoprim-sulfamethoxazole, and cephalosporins are effective against β-lactamase production by strains of *H. influenzae* and *M. catarrhalis*. Penicillin V potassium (Pen-Vee K) and metronidazole are not effective in the group. Cephalexin, cefuroxime, or cefixime can be used as alternatives.

58. **(2)** The decision to prescribe prophylactic antibiotics is individualized but should be considered for children who have experienced three documented episodes of AOM in a 6-month period. The risks and benefits should be explained to the parents. Antibiotic prophylaxis has been found to be as effective as ventilating tubes in preventing new cases of AOM.

59. **(1)** The treatment of mononucleosis includes bed rest while the client has fever and myalgia (10–14 days), supportive acetaminophen or ibuprofen, warm saline gargles, and throat lozenges or spray. The client must avoid strenuous exercise and contact sports for the first 2–3 weeks. Corticosteroids are recommended only in clients with impending airway obstruction. Ampicillin is not recommended, due to allergic reaction and rash reaction. About 95% of clients with mononucleosis recover uneventfully with supportive treatment.

60. **(4)** The client is experiencing symptoms of acute sinusitis. The first-line antibiotic to prescribe for this condition is amoxicillin, due to its safety and efficacy. Oral antihistamines such as diphenhydramine should not be used unless the client has allergies. Oral decongestants (pseudoephedrine hydrochloride) are not as effective in clients with sinusitis as are topical agent. Erythromycin is not a first-line antibiotic for sinusitis.

61. **(3)** The recommended treatment for otitis media in a toddler is amoxicillin, 40 mg/kg/day or, for this child, 250 mg, 1 tsp tid × 10 days. For a child under 20 kg the recommendation is ampicillin 50–100 mg/kg/day or, for this child, 250 mg, 1 tsp qid × 10 days. Erythromycin or trimethoprim-sulfamethoxazole (Bactrim) are other alternatives.

Integumentary & Childhood Diseases

Physical Examination & Diagnostic Tests

1. The nurse practitioner describes an annular skin lesion as usually arranged in:

   1. Groups of vesicles erupting unilaterally.

   2. A line.

   3. A pattern of merging together, not discrete.

   4. A circle, or ring shaped.

2. A client has pitting of the nails. The nurse practitioner understands this is associated with:

   1. Psoriasis.

   2. Iron deficiency anemia.

   3. Malnutrition.

   4. Hyperthyroidism.

3. The nurse practitioner is inspecting a dark-skinned individual for signs of jaundice. The best place to observe is:

   1. Sclera of the opened eye.

   2. Palms and soles of the hands and feet.

   3. Oral mucosa.

   4. Nail beds.

4. When assessing the hydration status of a client, the best place to evaluate skin turgor on an adult is:

   1. Just below the clavicle.

   2. Below the scapula on the back.

   3. On the inside of the forearm.

   4. On the back of the hand.

5. The Wood's lamp is used to evaluate skin lesions. When the light is shone on the client's skin, a green-yellow fluorescence indicates:

   1. Presence of fungi.

   2. Lichenification.

   3. Keratinized cells.

   4. Bacterial colonies.

6. On examination of a client's skin, the nurse practitioner finds a lesion that is about 0.75 cm in diameter, brown, circumscribed, flat, and nonpalpable. The correct term for this lesion is:

   1. Macule.

   2. Papule.

   3. Nodule.

   4. Wheal.

7. The history and physical of a client indicates past occurrences of lichenification. The nurse practitioner identifies the characteristics of this lesion as:

   1. Dried, crusty exudate, slightly elevated.

   2. Rough thickened epidermis, accentuated skin markings.

   3. Keratinized cells shaped in an irregular pattern with exfoliation.

   4. Loss of epidermis with hollowed-out area and dermis exposed.

8. Clubbing of the nails occurs in clients with chronic respiratory conditions. The nurse practitioner assesses for this condition by:

   1. Evaluating the nail for transverse depressions and ridges.

   2. Placing both of the client's hands together with palms inward and index fingers aligned.

   3. Placing nail beds of each index finger together to determine angle of nail plate.

   4. Determining if there is diffuse discoloration of the nail bed from decreased oxygenation.

9. A circumscribed, elevated lesion >1 cm in diameter and containing clear serous fluid is best described as a:

   1. Papule.

   2. Vesicle.

   3. Bulla.

   4. Pustule.

10. In performing a skin assessment, the nurse practitioner understands that the following characteristic of a mole would necessitate immediate intervention:

    1. A 5-mm, symmetrical, uniformly brown mole on the thigh that has been present and has not changed in appearance for over 5 years.

    2. Multiple small (1–3 mm), flat moles across the upper back that are dark brown in color, round, and have smooth edges.

    3. A 3-cm waxy papule, with a "stuck-on" appearance, noted on the face.

    4. A new 2-mm mole that is brown with a red, irregular border, and is occasionally pruritic.

11. Dermatophyte skin infections can be diagnosed from skin scrapings and prepped with which solution for microscopic exam:

    1. Hydrochloric acid.

    2. 20% potassium hydroxide (KOH) solution.

    3. Gram's stain.

    4. Distilled water.

12. When administering skin tests to an immunocompromised client, the nurse practitioner must consider:

    1. The importance of not applying more than one skin test at a time.

    2. That the skin test may react more aggressively than expected.

    3. Identifying a known allergen for the client and utilizing it as a control.

    4. That the immunocompromised client should not be skin tested.

13. The nurse is examining a 6-week-old infant of Latin American descent. There are irregular areas of deep blue pigmentation across the infant's buttocks. The nurse would identify this as characteristic of:

    1. Child abuse.

    2. Telangiectatic nevi.

    3. Cutis marmorata.

    4. Mongolian spots.

Skin Disorders

14. A client complains of intolerable itching in the pubic hair. On examination the nurse practitioner notes erythematous papules and tiny white specks in the pubic hair. The differential diagnosis includes all **except**:

    1. Pediculosis pubis.

    2. Scabies.

    3. Impetigo.

    4. Atopic dermatitis.

15. An elderly lady has an area of vesicles in clusters with an erythematous base that extend from her spine, around and under her arm and breast, to the sternum on her left side. She says the area was very tender last week and the vesicles started erupting yesterday. She is complaining of severe pain in the area. The diagnosis for this condition is:

    1. Psoriasis.

    2. Herpes zoster.

    3. Contact dermatitis.

    4. Cellulitis.

16. A chronic skin condition sometimes associated with arthritis is:

    1. Eczema.

    2. Psoriasis.

    3. Neurodermatitis.

    4. Pityriasis rosea.

17. Which is a true statement about psoriasis?

    1. It is usually worse in the summer.

    2. It is highly contagious.

    3. It can be aggravated by stress.

    4. All clients have accompanying pruritis.

18. A mother brings her school-age child in for examination. She reports the child has been noted to be frequently scratching and the itching seems to be worse at night. Upon examination, the family nurse practitioner notes lesions on the sides of the fingers and inner aspect of the elbows. These lesions are short, irregular runs approximately 2–3 mm long and the width of a hair. The nurse practitioner tells the mother she suspects:

    1. Scabies.

    2. Hives.

    3. Fleas.

    4. Ticks.

19. A client with actinic keratosis should be told:

    1. These are a normal part of aging and are benign.

    2. These lesions can develop into squamous cell carcinomas.

    3. This is part of an allergic reaction and the offending allergen needs to be identified.

    4. This skin condition responds well to sunlight, which will help alleviate the symptoms.

20. The following are all true statements regarding urticaria **except**:

    1. Most cases of acute urticaria are mediated by immunoglobulin E mast cell degranulation after exposure to certain substances.

    2. Chronic urticaria may be related to occult infections.

    3. Urticaria is characterized by itchy, red swellings of a few millimeters to a few centimeters in size.

    4. Laboratory studies are necessary to identify the causative agent.

21. A client who is known to be human immunodeficiency virus (HIV) positive presents with several painless, persistent, raised purple lesions on the face. The most likely cause is:

    1. Seborrheic dermatitis.

    2. Molluscum contagiosum.

    3. Kaposi's sarcoma.

    4. Fungal infection.

22. In making a differential diagnosis between nummular eczema (dermatitis) and dyshidrotic eczematous dermatitis, the nurse practitioner knows:

    1. Nummular eczema is characterized by flushing and clusters of papulopustules on the cheek and forehead.

    2. Dyshidrotic eczematous dermatitis is a chronic vesicular type of hand and foot eczema characterized by vesicles (tapioca-like), scaling, lichenification, and pruritius.

    3. Nummular eczema is a hereditary disorder characterized by chronic scaling plaques that are usually bilateral appearing on exposed areas (knees, elbows).

    4. Dyshidrotic eczematous dermatitis affects primarily young adults, is contagious, and is characterized by firm papules with a clefted surface and multiple conical vegetations.

23. A middle-aged male client presents to the clinic with a complaint of being bitten last night by another individual during a fight. He has a bite mark on his forearm and the skin has been broken. He reports he has had a tetanus shot about 8 years ago. Recommended treatment by the family nurse practitioner should include all **except**:

    1. Administration of 0.5 ml of tetanus toxoid IM.

    2. Instruct client to watch for signs of infection.

    3. Initiate treatment with penicillin plus a penicillinase-resistant penicillin.

    4. Close wound with sutures or steri-strips.

24. Nail involvement secondary to primary foot and hand tinea, which is characterized by accumulation of subungual keratin that produces thickened, distorted, crumbling nails, is termed:

    1. Hippocratic nails.

    2. Onychomycosis.

    3. Koilonychia.

    4. Anonychia.

25. A middle-aged client presents for an office visit with a complaint of a measles-like rash on his trunk and spreading to his extremities. He was seen several days ago for bronchitis and started on trimethoprim-sulfamethoxazole (Bactrim DS) 1 tab PO bid. The recommended action for the family nurse practitioner is to:

    1. Instruct client to continue Bactrim and see if any change occurs in the rash.

    2. Discontinue Bactrim.

    3. Take client off Bactrim for 3 days and restart the medication.

    4. Decrease Bactrim to half dose.

26. When treating atopic dermatitis in children, all of the following instructions are applicable **except**:

    1. Eliminate one food at a time that is thought to induce flares.

    2. Avoid use of bubble bath.

    3. Avoid overheating.

    4. Encourage bathing two to three times a day.

27. A client complaining of hyperhidrosis should be counseled that:

    1. This is a normal occurrence.

    2. There are no therapies for this complaint.

    3. Bathing in a 20% alcohol solution of aluminum chloride hexahydrate (Drysol) on a nightly basis may be beneficial.

    4. A history and physical exam needs to be completed so that any medical etiologies can be ruled out.

28. During the physical examination, the nurse practitioner assesses a macular-papular skin lesion on a client's back that is warty, scaly, greasy in appearance, and light tan in color. The nurse practitioner would make the diagnosis of:

    1. Actinic keratosis.

    2. Basal cell carcinoma.

3. Seborrheic keratosis.

4. Senile lentigines.

29. The nurse practitioner would expect to make which assessment with an older client diagnosed with herpes zoster (shingles) during the prodromal stage?

1. Erythematous lesions present over 4 different parts of the body.

2. A red, pinpoint, painless rash.

3. A burning pain in a line on only half of the client's chest that does not cross the midline.

4. Painless purulent lesions for 2 days followed by complaints of itching, burning, and nausea.

30. What would be the appropriate management for a client with herpes zoster (shingles)?

1. Acyclovir (Zovirax).

2. Miconazole (Monistat-Derm).

3. Clotrimazole (Lotrimin).

4. Corticosteroid (prednisone).

31. An elderly retired farmer presents with a dome-shaped, pearly, firm nodule with telangiectasia on his nose. In making a diagnosis, the nurse practitioner recognizes this to be:

1. Compound nevus.

2. Melanoma.

3. Bullous pemphigoid.

4. Basal cell carcinoma.

32. An adult female presents with an irregular variegated nevus on her lower left back that has doubled in size in the past 3 months. The nurse practitioner should:

1. Do a punch biopsy to confirm the diagnosis.

2. Take a photograph of the lesion and recheck it in 1 month.

3. Refer immediately to a dermatologist.

4. Reassure the client that these are normal changes related to hormone variations.

33. A client presents with pain in his right chest wall for the past 48 hours. Upon examination, the nurse practitioner notices a vesicular eruption along the dermatome and identifies this as herpes zoster. The nurse practitioner informs the client that:

1. All symptoms will disappear in 3 days.

2. Oral medication can dramatically reduce the duration and intensity of symptoms.

3. He has chickenpox and can be contagious to his grandchildren.

4. The eruptions will recur at regular intervals.

34. A young adult female presents to the nurse practitioner's office, stating that she has a red rash over her trunk that itches and has been present for 2 weeks. She has tried over-the-counter lotions and creams, with no relief of symptoms. She states that it started as a small, round red patch on her chest and has since spread across her chest, back, arms, and legs. Physical exam reveals a generalized distribution of erythematous, scaly macular lesions that run parallel to each other, creating a "Christmas tree" pattern. The nurse practitioner should:

1. Do a thorough medication history, investigate any potential allergens, and send the client to an allergy specialist.

2. Prescribe traimcinolone acetonide 0.025% (Aristocort A) cream bid for 2 weeks.

3. Teach the client to expose herself to modest amounts of sunlight without burning, and use calamine lotion or oatmeal baths for symptom relief.

4. Refer the client to a dermatologist for a biopsy.

35. An adult male client presents to the nurse practitioner's office complaining of flu-like symptoms, a large red spot in the right groin, headaches, and generalized muscle pain. These symptoms have persisted for approximately 4–5 weeks. In taking the client's history, it would be most important to determine whether the client:

    1. Was using new skin care products, detergents, etc.

    2. Was taking any new medications, vitamins, herbal therapies, etc.

    3. Has had a recent insect bite, or was potentially exposed to insects such as ticks (i.e., camping trips, travel to heavily wooded areas).

    4. Has been exposed to anyone who has tuberculosis.

36. A nurse practitioner is teaching the mother of a child how to use permethrin 1% creme rinse (Nix) for treatment of pediculosis capitis. What is the most important information the nurse practitioner should give to the mother?

    1. Shampoo the child's hair daily for one week with permethrin 1% (Nix).

    2. After hair is shampooed and towel-dried, apply permethrin 1% (Nix) creme rinse to scalp and hair, leaving on for 10 minutes before rinsing.

    3. The shampoo should not be used again, as it is toxic and may absorb systemically and cause acute respiratory problems.

    4. It is not necessary to treat other children in the family or launder bedding or clothing.

37. The nurse practitioner understands that most accidental scaldings in young children occur:

    1. On the back of the body.

    2. On the front of the body.

    3. In a circular or glove pattern.

    4. With no specific pattern.

38. An infant has pruritus due to eczema. The nurse practitioner teaches the mother the following regarding the infant's care:

    1. Dress the infant in cotton shorts and short-sleeved shirts.

    2. Dress the infant in wool blend long-sleeved jump suits.

    3. Give the infant cornstarch or Aveeno baths.

    4. Give the infant salt baths three times a day.

39. A new mother is concerned about the hemangioma on her infant's neck. What is the treatment choice for the majority of infants with hemangioma?

    1. Cryosurgery.

    2. Intralesional injection of steroids.

    3. Observation.

    4. Injection of a sclerosing agent.

40. The nurse practitioner is examining an infant with atopic dermatitis. The physical exam reveals:

    1. Dry, scaly rash with pruritus.

    2. Distribution of rash on face and extensor surfaces.

    3. Erythematous raised areas on flexor surfaces.

    4. Moist, crusting rash with no pruritus.

41. The practitioner is examining a 6-year-old child and identifies eight to ten patches of coffee-colored areas on the trunk. The areas are nontender, the border is irregular, and most of the areas are >1.5 cm and are nonpalpable. What is the best recommendation to the parents of this child?

    1. The child should be further evaluated by a pediatrician.

    2. These areas are normal pigmentation and will disappear.

3. A dermatologist should be consulted for removal of lesions.

4. Emollients should be applied to keep skin moist and sunlight on the areas should be avoided.

42. An infant is noted at his well-child visit to have a yellowish, greasy scaly rash on his scalp, forehead, and ears. The most likely diagnosis would be:

1. Seborrheic dermatitis.

2. Atopic dermatitis.

3. Erythema toxicum.

4. Eczema.

43. A 1-month-old is being seen by the nurse practitioner for a diaper rash. Upon examination, the practitioner notes moderate erythema and poorly marginated, dry patches of skin that are localized to the buttocks. The deep folds are not affected. There are no satellite lesions. The most likely diagnosis would be:

1. Infantile seborrheic dermatitis.

2. Allergy to disposable diapers.

3. Contact dermatitis.

4. Candidal diaper rash.

44. The mother of a preschooler brings the child to see the nurse practitioner because of sores on his arms and legs. Upon examination, the nurse practitioner notes several honey-colored crusted lesions with an erythematous base on the arms and legs. There is a history of exposure to mosquitoes. The rest of the physical examination is essentially negative. The most likely diagnosis would be:

1. Scabies.

2. Impetigo.

3. Pityriasis rosea.

4. Varicella.

45. A 6-month-old infant returns to the clinic to have his ears rechecked after a 10-day course of antibiotics for an ear infection. During the visit the mother states that the child is now eating better and appears to be recovering, but he now has a bad diaper rash. The most likely cause of this rash is:

1. Poor hygiene.

2. Contact dermatitis.

3. Seborrheic diaper dermatitis.

4. *Candida albicans.*

46. A school-age child presents with erythematous papular lesions and scaly plaques in the antecubital and popliteal fossae, and on the neck, wrists, and ankles. The mother states that the child has been scratching the areas, especially at night. History reveals that the child also has been treated for asthma. The nurse practitioner would make the diagnosis of:

1. Scabies.

2. Atopic dermatitis.

3. Tinea corporis.

4. Contact dermatitis.

Childhood Diseases

47. Anticipatory guidance for the parents of a child with measles would include reporting the onset of which symptoms after the child begins recovery?

1. Fever, drowsiness, vomiting.

2. Skin desquamation.

3. Abdominal pain and diarrhea.

4. Worsening conjunctivitis.

48. A 6-year-old client with a rash on the face and Forschheimer spots on the soft palate will usually be diagnosed within 24 hours of the rash spread. The initial diagnosis may include possible:

1. Rubella.

2. Mononucleosis.

3. Scarlet fever.

4. All of the above.

49. Phone consultation with a mother reveals that her child has been on trimethoprim-sulfamethoxazole (Bactrim) for 3 days for a urinary tract infection. She has been treated with the drug previously with no problems. Currently, the child is experiencing blister-like sores in the skin-fold areas (i.e., axilla and groin), also oral ulceration and a few in the genital area. Her temperature is 40°C and she is very weak. Differential diagnosis includes:

    1. Kawasaki disease.

    2. Erythema multiforme (major).

    3. Viral exanthem.

    4. Early scalded skin syndrome.

50. A child's day-care center director calls to confirm when the child can return to the center, since they have fifth disease (erythema infectiosum). The nurse practitioner's response is based on the knowledge that the period of communicability lasts until:

    1. The rash is gone.

    2. The rash appears.

    3. Upper respiratory symptoms are gone.

    4. The transient joint pain disappears.

51. Examination of an ill-appearing 6-year-old reveals vesicular and a few ulcerative oral lesions, an erythematous rash on the legs and buttocks, and a maculopapular rash on the hands and feet; temperature is 38°C (100.4°F) and the child has feelings of malaise. Differential diagnosis includes:

    1. Hand-foot-and-mouth disease.

    2. Coxsackievirus, group B.

    3. ECHO virus 11.

    4. Varicella.

Pharmacology

52. An obese woman presents to the clinic with complaints of tenderness and irritation under both of her breasts. The examination reveals a very irritated, moist, inflamed area with macules and papules present. The best treatment for this woman is:

    1. Nystatin cream two to three times a day for 10 days; encourage thorough drying of the area and exposure to light and air.

    2. Systemic anti-staphylococcal antibiotics (dicloxacillin) and soaking with moist pads of normal saline three times a day.

    3. Gentle washing of the area and removal of crusts, then application of antibiotic ointment.

    4. Antiviral treatment (acyclovir) and topical ointment to prevent secondary infection.

53. Which classification of drugs has the potential to aggravate psoriasis?

    1. β-Blockers.

    2. Thiazide diuretics.

    3. Vasodilators.

    4. Monoamine oxidase (MAO) inhibitors.

54. In treatment of severe inflammatory acne for a female adolescent, the nurse practitioner understands that:

    1. Isotretinoin (Accutane) provides an effective first-line therapy.

    2. The benefits of treatment will be noted in 5–7 days.

    3. Counseling on stringent dietary changes is important.

    4. Systemic antibiotics are effective treatments.

55. A young mother brings her infant to the family nurse practitioner with a complaint of difficulty with diaper rash. She reports the infant has had it for about a week. Upon exam the diaper area appears beefy red with sharply marginated dermatitis. Satellite lesions are also noted. The family nurse practitioner recommends:

    1. Change from disposable diapers to cloth diapers with plastic pants.

    2. Application of nystatin (Mycostatin) after each diaper change.

3. Apply wet soaks tid.

4. Liberally apply oil after bathing.

56. All of the following are true of postherpetic neuralgia **except**:

    1. Capsaicin (Zostrix) cream may alleviate some of the discomfort.

    2. The majority of clients who have postherpetic pain lose it gradually, day by day, week by week.

    3. Acyclovir (Zovirax) 200 mg, 5 capsules a day PO in divided doses, is an effective therapy.

    4. It is more common in clients over age 60.

57. When treating genital warts with topical podophyllin, it is important for the family nurse practitioner to:

    1. Apply preparation directly to the wart and approximately 5 mm around base of wart.

    2. Cover with a dressing so the solution remains moist and caution client not to remove for 24 hours.

    3. Instruct client to wash off medication in 4–6 hours.

    4. Treat with liquid nitrogen before applying podophyllin.

58. What is the recommended treatment of rosacea?

    1. Oral hydrocortisone.

    2. Oral ketoconazole.

    3. Low-dose tetracycline.

    4. Topical 5-fluorouracil.

59. When using lidocaine with epinephrine 1–2% as a local anesthetic in the repair of an injury, it is essential to keep in mind that the maximum allowable dose is:

    1. 7 mg/kg.

    2. 2 mg/kg.

    3. 10 mg/kg.

    4. 5 mg/kg.

60. An elderly client presents to the nurse practitioner complaining of a painful, tingling rash across the right side of his abdomen. Exam reveals vesicles with erythematous bases; some of the vesicles are draining cloudy fluid, while others are crusted. The nurse practitioner makes the diagnosis of herpes zoster infection, and places the patient on antiviral therapy. The patient states that the painful rash has kept him from sleeping for the past four nights. Appropriate therapy for this client's pain would include:

    1. Amitriptyline (Elavil) 10 mg PO qhs, nonsteroidal anti-inflammatory drugs (NSAIDs) prn as directed, along with application of cool compresses to the lesions for 30 minutes, several times a day.

    2. High-dose corticosteroid therapy.

    3. Application of heat directly to the area involved.

    4. There is no appropriate therapy currently available to treat neuropathic pain.

61. On a return visit to the clinic, a client who is receiving sulfonamide therapy exhibits the following symptoms: generalized rash, mucous membrane lesions, sloughing of the skin of the palms and feet, high fever, and generalized malaise. These findings would alert the nurse practitioner to consider:

    1. Hepatitis B.

    2. Stevens-Johnson syndrome.

    3. HIV infection/acquired immunodeficiency syndrome.

    4. *Pneumocystis carinii* pneumonia.

62. The nurse practitioner is examining lesions on a child's face around his nose and mouth. The mother states the lesions began several days ago and seem to be getting worse. The lesions are vesicular, edematous, red, and tender. Some have yellow crusts and an erythematous base. The treatment for this child is:

    1. Mupirocin ointment (Bactroban) qid × 10 days.

    2. Gently soaking the lesions with antibacterial soap and removing the crust.

    3. Dicloxacillin (Dynapen) at 15 mg/kg/day divided into four doses × 10 days.

    4. Diphenhydramine HCl (Benadryl) 5 mg PO q6h to decrease itching and spreading.

63. The mother of a 1-year-old child brings the child to the clinic for problems with a "rash." She states the child has not been feeling well since the rash started 2 days ago. The nurse practitioner observes numerous macules and vesicles in clusters over the child's trunk and mucous membranes; some are clear, some are crusting. The child is irritable, but does not have a fever. The diagnosis and treatment for this child includes:

    1. Varicella: immunize with varicella zoster vaccine to decrease symptoms and begin acyclovir (Zovirax) therapy to decrease incidence of severe complications.

    2. Impetigo: treat with antibiotics for 10 days and return to clinic in 2 weeks.

    3. Contact dermatitis: thoroughly review with mother any changes in care, diphenhydramine HCl (Benadryl) spray over the rash; cut child's fingernails to decrease scratching.

    4. Varicella: treat with hydroxyzine (Atarax) 2 mg/kg/day in three divided doses for itching; daily bathes with baking soda to relieve itching and prevent superinfection.

64. A six-month-old is brought to the clinic for a rash on the face and diaper area that consists of linear erythematous burrows. An older sibling has a similar rash on his wrists and between his fingers. An appropriate intervention would be:

    1. Neosporin ointment.

    2. Mycitracin ointment.

    3. Acitretin (Soriatane).

    4. Permethrin 5% cream (Elimite).

65. A mother brings her school-age child to the nurse practitioner's office. She states that the child developed a blistering rash on his face 2 days ago, that has since spread to his hands and forearms. Examination reveals the presence of multiple, small vesicular lesions across the child's face, arms, and hands. Some of the lesions are covered with a honey-colored crust. The nurse practitioner diagnoses impetigo and recommends:

    1. Frequent scrubbing of the lesions with a stiff-bristled brush.

    2. Keep the child isolated for 7 days and discard clothing the child has been wearing since the lesions appeared.

    3. Prescribe dicloxacillin (Dynapen) suspension, 25 mg/kg/day, divided into four doses × 10 days, recommend gentle washing of the lesions to remove any loose crusts, and wash the child's clothing and linen separately in hot water.

    4. Refer the child to a dermatologist and counsel the mother that she needs to practice better personal hygiene.

66. An adolescent female presents to the nurse practitioner's office with a prolonged history of facial acne. She has been seen by several dermatologists and has been treated over the past 3 years with multiple therapies, including topical antibiotics, drying agents, intralesional injections of corticosteroids, and multiple systemic antibiotics, without success. After consulting with the collaborating physician, the nurse practitioner prescribes isotretinoin (Accutane). Teaching/counseling related to the use of this medication includes:

    1. No dietary/alcohol restrictions are necessary.

2. Exposure to sunlight without burning can be helpful in hastening the healing process.

3. Eliminate all fat from the client's diet.

4. Emphasize the importance of using effective contraception if the client is sexually active, due to the teratogenicity of the drug.

67. Indications for the use of oral acyclovir within 24 hours of rash eruption in children with chickenpox are:

   1. Child over the age of 6.

   2. History of chronic neurologic disorders.

   3. Use of aerosolized corticosteroids.

   4. Concomitant otitis media.

8 Answers & Rationales

Physical Examination & Diagnostic Tests

1. **(4)** Annular skin lesions may be arranged in a circular manner or in an arciform (arc-shaped) pattern (i.e., tinea corporis). Multiple groups of vesicles erupting unilaterally following the course of cutaneous nerves is herpetiform or zosteriform (i.e., herpes zoster). Linear lesions are arranged in a line (i.e., allergic contact dermatitis to poison ivy). Confluent lesions become merged together and are not discrete (i.e., scarlet fever rash).

2. **(1)** Psoriasis, peripheral vascular disease, diabetes, tuberculosis, and other infectious diseases such as syphilis are associated with pitting deformities of the nail that may vary from pinpoint to pinhead size and may be linear or irregular in distribution. Iron deficiency anemia, eczema, malnutrition, and pellagra are associated with koilonychia (spoon nails). Hyperthyroidism and hypothyroidism are associated with onycholysis, which is a separation of the nail from the nail bed, originating at the free edge and progressing proximally.

3. **(1)** The place to inspect is in that portion of the sclera that is observed when the eye is open. If jaundice is suspected, the posterior portion of the hard palate should be examined for a yellowish cast. Pallor and cyanosis can be noted in the nail beds, palms, and soles.

4. **(1)** Just below the clavicle or on the abdomen for an adult and on the abdomen for infants and children are the most reliable areas for indication of hydration status.

5. **(1)** Fungal lesions will be visualized as a green-yellow fluorescence when viewed with the Wood's lamp in a dim room.

6. **(1)** A macule is <1 cm in diameter; nonpalpable; and brown, red, purple, or tan (freckles, flat moles, rubella). A papule is elevated and palpable (warts, pigmented nevi). A nodule is 1–2 cm in diameter, elevated, and deeper (lipoma). A wheal is elevated and irregular, and has a variable diameter (insect bites, urticaria).

7. **(2)** Lichenification occurs with chronic irritation, often of an exposed extremity (chronic dermatitis). Crusts are dried exudate; scales are heaps of keratinized cells from exfoliation (psoriasis); and loss of epidermis is excoriation, as seen in an abrasion.

8. **(3)** The angle of the nail beds should form a diamond when the nail beds are approximated. Transverse ridges and grooves may occur from trauma. Placing the palms together provides no assessment data, and diffuse discoloration may be from a fungal infection or an injury.

9. **(3)** Bulla is the correct term. A papule is solid, a vesicle is <1 cm in diameter, and a pustule contains a purulent exudate.

10. **(4)** The appearance of a new mole with high-risk features, including irregular border, color changes, and changes in sensation (i.e., pruritis), would necessitate immediate biopsy to rule out melanoma, and/or referral to a dermatologist. Uniform moles, those that are symmetrical and have smooth borders, and those that are not showing signs of change are those that can be followed with annual skin assessments. Seborrheic keratosis is a benign skin growth that usually presents on sun-exposed areas, and appears waxy or "stuck-on," requiring no treatment.

11. **(2)** Under microscope exam, fungal scrapings in KOH solution will appear as thread-like hyphae crossing cell walls. The other solutions are not indicated for use to identify dermatophytes.

12. **(3)** It is important to remember to apply controls when skin testing the immunocompromised client. Ask clients what diseases they believe they have immunity to, such as measles. Apply the "known" allergen and the skin test to be tested. If the client is unable to mount an immune response at all, the known allergen will not react. By not applying the controls, the nurse practitioner may assume a skin test is negative, when in fact the client's immune system is unable to respond.

13. **(4)** This best describes mongolian spots that are characteristic in newborns of African, Asian, or Latin descent. When closely evaluated, these do not have the appearance of ecchymoses that occur with trauma. Telangiectatic nevi are commonly known as "stork bites" and are deep pink lesions most often found on the back of the neck. Cutis marmorata is the transient mottling that occurs when an infant is cold.

Skin Disorders

14. **(3)** Intense itching is characteristic of pediculosis pubis, scabies, and atopic dermatitis. Impetigo starts out as a tender, erythematous papule and progresses through a vesicular to a honey-crusted stage with no itching.

15. **(2)** Herpes zoster typically presents with a history of tenderness followed by eruptions and vesicles that follow a dermatome on one side of the body. This is very painful. Other symptoms may include fever, headaches, and malaise.

16. **(2)** Approximately 10–30% of people with psoriasis develop an accompanying form of arthritis called psoriatic arthritis. The other options are dermatologic conditions but are not directly associated with arthritis.

17. **(3)** Stress can aggravate psoriasis. Sunlight helps psoriasis, so it is usually better in the summer. It is not contagious, and only about 30% of clients with psoriasis itch.

18. **(1)** The location and appearance of the lesions is typical of scabies—short, irregular runs approximately 2–3 mm long and the width of a hair.

19. **(2)** Actinic keratoses are potentially precancerous lesions and are found in areas of skin exposed to sunlight. Due to the increasing popularity of sunbathing, they can even be seen in persons in the 30- to 50-year-old age group.

20. **(4)** Laboratory studies are not likely to be helpful in evaluation of urticaria. Identification of causes is usually based on history and physical findings. The other statements are true of urticaria.

21. **(3)** Although any one of these skin conditions can affect the skin, particularly of an HIV-positive client, the description relates most closely to Kaposi's sarcoma and warrants a biopsy.

22. **(2)** Despite the name, dyshidrotic eczematous dermatitis (bullous form called pompholyx), there is no evidence of sweating. Most clients have an atopic history, and emotional stress is often a precipitating factor in the appearance of the vesicles. Nummular (discoid) eczema is a chronic, pruritic, inflammatory dermatitis that occurs in the form of coin-shaped plaques composed of grouped small papules and vesicles on an erythematous base. Option #1 describes rosacea. Option #3 describes psoriasis. Option #4 describes a verruca or common wart.

23. **(4)** Delay wound closure until determination of no infection in approximately 24–48 hours. Mouth flora of humans is abundant, and with a bite there is the possibility of heavy bacterial inoculum and potential severe infection. Tetanus toxoid is indicated, since there has been no booster in the last 5 years.

24. **(2)** Onychomycosis is the correct term. Hippocratic nails are clubbed nails and fingers associated with chronic heart and lung disorders; koilonychia is a concavity of the nail plate often associated with iron deficiency anemia; and anonychia is a total congenital absence of the nail.

25. **(2)** In case of suspected drug reactions, it is recommended that the drug be eliminated and documented in the client's record so it is not reintroduced.

26. **(4)** Excessive bathing dries the skin, which irritates the atopic dermatitis. Food allergies along with any other causative triggers should be identified and avoided. Bubble bath can irritate skin, as can sweating.

27. **(4)** Excessive sweating can be normal but the client needs to have history and physical to rule out any underlying causes. There are therapies that can be offered. The Drysol is only for use on the feet and axilla. Full bathing is not recommended with this solution.

28. **(3)** The assessment describes a seborrheic keratosis. The actinic keratosis is an irregular, rough, scaly, white to erythematous macular lesion found most commonly on the dorsal surface of the hands, arms, neck, and face. It has malignant potential. The basal cell carcinoma is a smooth, round nodule with a pearly gray border and central induration. Senile lentigines are gray-brown, irregular, macular lesions on sun-exposed areas of the face, arms, and hands.

29. **(3)** Herpes zoster (shingles) is a vesicular dermatomal eruption related to a reactivation of latent varicella virus. It increases with advanced age and is characterized by burning pain and paresthesia along one or two dermatomes. This will not cross the midline. This discomfort may be accompanied by fever, malaise, or headache. The vesicular stage lasts 2–3 weeks. The vesicles are initially clear or blood-filled and become purulent. The area along the dermatome is erythematous, and the vesicles crust and then scab, which may leave hypopigmented scars. The other options discuss painless lesions and are not specific to this prodromal stage.

30. **(1)** Antiviral therapy with acyclovir 800 mg five times per day for 7 days may speed healing if started within 2–3 days of onset, especially in immunocompromised individuals. Miconazole and clotrimazole are antifungal creams, and the prednisone would only be used to decrease the incidence of postherpetic neuralgia. Prednisone may increase the incidence of disseminated infection.

31. **(4)** These are classic signs of a basal cell carcinoma, also supported by the employment history of the client. Melanoma would be pigmented, compound nevus would not be firm or have telangiectasia, and bullous pemphigoid results in bullous lesions.

32. **(3)** Refer immediately to a dermatologist, since these findings are highly suspicious for a melanoma. Biopsy should never be done on a melanoma, and any delay could be detrimental to the outcome.

33. **(2)** Oral acyclovir is very effective in reducing intensity and duration of symptoms if started early in the course of the disease. Herpes zoster does not usually recur at regular intervals but frequently lasts for several weeks.

34. **(3)** This client presents with a classic case of pityriasis rosea, a benign, self-limiting skin eruption of unknown etiology. Although a medication/allergen history would be warranted, referral to an allergy specialist or dermatologist would not be necessary. Triamcinolone would not be indicated, as the treatment is mainly symptomatic. Sunlight in moderate amounts has been shown to hasten healing in some cases.

35. **(3)** The signs and symptoms presented are classic for Lyme disease, which is transmitted by ticks. Therefore, it would be

important to inquire about potential exposure to ticks in the time period prior to the development of signs and symptoms. Exposure to new skin care products would be important if the practitioner suspected an allergic reaction, which is not consistent with the signs and symptoms presented. Although a thorough medication history should always be done, it is most likely not going to reveal the cause of the signs and symptoms in this case. Tuberculosis does not present in this manner.

36. **(2)** This is the correct procedure for the shampoo, e.g., after hair is shampooed and towel-dried, apply permethrin 1% (Nix) creme rinse to scalp and hair, leaving on for 10 minutes before rinsing. After the rinse, remove nits with a nit comb. Repeat shampoo treatment after 7 days, if living lice still observed. Clothing and bedding should be washed or drycleaned. Family members should also be treated.

37. **(2)** Accidental scalding is usually splash-related and occurs on the front of the body. The nurse practitioner should be suspicious of any burns on the back of the body or any well-defined, uniform burn areas on the buttocks or extremities, as they may indicate physical abuse. Immersion burns on the buttocks may be seen as punishment for toileting or wetting "accidents."

38. **(3)** The cornstarch or Aveeno baths will temporally help relieve the itching. The shorts and short-sleeved shirt would expose too much skin, which would be scratched by the infant. Wool irritates the skin. Salt would also be an irritant.

39. **(3)** The most common treatment is observation, as the majority of hemangiomas resolve within time, usually beginning around 18 months of age. The other treatments may be performed, especially for those that are proliferating at a fast rate.

40. **(2)** Infantile atopic dermatitis, as contrasted to atopic dermatitis in older children and adolescents, is a moist, oozing, crusting rash with pruritus found mainly on the extensor surfaces of the body and the face. It usually begins around 2 months of age, and often there is a family history of atopy.

41. **(1)** In prepubertal children, café au lait spots that are >1 cm and are present in more than five areas are of concern and may be associated with neurofibromatosis. The child should be referred to a pediatrician for further evaluation.

42. **(1)** Seborrheic dermatitis is usually salmon in color and has a yellowish, greasy appearance. It occurs in infants <6 months of age. It does not itch. The distribution is mainly to the face, postauricular scalp, axillae, and groin. Atopic dermatitis and eczema is pink or red if inflamed and has a whiter, nongreasy appearance. It may begin at 2–12 months and continues through childhood and is associated with a family history of allergy. The distribution is to the cheeks, trunk, and extensors of extremities. Itching may be severe. Erythema toxicum consists of yellow or white papules on the face. It occurs in 30–50% of term infants and disappears in 2 weeks.

43. **(3)** Given the distribution of the rash, the most likely cause is a contact dermatitis such as that caused by the use of baby wipes. Allergy to disposable diapers would involve the entire diaper area. Seborrheic dermatitis presents as large confluent sharply marginated bright plaque on the anterior surface of the groin. Candidal rashes are bright red with satellite lesions that involve the deep folds and may spread to the entire diaper area.

44. **(2)** Impetigo presents with honey-colored crusted lesions with an erythematous base. Staphylococci and group A streptococci are important pathogens in this disease. Scabies presents with linear burrows about the wrists, ankles, finger webs, areolars, anterior axillary folds, genitalis, or face (in infants). Pityriasis rosea presents as erythematous papules that coalesce to form oval plaques preceded by a large oval plaque with central clearing and a scaly border (the herald patch). Varicella presents as crops of red macules that rapidly become tiny vesicles with surrounding erythema that form pustules. The pustules become crusted and then scab over. The rash appears predominantly on the trunk and face.

45. **(4)** After a course of antibiotics, the normal flora is destroyed, making the child a prime target for *Candida albicans*. The classic signs of a yeast infection include a beefy red, sharply marginated, maculopapular rash with satellite lesions. Poor hygiene and a contact dermatitis would present as erythema and thickening of the skin in the perianal area. Seborrheic dermatitis consists of an erythematous scaly dermatitis accompanied by overproduction of sebum occurring in areas rich in sebaceous glands (i.e., the face, scalp, and perineum).

46. **(2)** Atopic dermatitis commonly presents in the flexural areas of children. The lesions are characteristically erythematous and papular, with scales and pruritis commonly noted. A personal or family history of atopy is noted in about 70% of clients with atopic dermatitis. Scabies lesions appear as gray or skin-colored ridges, vesicles, and papules. Tinea corporis lesions are generally distributed over the entire body and face, and have an area of clearing in the center of the lesion. Contact dermatitis usually produces lesions in the shape of the object causing the reaction, and are usually vesicular in nature.

Childhood Diseases

47. **(1)** Fever, drowsiness, vomiting, headache, convulsions, and possible coma are signs of neurologic complications that present as the child appears to recover.

48. **(4)** Rubella may be difficult to diagnose and the rash is often confused with infectious mononucleosis and scarlet fever.

49. **(2)** Kawasaki disease presents with a more diffuse erythematous rash. Viral exanthems are centrally located and not blister-like. Scalded skin syndrome, staphylococcal in origin, causes the skin to peel off and be very red. Erythema multiforme is a major side effect of sulfa drug use that presents with a sudden onset of high fever, weakness, blisters, bulla, and ulcerations of the mucous membranes.

50. **(2)** The incubation period for erythema infectiosum is 4–14 days, with communicability until the rash appears.

51. **(1)** The symptoms are indicative of coxsackievirus 5 or 16 group A, which is called "hand-foot-and-mouth disease." Varicella lesions begin on the trunk with classic "teardrop vesicles."

Pharmacology

52. **(1)** The description is consistent with candidiasis intertriginous, which is treated with an antifungal ointment or oral medication. It is not a staphylococcal infection; the area does not need to be kept moist but needs to be kept dry. An antibiotic ointment will not relieve the problem. Herpes zoster is treated with antiviral medications; this is not described as particularly painful, and it is bilateral.

53. **(1)** β-Blockers can exacerbate psoriasis. They are believed to decrease cyclic-AMP–dependent protein kinase (an inhibitor of cell proliferation). No known effect on psoriasis with drugs in the other stated classifications.

54. **(4)** Systemic antibiotics (such as tetracycline) offer the most effective treatment in inflammatory acne. Accutane is also very effective but, because of serious teratogenic side effects, it is not first-line treatment. Improvement in acne will not be noted for 4–8 weeks and dietary changes have not been demonstrated to have any beneficial effect.

55. **(2)** Appearance is indicative of *Candida albicans* which is best treated with nystatin. The other choices would aggravate the diaper rash, due to promotion of overhydration.

56. **(3)** Acyclovir offers no benefit for postherpetic pain, since this is a treatment for the acute phase during initial eruption of vesicular lesions.

57. **(3)** Clients need to be instructed to wash off podophyllin. It is to be applied sparingly, only to the wart, while avoiding normal skin, and allowed to dry thoroughly before the client dresses. There is no rationale to treat with both liquid nitrogen and podophyllin.

58. **(3)** Systemic treatment with low-dose tetracycline is very effective for rosacea; topical treatment with metronidazole or low-dose hydrocortisone may also be useful. Oral cortisone and antifungal agents are not known to be effective. Topical 5-fluorouracil is used in the treatment of actinic keratosis, a precancerous skin condition.

59. **(1)** The maximum allowable dose for adults is 7 mg/kg of lidocaine with epinephrine and 5 mg/kg of lidocaine without epinephrine. Although local anesthetics are commonly used, the maximum allowable doses are rarely emphasized, and overdose can result in anaphylactic shock.

60. **(1)** Amitriptyline in low doses has been shown to be effective in treating neuropathic pain. NSAIDs can also be effective in treating the inflammatory component of herpes zoster pain. The most effective nonpharmacologic method of treating pain from shingles is the application of cool compresses. Heat has been shown to exacerbate neuropathic pain in some cases. Antidepressants and anticonvulsants have been shown to be effective adjuvant therapy in the treatment of neuropathic pain.

61. **(2)** Stevens-Johnson syndrome is a severe form of erythema multiforme that can be fatal. The clinical picture of this syndrome is mucous membrane lesions, conjunctival and corneal lesions, fever, malaise, arthralgia, and sloughing of the skin of the hands and feet. The distinguishing characteristics that differentiate this condition are the eruption of vesicles, ulcerations of the mucosa, and the sloughing skin.

62. **(3)** The child's lesions are characteristic of impetigo and should be treated with an antibiotic, if they are present on the child's face; dicloxacillin is the drug of choice. The ointment, the soaking, and the Benadryl will not stop the spread of the infection, which could lead to poststreptococcal glomerulonephritis.

63. **(4)** Varicella (chickenpox) should be treated symptomatically unless the child is at high risk secondary to other medical problems.

Acyclovir is not recommended for routine treatment of uncomplicated varicella. Impetigo commonly occurs on the face and neck and usually does not have diffuse lesions over the trunk. Contact dermatitis is characterized by erythema and scaling, and it may have weeping vesicles. The area of distribution of rash offers clues to diagnosis.

64. **(4)** Permethrin 5% cream (Elimite) is used in infants, however it is not recommended in under 2 months of age. Neosporin could be used to treat secondary infections but would do nothing to irradicate the scabies. Mycitracin is also not effective for the treatment of scabies. Acitretin (Soriatane) is used for the treatment of psoriasis.

65. **(3)** Impetigo is communicable until the client has been on antibiotic therapy for 48 hours. Washing clothing and linens separately with hot water is recommended, along with surveillance of close contacts for the appearance of lesions. Isolation is not necessary, except to keep the child home from school until 48 hours of antibiotic therapy has been completed. Dicloxacillin is considered to be the drug of choice. Gentle washing is recommended to keep the lesions clean and to prevent scarring (potentially caused by vigorous scrubbing).

66. **(4)** Isotretinoin is extremely teratogenic; therefore, a sexual assessment, along with a pregnancy test in women with child-bearing capacity, and contraceptive counseling should be done for all clients. The combination of alcohol and isotretinoin can cause a disulfuram-like reaction; therefore, the use of alcohol should be avoided. Isotretinoin can cause photosensitivity, so the nurse practitioner should counsel the client to avoid sunlight, wear protective clothing and sunglasses, and apply sunscreen to all sun-exposed areas without acne. No conclusive relationship between diet and acne has been established.

67. **(3)** The indications for use of oral acyclovir in chickenpox are that the child is over age 12, has a chronic pulmonary disorder, is on chronic salicylate therapy, or is receiving intermittent or short courses of aerosolized corticosteroids.

9 Endocrine

Physical Examination & Diagnostic Tests

1. What is the correct procedure for palpation of a client's thyroid gland?

    1. Stand behind the client, hyperextend the head, and palpate both sides simultaneously.

    2. Have the client lower his chin and lean his head slightly toward the side being evaluated.

    3. Hyperextend the head and have the client lean away from the side being evaluated.

    4. Have the client lean away from the side being examined and take a swallow of water.

2. When a client sips water and swallows, the thyroid gland:

    1. Moves downward and slightly posterior and feels smooth on palpation.

    2. Elongates and enlarges during the swallow and immediately returns to a resting position at the end of palpation.

    3. Moves slightly out during the sipping and backward during the swallowing.

    4. Moves upward during the swallow and feels symmetrical and smooth to palpation.

3. Which question is **not** part of the Carville Diabetic Foot Screen?

    1. Has there been a change in the foot since the last evaluation?

    2. What was the last fasting blood sugar (FBS) and glycosylated hemoglobin ($HgbA_{1c}$)?

    3. Does the foot have an abnormal shape?

    4. Are the nails thick, too long, or overgrown?

4. While conducting the interview for a physical examination, the nurse practitioner identifies what finding in the client's history as being commonly associated with thyroid carcinoma?

    1. Family history of thyroid cancer.

    2. History of hyperthyroidism.

    3. Irradiation of the neck.

    4. Smoking for 15 years.

5. When doing a physical examination on a client with hyperthyroidism, a common neurologic finding is:

   1. Memory, attention, and problem-solving deficits.

   2. Diminished deep tendon reflexes.

   3. Severe cognitive impairment.

   4. Delusions and psychosis.

6. The treatment goal for glycemic control in a type II diabetic is to achieve and maintain an HgbA$_{1c}$ of:

   1. <10%.

   2. Between 6% and 9%.

   3. <7%.

   4. >8%.

7. Which finding would alert the nurse practitioner that a client might be experiencing a problem with the endocrine system?

   1. Coagulation abnormalities and fatigue.

   2. Growth abnormalities and glucose intolerance.

   3. Hypoxia and jaundice.

   4. Steatorrhea and abdominal distention.

8. The nurse practitioner notes a solitary thyroid nodule on a client during a routine physical examination. The preferred diagnostic test of choice is:

   1. Thyroid scan and antibody level.

   2. Thyroid-stimulating hormone (TSH) level and ultrasound.

   3. X-ray of the thyroid.

   4. Fine-needle aspiration (FNA) biopsy.

9. An adult female client presents to the nurse practitioner's office, complaining of fatigue, weakness, and weight gain over the past 4 months. Physical examination reveals an elevated blood pressure, facial and supraclavicular fullness, hirsutism noted on the face, proximal muscle weakness, and facial and truncal distribution of acne.

Appropriate laboratory tests the nurse practitioner should order include:

   1. Antinuclear antibody test (ANA) and rheumatoid factor (RF).

   2. 3-hour glucose tolerance test and lipid profile.

   3. Red blood cell count and a calcium level.

   4. Dexamethasone suppression test, a urine free cortisol level, and TSH/thyroxine (T$_4$).

10. In evaluating the laboratory values taken from a client with Graves' disease, one should expect:

    1. TSH levels to be increased.

    2. TSH levels to be decreased.

    3. TSH levels to be within normal limits (WNL).

    4. T$_4$ levels to be decreased.

11. What information is correct regarding foot screening using a nylon filament (5.07 Semmes-Weinstein)?

    1. Use a 25-gm filament and apply along perimeter of any scar or ulcer tissue.

    2. Apply the filament at a 45-degree angle to the skin surface.

    3. Apply sufficient force for approximately 1.5 seconds to cause the filament to bend.

    4. Slide the filament across the skin and make repetitive contact to each of the ten sites.

Disorders

12. The etiology of type I diabetes can be best described as:

    1. An autosomal dominant genetic disorder.

    2. Autoimmune destruction of the β cells.

    3. Overnutrition and resulting obesity as the major risk factor.

    4. Prevented by exercise, which increases the concentration of insulin receptors.

13. The nurse practitioner should do an annual referral for the client who has had diabetes for over 5 years to:

    1. A cardiologist.

    2. A dietitian.

    3. A vascular surgeon.

    4. An ophthalmologist.

14. Hirsutism presenting in a female with normal menstruation and normal plasma androgens is most likely:

    1. An ovarian tumor.

    2. Cushing's syndrome.

    3. Idiopathic.

    4. Polycystic ovary disease.

15. Pathophysiologic reasons for decreased testosterone levels develop in the:

    1. Hypothalamus.

    2. Anterior pituitary.

    3. Testes.

    4. All of the above.

16. The most common cause of poor control of type I diabetes during the adolescent period is:

    1. Emotional disturbance.

    2. Noncompliance with dietary restrictions.

    3. Poor adherence to blood testing and insulin injections.

    4. All of the above.

17. When counseling a diabetic client on foot care, it is important to emphasize:

    1. Daily foot soaks in warm, soapy water.

    2. Careful daily foot inspections.

    3. Trimming corns and calluses regularly.

    4. Trimming toenails as close to the bed of the nail as possible and rounding nails to avoid scratching other toes.

18. An adult client presents to the nurse practitioner for evaluation of polyuria, polydipsia, and weight loss. Which lab result would require immediate intervention by the nurse practitioner?

    1. An HgbA$_{1c}$ of 14%.

    2. A serum glucose of 150 mg/dl.

    3. An HgbA$_{1c}$ of 6.0%.

    4. A serum glucose of 65 mg/dl.

19. An adult client is being evaluated for hypoglycemia due to a blood sugar of 58 mg/dl on a screening SMAC-20. The nurse practitioner can begin her differential diagnosis by:

    1. Deciding if the hypoglycemia is fasting or postprandial.

    2. Ascertaining if it is related to alcohol use.

    3. Deciding if the client has other medical problems.

    4. Reassuring the client that it is a benign problem.

20. An older adult male client complains of lethargy, cold intolerance, weight gain, and yellowing of the palms. The most important laboratory study ordered by the nurse practitioner in diagnosing this condition is:

    1. Complete blood count.

    2. Liver enzymes.

    3. Thyroid panel.

    4. Cardiac enzymes.

21. A middle-aged, normally healthy female presents for evaluation of intermittent palpitations. She originally thought it was related to job stress. She also reports mood variability, tremulousness, difficulty falling asleep, and a 10-lb weight loss despite a normal appetite. She feels warm most of the time and wonders if she is perimenopausal. She has no history of heart disease. The objective data that would yield the most useful information would be:

    1. Electrocardiogram (ECG).

    2. TSH, free T$_4$.

    3. Electrolytes.

    4. Holter monitor.

22. An adult client presents to the clinic complaining of fatigue, weakness, weight gain in spite of lack of appetite, and feelings of depression. Her physical examination reveals an obese, alert female with thinning hair, bilateral chest puffiness, increased facial hair, supraclavicular fat pad, thin arms and legs, purple striae on the abdomen, and multiple ecchymotic areas on extremities. Her vital signs are blood pressure (BP) 158/96, pulse 88, respirations 22. Laboratory studies an FBS of 200 mg/dl, electrolyte panel WNL except for potassium 3.0 mEq/L, hemoglobin 11.8 gm, and hematocrit 34%. The nurse practitioner suspects:

    1. Addison's disease.

    2. Pheochromocytoma.

    3. Cushing's syndrome.

    4. Hypoaldosteronism.

23. Which of the following is the best alternative for treating hyperthyroidism diagnosed during the first trimester of pregnancy?

    1. Radioactive iodine in smaller than usual dose during the first trimester.

    2. Propylthiouracil during the first trimester, subtotal thyroidectomy during the mid trimester, no thyroid replacement.

    3. Propylthiouracil during the first trimester, subtotal thyroidectomy during the mid trimester, thyroid replacement.

    4. No treatment until after delivery.

24. Clinical findings in a client with hypothyroidism include:

    1. Hyperactive bowel sounds.

    2. Oily skin and acne.

    3. Postural tremors of the hands.

    4. Edema of the face and eyelids.

25. A young adult male reports anxiety, tremulousness, headaches, palpitations, and sweating 2–4 hours after eating. Physical exam is normal. No labs are currently available. No history of any medical

conditions are noted. What is the most likely diagnosis?

    1. Dumping syndrome.

    2. Hypoglycemia.

    3. Alcohol abuse.

    4. Hyperthyroidism.

26. Which of the following is the most likely etiology for hypercalcemia in the medically well asymptomatic adult?

    1. Hyperthyroidism.

    2. Hyperparathyroidism.

    3. Hyperpituitarism.

    4. Hypothyroidism.

27. A middle-aged male with no previous medical history presents with a 30-lb weight gain in 2.5 months. He denies any medication use or allergies. He was recently laid off of a very active job and has been sedentary. Physical exam reveals BP 172/111, central obesity, FBS 200 mg/dl. What is the most likely cause of client's weight gain?

    1. Cushing's disease.

    2. Hypothyroidism.

    3. Depression.

    4. Diabetes.

28. A middle-aged female, accompanied by her daughter to the clinic, presents with agitation, confusion, fever, tachycardia, and diaphoresis. The daughter states these symptoms were preceded by nausea, vomiting, and abdominal pain. There is no history of cardiac disease, diabetes, or substance abuse. She was started on some "anti drug" 2 weeks ago and is scheduled for some kind of throat surgery next week (per daughter). Based upon this history, the nurse practitioner immediately orders:

    1. TSH, T_4.

    2. Urinalysis.

    3. Spinal tap.

    4. Computed tomography of the head.

29. A 45-year-old female client presents to the nurse practitioner's office, complaining of a

6-month history of fatigue, 15-lb weight gain, lethargy, an inability to tolerate cold temperatures, forgetfulness, hair loss, and constipation. Physical findings include dry coarse skin, periorbital edema and puffy facies, bradycardia, hyporeflexia and muscle weakness, and a smooth goitrous thyroid. The nurse practitioner would make the diagnosis of:

1. Congestive heart failure (CHF).

2. Diabetes mellitus (DM).

3. Hypothyroidism.

4. Thyroid cancer.

30. A diabetic client has been taking 6 U of regular insulin and 12 U of Lente insulin in the morning. In the evening she has been taking 3 U of regular insulin and 8 U of Lente insulin. The client has been monitoring her blood glucose levels and she shows the nurse practitioner the following chart.

	7 AM	Noon	5 PM	Bedtime
Monday	100	76	98	109
Tuesday	119	75	88	110
Wednesday	119	66	86	100
Thursday	123	70	111	122
Friday	128	60	99	110

The nurse practitioner adjusts the client's insulin by:

1. Increasing the regular insulin.

2. Decreasing the regular insulin.

3. Decreasing the Lente insulin.

4. Increasing both insulins.

31. The role of the nurse practitioner in the initial management of a client with a thyroid nodule involves:

1. Referring the client to an endocrinologist for further evaluation.

2. Obtaining an FNA of the nodule and sending to cytology.

3. Ordering an ultrasound and a thyroid scan.

4. Ordering levothyroxine (Synthroid) to reduce the size of the nodule.

32. When teaching a diabetic client about "sick day" guidelines, the nurse practitioner explains that the client should:

1. Stop measuring blood glucose and only check urine for ketones.

2. Not take your usual dose of insulin at the usual time.

3. Be sure to take metformin (Glucophage) and acarbose (Precose), even if nausea and vomiting are present.

4. Administer extra doses of regular insulin according to instructions for blood glucose levels above 240 mg/dl.

33. A young adult female client presents to the clinic with complaints of nervousness, tremulousness, palpitations, heat intolerance, fatigue, weight loss, and polyphagia. After a complete history and physical examination, along with thyroid function tests, the nurse practitioner makes the diagnosis of hyperthyroidism, recognizing that the most common cause of this condition is:

1. Thyroid cancer.

2. Graves' disease.

3. Pituitary adenoma.

4. Postpartum thyroiditis.

34. A young adult male client presents to the nurse practitioner's office, stating that he found a lump in his neck while shaving. Physical examination reveals a firm, 2-cm nodule that is fixed and nontender located on the right lobe of the thyroid gland. Right posterior cervical lymphadenopathy is also noted. The nurse practitioner should:

1. Order a TSH level to determine thyroid function, and refer the client to a surgeon for a fine-needle biopsy of the nodule.

2. No intervention is necessary at this time; schedule a follow-up visit in 6 months.

3. Prescribe levothyroxine (Synthroid) 0.1 mg PO daily and schedule a 6-week follow-up visit.

4. The client's thyroid should immediately be ablated with radioactive iodine, and the patient should be referred to an endocrinologist.

35. A client with Graves' disease is to have radioactive I^{131} therapy. When teaching about this treatment, it is important for the nurse practitioner to include what information?

    1. Clients are highly radioactive for approximately 7 days following treatment and need to be isolated.

    2. Clients should not become pregnant during or after receiving this therapy because of the teratogenic effects to the fetus that occur due to chromosomal abnormalities.

    3. Clients may become hypothyroid after this treatment, and will therefore need to have regular TSH and T_4 levels drawn, with the potential for thyroid hormone replacement therapy.

    4. This therapy is contraindicated in clients with cardiac disease.

36. An infant with congenital hypothyroidism is being discharged home. The nurse would instruct the parents to:

    1. Watch for constipation and slow pulse as signs of toxicity.

    2. Reduce the medication as symptoms decrease.

    3. Give the medication as a single dose in the early morning.

    4. Expect weight loss, until the child adjusts to the dose.

37. A goal in the management of a 7-year-old child with diabetes would be to maintain the blood sugars in what range?

    1. 100–200 mg/dl.

    2. 80–180 mg/dl.

    3. 70–150 mg/dl.

    4. 80–120 mg/dl.

38. A mother presents her school-age child to the nurse practitioner and expresses her concern that her son is the shortest child in his class and asks if something is the matter with him. Initial differentiation of

cause by the nurse practitioner of the child's short stature would include:

    1. History, physical exam, including Tanner stage with possible skeletal maturation assessed by radiography, if indicated.

    2. History, physical exam, and trial treatment with growth hormone.

    3. Immediate referral to an endocrinologist.

    4. Physical exam and complete blood count (CBC), thyroid function panel, urinalyis, karyotyping, chemistry profile, and insulin sensitivity tests.

39. Which of the following findings would the nurse practitioner expect to find in a child with pubertal gynecomastia?

    1. Tanner stage of II with testes ≤4 cm in length.

    2. Breasts and nipples nontender and equal in size.

    3. Breast tissue enlargement mainly glandular, movable, and nonadherent to skin or underlying tissue.

    4. Lymphadenopathy, goiter, asymmetrical testes, and repaired hypospadias.

40. Which of the following is true regarding hyperthyroidism in children?

    1. Boys have a higher incidence of Graves' disease.

    2. Autoimmune response is most often triggered by the body's reaction to a bacterial or viral infection.

    3. Decreased production and secretion of thyroid hormone and presence of goiter.

    4. Common, endemic congenital disorder caused by iodine deficiency.

41. The nurse practitioner notes the following on physical examination of a 14-year-old adolescent who complains of amenorrhea: BP 138/90, pulse 98, broad chest with widely spaced nipples, Tanner stage I, webbing of neck, low hairline, and prominent, anomalous ears. The nurse practitioner suspects:

    1. Klinefelter's syndrome.

    2. Marfan's syndrome.

3. Fragile X syndrome.

4. Turner's syndrome.

42. The nurse practitioner understands that growth retardation that appears after age 12 in boys is usually due to:

    1. Chromosomal abnormalities.

    2. Hyperthyroidism.

    3. Hyperpituitarism.

    4. Hypogonadism.

43. Which of the following conditions is associated with growth failure?

    1. Fanconi's syndrome.

    2. Tourette's syndrome.

    3. Klinefelter's syndrome.

    4. Angelman's syndrome.

44. The nurse practitioner understands that blood glucose levels in children 5–12 years of age with diabetes need to be maintained in which range?

    1. 60–75 mg/dl.

    2. 100–175 mg/dl.

    3. 80–180 mg/dl.

    4. Over 180 mg/dl.

45. An adolescent male presenting with recent onset nocturia, polydipsia, polyphagia, weight loss, and blurred vision is most likely to be experiencing the symptoms of:

    1. Insulin-dependent diabetes mellitus (IDDM).

    2. Non–insulin-dependent diabetes mellitus (NIDDM).

    3. Urinary tract infection (UTI).

    4. Mononucleosis.

46. In which of the following groups of clients is tight glycemic control contraindicated?

    1. Adolescent males.

    2. Middle-aged females.

3. Middle-aged males.

4. Infants under 2.

47. An infant with an abnormally pitched cry may demonstrate a genetic disorder or other problems such as:

    1. Hypothyroidism.

    2. Hypertelorism.

    3. Cleft palate.

    4. Pyloric stenosis.

Pharmacology

48. Clients started on metformin (Glucophage) need to be monitored closely for the following potential side effect:

    1. Significant increase in weight.

    2. Elevation of low-density lipoprotein (LDL) cholesterol level.

    3. Lactic acidosis.

    4. Increase in insulin requirements.

49. The nurse practitioner has ordered a client with type II diabetes to take glipizide (Glucotrol) 10 mg PO bid. In evaluating the medication's effectiveness, it is thought to reduce blood glucose by:

    1. Delaying the cellular uptake of potassium and insulin.

    2. Stimulating insulin release from the pancreas.

    3. Decreasing the body's need and utilization of insulin at the cellular level.

    4. Interfering with the absorption and metabolism of fats and carbohydrates.

50. The nurse practitioner would expect which symptom to be a side effect of metformin (Glucophage)?

    1. Gastrointestinal upset.

    2. Photophobia.

    3. Hyperglycemia.

    4. Skin eruptions.

51. A client is receiving antithyroid medication. The nurse practitioner understands that:

    1. Lifelong daily treatment is necessary to keep TSH levels within the normal range.

    2. Antithyroid medications do not cross the placenta.

    3. The medications are somewhat expensive and have serious cardiac and hematologic side effects.

    4. Clients remain on the medications for 1–2 years and then the medication is gradually withdrawn.

52. When prescribing an antihypertensive medication for a type II diabetic client with hypertension, the drug classifications that would tend to reduce insulin sensitivity are:

    1. Diuretics and calcium channel blockers.

    2. Diuretics and β-blockers.

    3. Calcium channel blockers and angiotensin converting enzyme (ACE) inhibitors.

    4. α-Blockers and ACE inhibitors.

53. A 35-year-old female sees the nurse practitioner with a complaint of cold intolerance, fatigue, dry skin, weight gain, and heavy menstrual periods. Upon physical exam, she is found to have a pulse of 58; a "waxy," sallow complexion; and a firm goiter. Her TSH level is checked and found to be 176 mU/L. The best treatment choice for this client is:

    1. Begin levothyroxine (Synthroid) at 0.025 mg PO qd and repeat TSH in 2 weeks.

    2. Administer a "loading dose" of oral levothyroxine (Synthroid), as well as starting a full replacement dose of levothyroxine (Synthroid).

    3. Administer a "loading dose" of IV levothyroxine (Synthroid) and start on a half replacement dose of levothyroxine (Synthroid).

    4. Begin levothyroxine (Synthroid) at a dose of 0.1 mg PO qd and recheck TSH in 6 weeks.

54. The nurse practitioner is seeing a 64-year-old man for a preoperative evaluation and exam. He is hospitalized with severe coronary artery disease and scheduled to undergo coronary artery bypass grafting. Physical exam finds the client to have mild facial puffiness, hoarse voice, and dry skin. Thyroid function tests were done and the client was found to have a TSH of 34 mU/L. The recommended treatment for this client is:

    1. Give a loading IV bolus of levothyroxine (Synthroid) 0.5 mg and proceed with surgery.

    2. Cancel surgery and send him home to begin a dose of oral levothyroxine (Synthroid) 0.1 mg. Instruct him surgery will be rescheduled as soon as he is euthyroid.

    3. Begin oral levothyroxine (Synthroid) and monitor in the hospital until the client is euthyroid.

    4. Proceed with surgery and treat hypothyroidism postoperatively.

55. The nurse practitioner is seeing an obese, middle-aged female client for a follow-up visit. She was diagnosed as a type II diabetic 3 months ago and started on a regimen of diet and exercise. Today her fasting plasma glucose is 200 mg/dl and HgbA₁c is 10%. She has lost 2 lb. She reports her home monitoring gluose has ranged from 180–300 mg/dl. The rest of her chemistry profile is WNL. The best treatment choice for this client is:

    1. Review her diet and exercise plan, increase exercise regimen, and reduce caloric intake. Schedule her for another follow-up in 3 months.

    2. Start her on sliding-scale insulin and instruct her on recording glucose and insulin requirements. Schedule her to return in 1 week to be re-evaluated for long-acting insulin.

    3. Initiate treatment with metformin (Glucophage).

    4. Initiate treatment with an oral sulfonylurea agent (i.e., glyburide).

56. What is associated with chronic overtreatment with levothyroxine (Synthroid)?

    1. Tachycardia.

2. Severe osteoporosis.

3. Insomnia.

4. Sweating.

57. A middle-aged male presents for a diabetes follow-up exam. He has been in good health without identified complications of diabetes. His FBS is 100 and his personal records indicate that he is taking insulin in the prescribed amounts and times. Vital signs are BP 142/98, pulse 80, respirations 20. Today's plan would include:

    1. Begin diuretics and a β-blocker.

    2. Begin ACE inhibitor and consider a diuretic.

    3. Get an ECG and chest x-ray.

    4. Return for BP check in 5–7 days.

58. An adult male has recently been started on insulin. His regimen is two daily injections with two thirds of the total daily insulin in the morning and one third in the evening. He is using the 70/30 mixture of intermediate- and short-acting insulin in both injections. He presents for a follow-up visit with his log of blood glucose. The nurse practitioner notes that his recorded glucose levels before the evening meal have been in the 60–70 mg/dl range. Other checks during the day are in 100–120 mg/dl range. What adjustments need to be made?

    1. Intermediate insulin, change 70/30 combination to self-mix and reduce AM intermediate dose.

    2. Regular insulin, reduce AM dose of 70/30.

    3. Intermediate insulin, reduce AM dose of 70/30.

    4. Regular insulin, change 70/30 to self-mix and reduce AM regular dose.

59. A client on antithyroid drug therapy for hyperthyroidism presents with complaints of palpitations and dry mouth for the past 2 days. He has had a cough and cold symptoms for the past 3 days, which he has been treating with over-the-counter medications. Which medication would the nurse practitioner encourage the client to avoid?

1. Benzocaine (Chloraseptic) lozenge.

2. Guaifenesin (Robitussin).

3. Ibuprofen (Advil).

4. Pseudoephedrine (Sudafed).

60. What is the most frequent complaint of clients who use insulin pumps?

    1. Problems with elevated glucose after changing the catheter-type (nonneedle) infusion set.

    2. Skin and site problems related to dressing adhesive not sticking, redness and pain at infusion site, and allergic response to tape.

    3. Mechanical problems with the pump's digital readout.

    4. Understanding "sick day" management modifications.

61. The nurse practitioner understands that troglitazone (Rezulin) is indicated for:

    1. Prenatal clients with gestational diabetes.

    2. Brittle type I clients.

    3. Type II clients who require insulin who have poor glycemic control and insulin resistance.

    4. Type II clients to prevent the rapid postprandial blood glucose surges by delaying carbohydrate absorption.

62. An older client with a history of hypertension and coronary bypass surgery has been diagnosed with hypothyroidism. Appropriate medication management is:

    1. Levothyroxine (Synthroid) 0.1 mg daily and return in 6 weeks for follow-up.

    2. Desiccated thyroid extract 2 grains daily and return in 6 weeks for follow-up.

    3. Levothyroxine (Synthroid) 0.025 mg daily for 6 weeks with slow gradual increase in dosage every 4–6 weeks until therapeutic level is obtained.

    4. Methimazole (Tapazole) 15 mg daily in three divided doses, gradually increasing dose every 4-weeks until a therapeutic level is obtained.

63. A client is newly diagnosed as being hypothyroid and is placed on levothyroxine (Synthroid) 0.1 mg PO daily. Follow-up by the nurse practitioner should include:

    1. No follow-up visits are necessary.

    2. The client should return to the clinic in 4−6 weeks to evaluate the response to treatment, including a TSH level, and to determine if there has been symptomatic improvement.

    3. The client should have weekly levothyroxine levels drawn.

    4. The client should have monthly CBCs while on levothyroxine (Synthroid), because the medication has been found to be myelosuppressive.

64. Classes of medications commonly used to treat hyperthyroid conditions include:

    1. Antibiotics and corticosteroids.

    2. ACE inhibitors, anxiolytics, and antithyroid medications.

    3. β-Blockers, nonsteroidal anti-inflammatory drugs (NSAIDs), and antithyroid medications.

    4. Calcium channel blockers and corticosteroids.

65. A client with hypothyroidism has been receiving daily levothyroxine (Synthroid) for 3 weeks. The client now presents with complaints of chest pain. The nurse practitioner should:

    1. Discontinue the levothyroxine (Synthroid), as this is a contraindication to continuing this medication.

    2. Schedule the client for a stress test.

    3. Decrease the dose of levothyroxine (Synthroid), order an ECG, and consult with a collaborating physician.

    4. Prescribe an anxiolytic agent for the client.

66. An infant with congenital hypothyroidism is being given levothyroxine (Synthroid). The nurse practitioner would instruct the parents to:

    1. Watch for constipation and slow pulse as signs of toxicity.

    2. Reduce the medication as symptoms decrease.

    3. Give the medication as a single dose in the early morning.

    4. Expect weight loss, until the child adjusts to the dose.

67. A 6-year-old child with hypothyroidism diagnosed shortly after birth is seen by the nurse practitioner for a routine physical exam. His temperature is 96.8°F (36°C) and his pulse is 68. The mother states that she has noticed that the child has been constipated and seems to be more tired than usual. Based on the history of this child, the nurse practitioner should suspect:

    1. The child has been taking too much of his levothyroxine (Synthroid) and is exhibiting symptoms of toxicity.

    2. The child needs to add more fluids to his diet to correct his constipation.

    3. The child needs to have his dose of levothyroxine (Synthroid) increased because he is exhibiting signs of hypothyroidism.

    4. The child has "outgrown" his hypothyroidism and no longer needs levothyroxine (Synthroid).

68. A 6-year-old has been discharged home on DDAVP (desmopressin acetate) for diabetes insipidus after a pituitary tumor removal. Upon examination, it is noted that the child is lethargic but has 4+ deep tendon reflexes. The nurse practitioner suspects:

    1. Noncompliance with therapy.

    2. Water intoxication

    3. Increased vasopressor effect.

    4. Interaction with OTC cough medicine products.

69. When monitoring an adolescent's insulin therapy regimen, the nurse practitioner is aware that the NPH to regular insulin proportions are:

    1. 2:1 in the AM and 1:1 in the PM.

    2. 1:1 in the AM and 1:2 in the PM.

3. 1:2 in the AM and 2:1 in the PM.

4. 1:1 in the AM and PM.

70. The nurse practitioner understands that lispro insulin (Humalog):

    1. Can be injected just prior to eating.

    2. Is less costly than regular insulin.

    3. Increases the likelihood of late postprandial hypoglycemia due to its length of action.

    4. Has a long-term safety profile and does not cause any teratogenic effects.

9　Answers & Rationales

Physical Examination & Diagnostic Tests

1. **(2)** When examining the thyroid, it is important to have the client relax the sternocleidomastoid muscles. This can be done by having the client lean toward the side being evaluated.

2. **(4)** The thyroid gland is fixed to the trachea and thus ascends during swallowing. This assists the nurse practitioner to distinguish thyroid structures from other neck masses. The gland's size, degree of enlargement, consistency, surface characteristics, and presence of nodules or bruits are noted during the examination.

3. **(2)** There are five questions to the Carville Diabetic Foot Screen. They are as follows: Has there been a change in the foot since the last evaluation? Is there a foot ulcer now or history of foot ulcer? Does the foot have an abnormal shape? Is there weakness in the ankle or foot? Are the nails thick, too long, or overgrown?

4. **(3)** Papillary carcinoma is the most common form of thyroid cancer. It is associated with a history of exposure to radiation. Family history, history of hyperthyroidism, and smoking are not considered significant risk factors for this malignancy.

5. **(1)** The high level of thyroid hormone affects the nervous system, causing sympathomimetic symptoms such as brisk deep tendon reflexes, fine rapid tremor of the hands, restlessness, irritability, insomnia, dreams, nightmares, and rarely severe cognitive impairment and psychosis.

6. **(3)** The American Diabetes Association (ADA) recommends <7% as an important treatment goal to decrease risk of long-term complications. A lab result of >8% $HgbA_{1c}$ is an indication that action needs to be taken, either by a change of medication or a reinforcement of education.

7. **(2)** Growth abnormalities are associated with anterior pituitary dysfunction and glucose intolerance with diabetes related to pancreas dysfunction. Coagulation abnormalities and fatigue would be associated with hematologic dysfunction. Hypoxia would be associated with oxygenation problems and jaundice with liver or biliary problems. Steatorrhea is associated with malabsorption syndrome and cystic fibrosis.

8. **(4)** Although the primary care provider may obtain TSH and antibody levels, the preferred diagnostic tool for the endocrinologist is the FNA biopsy. Scans, sonography, and x-ray tests can be used in initial screening; they do not assist in the determination of whether the nodule is malignant or not. The aspirate is sent for cytology and interpretation.

9. **(4)** The dexamethasone suppression test is the best screening test for Cushing's disease and a 24-hour urine for free cortisol is the best confirmatory test for Cushing's. TSH/T_4

may also be appropriate to rule out a thyroid condition, as some of the client's signs and symptoms are consistent with thyroid dysfunction. ANA and RF are ordered when rheumatoid arthritis or systemic lupus erythematosus (SLE) are suspected; this client's clinical picture is not consistent with these conditions. A red blood cell count would be done to rule out anemia, a potential problem for this client based on the history of fatigue, but the rest of the clinical picture points to something more than anemia. There are no clinical findings to support a calcium level being drawn.

10. **(2)** TSH levels should be decreased in a client with Graves' disease, because thyroid-stimulating immunoglobulins bind to TSH receptors, which increase T_4 synthesis and release, subsequently suppressing TSH levels.

11. **(3)** Correct procedure is to use a 10-gm (5.07 Semmes-Weinstein) filament and apply it to ten sites on the foot (one on the top of the foot, nine on the heel, sole, and toes). The filament is to be applied perpendicular (90-degree angle) to the skin surface and have sufficient force applied for 1.5 seconds to cause the filament to bend. The filament should not be allowed to slide across the skin or make repetitive contact with each test site. Randomizing the selection of test sites (start with big toe→heel→instep area→little toe→etc.) and the time between successive tests to reduce client guessing, and having the client close their eyes, also helps.

Disorders

12. **(2)** Type I diabetes is caused by destruction of the β cells mediated through the immune system. The other three choices refer to type II diabetes.

13. **(4)** An annual eye exam with the pupils dilated should be done by a specialist who can recognize subtle abnormalities. Although the other referrals can offer important contributions to diabetic care, they would be done on an as-needed basis rather than annually.

14. **(3)** Because of the normal menstrual periods and androgen plasma level, this hirsutism would be considered idiopathic. Diseases related to the ovaries would cause changes in the menstrual cycle, and with Cushing's syndrome they would have adrenal androgen overproduction.

15. **(4)** Testosterone production is regulated by the hypothalamic-pituitary-testicular (HPT) axis. Thus abnormalities in any one of these areas can affect the production of testosterone.

16. **(4)** All of these contribute significantly to difficulty controlling diabetes in the teen years. Hormonal changes and the desire to become independent increase emotional conflicts. Teens have a great desire to be like their peers and do not want to be regimented in following a specific diet and adhering to a treatment plan.

17. **(2)** It is important for diabetics to have their feet inspected daily either per self-exam or by a family member. Feet should be washed daily but never soaked. Corns and calluses should be cared for by a professional. Nails should be trimmed straight across to avoid injury to the nail beds.

18. **(1)** The normal serum glucose for adults ranges from 70−120 mg/dl. Diabetic acidosis is not of concern until the glucose is >300 mg/dl. An HgbA$_{1c}$ of >8.0% indicates poor glucose control over the past few months.

19. **(1)** True hypoglycemia can be organized around whether it is fasting or postprandial. Postprandial hypoglycemia may be caused by early adult-onset diabetes or postgastrectomy syndrome. Fasting hypoglycemia is most commonly caused by excessive doses of insulin or sulfonylureas.

20. **(3)** The symptoms are suggestive of hypothyroidism, and thyroid studies (TSH) would be the most useful.

21. **(2)** This middle-aged female client presents with many of the classic symptoms of early hyperthyroidism. A suppressed TSH with an elevated free T_4 establishes the diagnosis of hyperthyroidism.

22. **(3)** The client's physical findings and habitus, along with hypertension and hypokalemia, are associated with Cushing's syndrome, which is a state of excessive cortisol production due to a pituitary tumor. A Cushing's-like syndrome is often associated with prolonged glucocorticoid administration. Obesity is the primary finding in Cushing's syndrome, along with the "moon face," "dowager" or "buffalo hump," truncal obesity, hirsutism in women, and impotence and loss of body hair in men. Addison's disease is characterized by hyperkalemia, hyponatremia, hypoglycemia, anemia, and hypercalcemia. Clients with hypoaldosteronism (impaired renin secretion) have hyperkalemia. Pheochromocytoma would be in the differential diagnosis of this client because of the hypertension; the other findings are not consistent with this diagnosis.

23. **(3)** Low-dose antithyroid drugs are considered a good alternative to prevent the ill effects of hyperthyroidism on the mother and developing fetus until surgery can be performed. It is noted that some opt to use an antithyroid drug until after delivery and then have surgery. Removal of the thyroid during the mid trimester can be performed safely and is the usual recommendation. Replacement is essential after removal of the gland.

24. **(4)** Accumulation of hyaluronic acid in interstitial tissues increases capillary permeability to albumin, and accounts for the interstitial edema that is noted in the face and eyelids of individuals with hypothyroidism.

25. **(2)** While alcohol abuse may be a cause of hypoglycemia, this client is presenting with classic symptoms of postprandial hypoglycemia. It would be a good idea to assess for alcohol abuse as the etiology of the diagnosis of hypoglycemia.

26. **(2)** Hyperparathyroidism accounts for more than 60% of clients and is likely to be the explanation for elevated serum calcium levels.

27. **(1)** While Option #3 may explain the weight gain, Cushing's disease is correct for the constellation of symptoms of rapid weight gain, hypertension (HTN), and elevated blood sugar. These symptoms suggest adrenal dysfunction. Serum cortisol and adrenocorticotropic hormone (ACTH) levels should be checked.

28. **(1)** This woman is likely experiencing the life-threatening syndrome that can occur in decompensated hyperthyroidism. The clues were her symptom presentation and progression, the new "anti drug," and upcoming throat surgery.

29. **(3)** The symptoms describe the classic presentation of a client with hypothyroidism. A client with CHF would exhibit jugular venous distention, and have rales and peripheral edema. The criteria for diagnosing DM are polydipsia, polyphagia, polyuria, and weight loss. Thyroid cancer commonly presents without physical symptoms, and often the only physical finding is a hard, fixed nodule on the thyroid gland.

30. **(2)** The client's blood sugars are low around lunch time, which is when the regular insulin is peaking (3–4 hours), so a reduction in the regular insulin would help this problem.

31. **(1)** The nurse practitioner's role in primary care for a client with a thyroid nodule involves initially the early identification of the thyroid nodule on physical examination, referring the client to an endocrinologist for further evaluation, and possibly obtaining some preliminary TSH and antibody testing. The endocrinologist performs the FNA. Levothyroxine may or may not be used to diminish the size of the nodule based on the findings from the FNA and the endocrinologist's chosen treatment plan.

32. **(4)** It is important for the diabetic client to understand that when they are sick their blood glucose level will probably increase, even when they are not eating. It is most important they monitor blood glucose levels every 2–4 hours and check urine for ketones, if glucose level is >240 mg/dl. The medications in Option #3 *should not* be given until the client's nausea and vomiting have subsided and he/she has resumed a normal diet (blood glucose monitoring is important during this period of time).

33. **(2)** Graves' disease, an autoimmune condition also known as diffuse toxic goiter, is the most common cause of hyperthyroidism in this age group. Much less common causes include cancer of the thyroid, adenoma of the pituitary gland, and postpartum (or silent) thyroiditis.

34. **(1)** The TSH should be ordered to determine whether the client is euthyroid, hypothyroid, or hyperthyroid. The client should also be sent to an endocrinologist/surgeon because all nodules of the thyroid should be biopsied to rule out malignancy. Watching and waiting is inappropriate without having a biopsy performed. Thyroid hormone replacement therapy would only be indicated in those clients found to be hypothyroid and in whom thyroid cancer has been ruled out. Thyroid ablation may be indicated in clients whose fine-needle biopsy results are positive for thyroid cancer, but this cannot be determined without a surgeon's intervention.

35. **(3)** Hypothyroidism often follows this treatment, with 50% of clients requiring replacement therapy in the first year, and nearly 100% within 10 years. For this reason, regular monitoring of TSH/T_4 levels should be performed. Clients emit a small amount of radioactivity after receiving the dose used to treat this condition, and do not require isolation for 7 days. Radioactive iodine is very safe without an increased risk of gonad chromosomal abnormalities; therefore, there is no contraindication to becoming pregnant after therapy, although clients are counseled to avoid pregnancy while on treatment and to avoid children and pregnant women after receiving the oral ablation dose. This therapy is recommended for those clients who have cardiac disease associated with their thyroid condition.

36. **(3)** Thyroid replacement is a lifelong maintenance and should be given as one dose in the morning. Weight loss, diarrhea, and tachycardia are signs of too much thyroid medication.

37. **(2)** Children between 5 and 12 years, 80–180 mg/dl; children <5, 100–200 mg/dl; ≥13 years, 70–150 mg/dl; and normal levels, 80–120 mg/dl.

38. **(1)** This is the best choice for the initial exam, since the history may reveal normal variation in pattern of growth related to race, heredity, size of other family members, and psychosocial status. Skeletal maturation "bone age" can be assessed through radiography, if child is less than or equal to the fifth growth percentile. Other choices are inappropriate without history and physical exam, and growth hormone would not be administered without lab evaluation.

39. **(3)** Pubertal (physiologic) gynecomastia is a visible or palpable glandular enlargement of the male breast that can occur in healthy adolescents. Typically, the breasts are unequal in size, may be tender, nipples are often irritated secondary to rubbing against clothing, and Tanner stages II to IV of pubertal development are noted. The symptoms in Option #4 are associated with pathologic gynecomastia.

40. **(2)** Hyperthyroidism in children most commonly affects girls and is an autoimmune (Graves' disease) disorder in which the body produces antibodies that stimulate TSH receptors, causing an overproduction of thyroid hormones and goiter. Hypothyroidism is associated with iodine deficiency.

41. **(4)** These findings are consistent with Turner's syndrome—short stature, gonadal dysgenesis, lymphedema (usually appearing in infancy), left-sided heart or aortic abnormalities, primary amenorrhea, and delayed onset of puberty. Fragile X syndrome is an inherited condition usually affecting males and characterized by long narrow face and prominent ears, mild to profound mental retardation, hyperactivity and poor attention span, and autistic type behavior. Marfan's syndrome is a connective tissue disorder in the adolescent who is tall and thin and is characterized by long limbs, narrow hands, long slender fingers, and nearsightedness. Klinefelter's syndrome is characterized by small testes, sterility, gynecomastia, and long legs.

42. **(4)** Hypogonadism characterized by delayed sexual development, sexual infantilism, and small testes is most often the contributing factor to growth retardation after age 10 years for girls and 12 years for boys. Other causes of decelerated growth or short stature include hypothyroidism, diabetes, and hypopituitarism. Chromosomal abnormalities would be noted at an earlier age.

43. **(1)** Fanconi's syndrome is most often a hereditary problem caused by an inborn error of metabolism, such as galactosemia or Wilson's disease, and usually presents as growth failure in children. Tourette's syndrome is a disorder characterized by multiple vocal or motor tics. Angelman's syndrome is a disorder characterized by mental retardation, seizures, wide-based ataxic gait, and a pleasant, happy disposition with limited vocabulary or absent speech. Klinefelter's syndrome is characterized by small testes, sterility, gynecomastia, and long legs.

44. **(3)** Option #1 is too low and may predispose the child to hypoglycemia. Options #2 and #4 are too high.

45. **(1)** IDDM usually appears before the age of 30 and is heralded by the trilogy of "Ps," polydipsia, polyuria, and polyphagia.

46. **(4)** Tight glycemic control is contraindicated in infants <2 years of age and should be instituted with extreme caution in children <7 years of age to avoid injuring the developing brain.

47. **(1)** Infants with hypothyroidism often have an abnormally pitched cry due to lethargy and delayed mental responsiveness. Hypertelorism does not produce an abnormal cry unless accompanied by microcephaly.

Pharmacology

48. **(3)** Lactic acidosis is a potentially severe and fatal reaction to metformin. Metformin does not contribute to weight gain; it often helps with weight loss, and decreases LDL, triglyceride levels, and insulin requirements.

49. **(2)** The sulfonylureas reduce blood glucose by stimulating insulin release from the pancreas. Also, over a long period of time, they may actually increase insulin effects at the cellular level and decrease glucose production by the liver. This is the reason why sulfonylureas are used in type II diabetics who still have a functioning pancreas.

50. **(1)** Anorexia, nausea, and a metallic taste in the mouth are common side effects. Over time, the gastrointestinal (GI) symptoms subside and can be relieved by taking the medication with food or by starting at a lower dose.

51. **(4)** Antithyroid medications (propylthiouracil or methimazole) are relatively inexpensive and do cross the placenta. The client remains on the medications for 1–2 years with the hope of a permanent remission of symptoms when they are withdrawn.

52. **(2)** Both of these drug classifications tend to reduce insulin sensitivity and can cause hyperglycemia. ACE inhibitors, calcium channel blockers, and selective α-blockers are metabolically neutral; some may actually have a beneficial effect.

53. **(4)** The client's symptoms indicate hypothyroidism along with the elevated TSH; the normal range for TSH is 0.5–4.7 mU/L. Full replacement dose of levothyroxine (Synthroid) should be started based on client's age, and TSH level should be checked in 6 weeks, since it can take that long for a given dose to become effective. Loading doses should never be given except for coma, which is treated by IV medication in the hospital.

54. **(4)** Coronary clients found to be mildly to moderately hypothyroid can safely undergo urgent surgery (including bypass procedures) without prior replacement. The rate of complications is no greater than for nonhypothyroid clients, and the cardiac risks are lessened compared to initiating replacement therapy preoperatively.

55. **(3)** Metformin is a better option in an obese client, as metformin is frequently associated with weight loss, whereas sulfonylureas may actually cause a weight gain. Insulin is also not a good choice, as it is an overly aggressive approach to mildly elevated glucose. Clients also tend to be less receptive to treatment requiring injections. Diet and exercise were unsuccessful, and the longer her blood sugar remains elevated, the greater the risk for end-organ damage.

56. **(2)** All but osteoporosis are related to acute overdosage of levothyroxine and can be relieved by omitting the dose for 3 days and then starting on a lower dose.

57. **(4)** In order to initiate treatment for elevated BP, it is recommended that three elevated readings be recorded on three separate occasions. There is no evidence to suggest that this gentleman had an elevated BP on prior visits.

58. **(1)** This is the best answer, as the AM intermediate dose affects the glucose level before dinner. Altering the regular insulin will affect levels before lunch and before bedtime; however, these levels are OK. In order to reduce the intermediate while maintaining the level of regular insulin, the client will need to self-mix the intermediate and regular insulin, using less of the intermediate.

59. **(4)** Pseudoephedrine (Sudafed) and other decongestant medications that contain sympathomimetics lead to adverse reactions of central nervous system (CNS) overstimulation, palpitations, headache, hypertension, nervousness, etc. Robitussin in combination (i.e., Robitussin-CF [dextromethorphan, phenylpropanolamine, guaifenesin] or Robitussin-PE [pseudoephedrine, guaifenesin]) can also cause palpitations and CNS overstimulation. Robitussin-DM (dextromethorphan, guaifenesin) usually has predominantly GI upset, drowsiness, headache, and rash as adverse effects.

60. **(2)** Infusion site problems and skin irritation are by far the most frequent complaints of a client who uses an insulin pump. Often, it is a major reason for the client's decision to discontinue using the pump. Clients also find it is more time consuming and costly. However, the Diabetes Control and Complications Trial (DCCT, 1993) reported a reduced risk of microvascular complications when insulin pumps and multiple daily injections were used.

61. **(3)** Prenatal clients are managed with insulin, not an insulin sensitizer. Troglitazone (Rezulin) acts by decreasing peripheral insulin resistance in skeletal muscle and adipose tissue without enhancing insulin secretion. It improves glucose tolerance and decreases insulin resistance in insulin-requiring type II diabetics. Option #4 refers to the action of α-glucosidase inhibitors (e.g., acarbose [Precose] and miglitol [Glyset]).

62. **(3)** Older clients, especially with heart disease, need to be started on the smallest amount of thyroid medication replacement (0.025 mg, not 0.1 mg) and gradually increased until a therapeutic level is achieved. If thyroid replacement occurs too quickly, the heart may decompensate. Two grains of thyroid extract is too much. Methimazole (Tapazole) is an antithyroid medication and is indicated for treatment of hyperthyroidism.

63. **(2)** The response to therapy is based on clinical symptomatology and a TSH assay approximately 4–6 weeks after initiation of therapy. This is continued until a stable does is obtained. TSH and a free T_4 level are the two standard tests that can be used to monitor the status of the thyroid; a levothyroxine level cannot be drawn. Levothyroxine (Synthroid) is not a myelosuppressive agent.

64. **(3)** β-blockers are initially prescribed to reduce the signs and symptoms of the condition and to reduce the peripheral conversion of T_4 to triiodothyronine (T_3); NSAIDs are indicated for reducing inflammation associated with thyroiditis; and antithyroid medications, such as propylthiouracil (PTU) or methimazole (Tapazole), are used to treat severe hyperthyroidism. Corticosteroids are sometimes used in the treatment of thyroiditis, but the remaining classes of medications (namely, antibiotics, ACE inhibitors, calcium channel blockers, and anxiolytics), are not routinely used in the management of hyperthyroidism.

65. **(3)** Decreasing the dose of levothyroxine and evaluating the cardiac status of the patient are the appropriate interventions in this situation, in addition to involving the collaborating physician regarding further work-up. Discontinuing the thyroid replacement would be inappropriate because the client remains hypothyroid and requires therapy to continue for life. An anxiolytic may be a helpful adjunct, but it is certainly not appropriate as the sole intervention, as it ignores the cardiac symptoms.

66. **(3)** Thyroid replacement is a lifelong maintenance and should be given as one dose in the morning. Weight loss, diarrhea, and tachycardia are signs of too much thyroid medication.

67. **(3)** A low temperature and pulse, constipation, and fatigue are all signs of hypothyroidism and, therefore, the dose of levothyroxine (Synthroid) needs to be increased. Synthroid toxicity would manifest with signs of hyperthyroidism. The constipation is a symptom of hypothyroidism and has nothing to do with the child's fluid intake. Congenital hypothyroidism is a lifelong condition and will require lifelong medication.

68. **(2)** DDAVP promotes reabsorption of water in the renal tubules, which can lead to water intoxication. The signs of water intoxication are lethargy, behavioral changes, disorientation, and neuromuscular excitability.

69. **(1)** Insulin injections for the child/adolescent are 2:1 proportion NPH/regular in the AM and 1:1 in the PM. Changes are made based on blood sugar level done four times a day. The proportion is based on the time periods of insulin activity.

70. **(1)** Lispro (Humalog) is the first analog of human insulin that has several advantages over regular insulin, including a more rapid onset and shorter duration of action. It reaches peak activity in 1–2 hours and has a 4-hour duration, as compared to 6–8 hours for regular insulin. It is convenient for many clients, as it can be injected immediately before eating (10–15 minutes). Because it has been on the market only since June 1996, there is no long-term safety profile established and the teratogenicity is unknown. In addition, it is more expensive than insulin and some third-party payers may not reimburse clients.

10

Musculoskeletal

Physical Examination & Diagnostic Tests

1. A goniometer is used in a routine physical examination of geriatric clients. The nurse practitioner utilizes this tool to determine:

   1. Strength of the muscles in the extremities.

   2. The degree of joint flexion and extension.

   3. Range of motion of the extremities.

   4. Point of joint flexion that is painful.

2. The nurse practitioner places a client in the prone position with the knee flexed to 90 degrees. The tibia is firmly opposed to the femur by exerting downward pressure on the foot. The leg is rotated externally and internally. If locking of the knee occurs, this is accurately called a positive:

   1. Drawer sign.

   2. McMurray's test.

   3. Apley's sign.

   4. Bulge sign.

3. A client has numbness and tingling in the thumb and first two fingers when pressing the backs of the hands together (flexes wrists at 90 degrees) for 60 seconds. This is a positive:

   1. Tinel's sign.

   2. Drawer sign.

   3. McMurray's test.

   4. Phalen's maneuver.

4. What is the name of the sign that occurs when compressing the suprapatellar pouch back against the femur and feeling for fluid entering the spaces?

   1. Drawer sign.

   2. Kernig's sign.

   3. Balloon sign.

   4. Bulge sign.

5. De Quervain's disease can be diagnosed in part by a positive:

   1. Finkelstein's sign.

   2. Tinel's sign.

   3. Phalen's sign.

   4. Lachman's sign.

6. The primary examination techniques to use for assessing the musculoskeletal system are:

   1. Inspection and percussion.

   2. Auscultation and palpation.

   3. Inspection and palpation.

   4. Palpation and percussion.

7. What can the nurse practitioner use to confirm a diagnosis of polymyalgia rheumatica (PMR)?

   1. Chest radiograph.

   2. Serum protein electrophoresis.

   3. Corticosteroid challenge.

   4. Erythrocyte sedimentation rate (ESR).

8. When performing an assessment, the nurse practitioner understands that the metacarpophalangeal (MCP) joints are frequently involved with:

   1. Gout.

   2. Rheumatic fever.

   3. Rheumatoid arthritis (RA).

   4. Osteoarthritis (OA).

9. In the evaluation of polyneuropathy, which study would not be recommended?

   1. Sedimentation rate.

   2. Complete blood count (CBC).

   3. Hemoglobin A_{1c} (HgbA$_{1c}$).

   4. Electromyography (EMG).

10. In accurately assessing a client who reports back injury, it is critical to question:

    1. Family history of back problems.

    2. Previous injury.

    3. Personal history of chronic illness.

    4. Mechanism of injury.

11. Tinel's sign and Phalen's maneuver are used in identifying a common workplace illness that the nurse practitioner recognizes as:

    1. Lateral epicondylitis.

    2. Carpel tunnel syndrome.

    3. Dupuytren's disease.

    4. Thoracic outlet syndrome.

12. An elderly client complains of fatigue, weakness, lightheadedness, and anorexia. He also complains of hot, swollen proximal interphalangeal (PIP) and metacarpophalangeal (MCP) joints. These symptoms occurred 5 months ago and have reoccurred a few days ago. Which lab findings would be most conclusive of these assessments?

    1. Mean corpuscular volume (MCV) 104, low serum ferritin.

    2. MCV 92, high serum ferritin.

    3. Elevation in the uric acid level.

    4. Elevation in the white blood cell (WBC) count.

13. In the talar tilt test:

    1. The examiner grasps the tibia with one hand and the heel with the other hand. The client's foot is held while backward pressure is applied to the tibia. Laxity of the ligament is graded.

    2. The ankle is gently inverted and laxity of the ligament is graded.

    3. The examiner passively inverts, everts, dorsiflexes, and plantar flexes the ankle.

    4. The client actively inverts, everts, dorsiflexes, and plantar flexes the ankle.

14. Varus pressure on a knee that is slightly flexed (30 degrees) tests:

    1. Medial collateral ligament stability.

    2. Lateral collateral ligament stability.

    3. Medial cruciate ligament stability.

    4. Lateral meniscus tear.

15. The nurse practitioner is assessing a preadolescent girl for scoliosis. She would:

    1. Have the girl bend at the waist and look for asymmetry in the back and hip area.

    2. Examine the child fully clothed, paying particular attention to the hips and back.

    3. Have the child walk heel-to-toe and observe the gait and pelvis.

    4. Place the child on her back and flex the knees and observe for misalignment.

16. In doing a physical assessment on a newborn, the nurse notes a "hip click." What other findings are associated with this condition?

    1. Shortened quadriceps.

    2. Lateral deviation of patella.

    3. Limited adduction.

    4. Lax hamstrings.

Disorders

17. An adolescent complains of right knee pain immediately after running in track practice. On exam, the knee is warm to touch, and a tender, swollen tibial tuberosity is noted. The nurse practitioner suspects:

    1. Osgood-Schlatter disease.

    2. Rheumatoid arthritis.

    3. Acute tendinitis.

    4. Posttraumatic knee effusion.

18. The nurse practitioner realizes that the most common cause of shoulder pain is:

    1. Frozen shoulder.

    2. Thoracic outlet syndrome.

    3. Impingement syndrome.

    4. Osteoarthritis.

19. A 45-year-old female complains of knee pain when kneeling and a "clicking" noise when walking up steps. On exam, there is a slight knee effusion and tenderness when palpating the patella against the condyles. The diagnosis for this client is:

    1. Anterior cruciate tear.

    2. Dislocated patella.

    3. Chondromalacia patella.

    4. Tendinitis.

20. A client has been diagnosed with a complete rotator cuff tear of the left shoulder. The nurse would expect the client to have difficulty in:

    1. Abducting the left arm.

    2. Supinating the left forearm.

    3. Shrugging the shoulders.

    4. Touching the left hand to the right shoulder.

21. Night-time extremity pain in school-aged children that is deep but not present in the joints and is thought to be due to inflammation of the muscle bodies in tight fascial sheaths and to periods of high activity is:

    1. Osgood-Schlatter disease.

    2. Patellofemoral stress syndrome.

    3. Growing pains.

    4. Shin splints.

22. A client has been diagnosed with polymyalgia rheumatica (PMR). The nurse practitioner understands that this disorder is:

    1. An autoimmune, multisystem problem where the body makes antibodies to its own proteins.

    2. A degenerative disorder with no inflammatory changes, and where joint cartilage wears away with age and eventually causes bone spurs.

    3. An inflammatory disorder involving the axial skeleton and large peripheral joints.

    4. An inflammatory connective tissue disorder that primarily affects older women and is associated with giant cell (temporal) arteritis.

23. In teaching a client about fibromyalgia, the nurse practitioner includes what information?

    1. Diagnostic studies such as ESR and CBC are important tools to confirm the progress of the syndrome.

    2. Avoid stretching exercises and daily low-impact aerobics.

    3. Take ibuprofen (Motrin) 200 mg q4–6h prn for pain and amitriptyline (Elavil) 10 mg 1–2 hours before bedtime.

    4. Apply heat or massage "trigger points" to reduce pain.

24. The nurse practitioner understands that chronic synovitis with pannus formation is the basic pathophysiologic finding in clients with:

    1. Systemic lupus erythematosus (SLE).

    2. Ankylosing spondylitis (AS).

    3. Rheumatoid arthritis.

    4. Osteoarthritis.

25. The nurse practitioner is examining a client who is complaining of pain in her hips and knees. She has a history of osteoarthritis. On examination, the joints are painful to movement and are warm to touch. The best immediate therapy for this client is:

    1. Physical therapy for range of motion of affected areas.

    2. Decreased physical activity and immobilizing splints for affected joints.

    3. Moist heat and/or cold therapy on painful joints.

    4. ESR to determine level of activity.

26. The history of a client who may have contracted Lyme disease includes:

    1. Erythematous rash on bridge of nose and cheeks with discoid patches on the trunk.

    2. Immediate development of arthritis symptoms, especially in the knees.

    3. Expanding rash with central clearing occurring within a month of being bitten.

    4. Early symptoms of meningitis and myocarditis.

27. The nurse practitioner understands that finding Heberden's nodes on a physical exam of a client is a cardinal sign of:

    1. Septic arthritis.

    2. Rheumatoid arthritis.

    3. Gouty arthritis.

    4. Osteoarthritis.

28. The nurse practitioner is teaching an adolescent with a lower leg cast for a fractured tibia to begin crutch walking. Instructions for assisting the adolescent to walk up the stairs with the crutches would include:

    1. Place both crutches on the upper step and step up with unaffected leg while balancing on crutches.

    2. Position the affected leg on the upper step and use the crutches to move up.

    3. Place the unaffected leg on the upper step and move affected leg and crutches up together.

    4. Position the affected leg and the crutch on the upper step and bring the unaffected leg up with the crutch.

29. Competing diagnoses for an adult male who presents with acute onset of unilateral inflammation, pain, and erythema of the first metatarsophalangeal joint could be:

    1. Gout, cellulitis, and osteoporosis.

    2. Cellulitis, rheumatoid arthritis, and gout.

    3. Osteoporosis, fibromyalgia, and cellulitis.

    4. Septic arthritis, rheumatoid arthritis, osteoarthritis.

30. Diseases that often present as polyarthritic diseases include:

    1. Lyme arthritis, rheumatic heart disease, ankylosing spondylitis, and psoriatic arthritis.

    2. Rheumatoid arthritis, gout, Reiter's syndrome, and osteoarthritis.

    3. Gonococcal arthritis, systemic lupus erythematosus, and septic arthritis.

    4. Polymyalgia rheumatica, Lyme arthritis, pseudogout, and psoriatic arthritis.

31. The circumstances under which a common injury that can cause a meniscus tear to occur are:

    1. The knee is almost completely extended and the tibia is externally rotated.

    2. An external force is applied that is strong enough to cause external rotation or hyperextension of the knee, or there is a forceful direct blow to the knee.

    3. Valgus or varus pressure on the knee occurs at full extension and at 30 degrees of flexion.

    4. An injury in which the knee is simultaneously twisted and flexed.

32. Pain in lumbosacral strain typically begins:

    1. Immediately with the injury.

    2. 1–2 hours after injury.

    3. 6–8 hours after injury.

    4. 12–36 hours after injury.

33. Acute onset of pain that shoots down to the lower leg and foot of a 25-year-old obese adult is likely to be a symptom of:

    1. Lumbosacral strain.

    2. Herniated intervertebral disc injury.

    3. Osteomyelitis.

    4. Osteoporosis.

34. In an event where a knee "gives out," usually associated with trauma, followed by severe pain and effusion, and later "locking" of the knee with pivoting or turning, the client has probably suffered:

    1. Patellofemoral stress syndrome.

    2. Growing pains.

    3. Shin splints.

    4. Patellar subluxation.

35. Quadriceps setting is one exercise recommended for clients suffering patellofemoral syndrome. Teach the client to:

    1. Lie supine on the floor with legs extended. Dorsiflex the foot. Push the thigh into the floor.

    2. Sit on the floor leaning back on the elbows. Flex one knee to 90 degrees and extend one completely. Raise the straight leg until the thigh is parallel to the flexed knee. Hold for 5 seconds. Repeat for opposite leg.

    3. Lie on the floor and flex both knees to about 20 degrees with a rolled up towel underneath them. Extend one leg and hold for 5 seconds. Repeat for the opposite leg.

    4. Use resistive exercises with an elastic band.

36. Which risk factor is associated with gout?

    1. Female.

    2. Age 20 years.

    3. Ingestion of salicylate medications.

    4. Overuse of the extremity.

37. In a third-degree ankle strain there is:

    1. Moderate ecchymosis, moderate edema, and a stable joint.

    2. Moderate ecchymosis, moderate edema, and an unstable joint.

    3. Marked ecchymosis, marked edema, and a stable joint.

    4. Marked ecchymosis, marked edema, and an unstable joint.

38. A client with rheumatoid arthritis presents for follow-up. One of the best evaluative questions the nurse practitioner can ask that will help determine the severity of disease is:

    1. "Were you able to drive the car to your appointment today?"

    2. "Were you able to fix your dinner last night?"

    3. "How long does it take for your joints to loosen up after you get up in the morning?"

    4. "How many pounds can you carry?"

39. A 35-year-old female is seen with a complaint of diffuse musculoskeletal pain, stiffness, and fatigue for the past 3 months. The pain is worse in the morning and also with changes in weather. She states she wakes up in the morning feeling tired and unrefreshed. Physical exam is normal except for pain on digital palpation in 12 tender points. Laboratory results are unremarkable. The most likely diagnosis is:

    1. Fibromyalgia.

    2. Myofascial syndrome.

    3. Rheumatoid arthritis.

    4. Depression.

40. When counseling a postmenopausal female client on prevention of osteoporosis, all the following are therapeutic recommendations **except**:

    1. Cessation of smoking.

    2. Daily intake of 200 mg of calcium and 40 IU of vitamin D.

    3. Continue hormone therapy indefinitely.

    4. Monitor bone loss by dual-energy x-ray absorptiometry (DEXA) every 1–2 years for women who are not on hormone replacement therapy but are at increased risk.

41. A client tells the nurse practitioner that she has a "whiplash injury." The nurse practitioner understands that this is:

    1. Cervical facet joint dysfunction.

    2. Cervical flexion injury.

    3. Cervical-thoracic injury.

    4. Cervical strain.

42. A client presents with a complaint of sudden pain and swelling in the knee. He also is complaining of chills and fever. Upon exam the knee is warm, tender, and swollen with evidence of effusion. The family nurse practitioner would:

    1. Splint the affected joint.

    2. Obtain aspiration of synovial fluid from the affected joint.

    3. Initiate treatment with nonsteroidal anti-inflammatory drugs (NSAIDs).

    4. Recommend rest, ice, compression, and elevation of affected joint.

43. When determining the specific etiology of polyarticular complaints, the clinical clues most helpful for diagnosis are:

    1. Lab identification of antinuclear antibodies (ANA) and sedimentation rate.

    2. X-ray of affected joints.

    3. Affected joint pattern and presence or lack of inflammation.

    4. Sexual history of client.

44. A client with ankylosing spondylitis needs to be educated to manage disease by all **except**:

    1. Regular exercise program.

    2. Maintenance therapy of systemic corticosteroids.

    3. Using indomethacin (Indocin) for discomfort.

    4. Watching for signs and symptoms of iritis.

45. An adolescent client is being evaluated by the nurse practitioner for knee pain. The client is active in sports in his school but can recall no specific injury to the knee. On exam the nurse practitioner finds unilateral swelling of the anterior aspect of the tibial tubercle that is tender. The most likely diagnosis is:

    1. Stress fracture.

    2. Patellar dislocation.

    3. Osgood-Schlatter disease.

    4. Neuman's syndrome.

46. An adult client comes to the office complaining of foot pain. He can recall no specific injury but gives a history of being an occasional runner who drinks about six to ten beers on weekends. What physical findings would the nurse practitioner expect to find?

    1. Redness, swelling, and warmth of the first metatarsophalangeal joint.

2. Swelling, ecchymosis, and decreased range of motion.

3. Swelling and decreased circulation.

4. Decreased range of motion and obvious bone deformity.

47. Which of the diet selections indicate that the older client understands the health education regarding the prevention of osteoporosis?

    1. Chicken and baked potato.

    2. A glass of skim milk and a toasted cheese sandwich.

    3. Hamburger and salad.

    4. Ice cream sundae with whipped cream.

48. During the history, which of the following questions would best assist the nurse practitioner in diagnosing osteoarthritis versus rheumatoid arthritis?

    1. "Is your joint pain symmetrical and localized?"

    2. "Does your morning stiffness usually last several hours?"

    3. "Have you experienced fatigue, weakness, and weight loss?"

    4. "Is your joint pain asymmetrical and worse with movement and relieved by rest?"

49. The number one cause of disability in adults under age 45 is:

    1. Cancer.

    2. Fracture.

    3. Low back pain.

    4. Migraines.

50. The following is the most accurate statement about juvenile rheumatoid arthritis (JRA):

    1. Symptoms present in much greater severity than adult rheumatoid arthritis.

    2. Complete remission occurs in three fourths of clients.

3. Over 90% progress to severe joint destruction.

4. Cytotoxic drugs should be initiated as early as possible in the treatment regimen.

51. Primary treatment of joint injury involves:

    1. Rest, ice, compression, and elevation.

    2. Narcotic pain control and x-ray.

    3. Specialist referral and magnetic resonance imaging.

    4. NSAIDs and exercise.

52. The most common complaint in a client with back injury who had cauda equina syndrome, a surgical emergency, is:

    1. Urinary retention.

    2. Numbness below the level of injury.

    3. Weakness in the lower extremities.

    4. Pain.

53. Recognition of anular tears is important in the diagnosis of back pain because:

    1. They require immediate surgery.

    2. They are often misdiagnosed as strain or sprain, leading to herniation.

    3. They result in rapid paralysis.

    4. X-ray would reveal them, but x-rays are usually not ordered initially.

54. A chronic musculoskeletal problem that may occur after an injury and that is characterized by a 3-month history of pain on both sides of the body above and below the waist and tenderness in at least 11 of 18 specified points is:

    1. Chronic osteoarthritis.

    2. Reflex sympathetic dystrophy.

    3. Tendinitis.

    4. Fibromyalgia.

55. Which client is at highest risk for osteoporosis?

    1. 55-year-old male, smoker, and retired athlete.

    2. 60-year-old white postmenopausal, female switchboard operator weighing 105 lb.

    3. 42-year-old African American female intensive care nurse who is lactose intolerant.

    4. 50-year-old white, obese female, wife of a dairy farmer, and mother of three.

56. A 38-year-old secretary complains of pain in her hands at night. On examination, the nurse practitioner notes wasting of the thenar eminence of both hands and dry skin on the thumb, index, and middle fingers. The nurse practitioner suspects:

    1. Carpal tunnel syndrome.

    2. Transient ischemic attack.

    3. Osteoarthritis.

    4. Raynaud's phenomenon.

57. A 53-year-old woman presents with complaints of morning stiffness in the neck and back. She has pelvic and shoulder pain, and fatigue. Her laboratory studies reveal an elevated ESR, a normal rheumatoid factor, a normal creatine phosphokinase, and normochromic, normocytic anemia. Physical examination reveals an elevated temperature, bilateral pain, and stiffness of the pectoral and pelvic muscles. Based on this information, the best diagnosis is:

    1. Polyarteritis nodosa.

    2. Wegener's granulomatosis.

    3. Polymyalgia rheumatica.

    4. Rheumatoid arthritis.

58. A 55-year-old woman with a prior diagnosis of PMR presents with headache, low-grade fever, aching, stiffness, fatigue, malaise, and anorexia. Based on this information, the nurse practitioner would make a preliminary diagnosis of:

    1. Influenza.

    2. Pneumonia.

    3. Temporal arteritis.

    4. Rheumatoid arthritis.

59. Children with JRA must be screened regularly for:

    1. Ulcerative colitis.

    2. Iridocyclitis.

    3. Diabetes mellitus.

    4. Adrenal insufficiency.

60. An adolescent twisted his knee while skateboarding. He complains of knee pain and also states that in the past few weeks his knee has "locked up" a couple of times. Upon examination, a positive McMurray's test is elicited. This is consistent with a diagnosis of:

    1. Anterior cruciate ligament tear.

    2. Dislocated patella.

    3. Medial meniscus tear.

    4. Chondromalacia patella.

61. In young children, a complaint of hip pain without a history of trauma suggests several differential diagnoses. The diagnosis that is considered a true orthopedic emergency is:

    1. Toxic synovitis of the hip.

    2. Legg-Calvé-Perthes disease.

    3. Increased femoral anteversion.

    4. Avascular necrosis of the femoral head.

62. Differentiation between structural and functional scoliosis can be done by placing the child in Adam's position. In this position:

    1. Structural scoliosis disappears and functional scoliosis is enhanced.

    2. Persistent functional scoliosis is indicated.

    3. Functional scoliosis disappears and structural scoliosis is enhanced.

    4. Curves >10 degrees are indicated.

63. A man comes into the clinic complaining of low back pain that radiates down the

lateral thigh. The pain began suddenly on the job after lifting a heavy object. The nurse practitioner would further evaluate the client for:

1. Compression fracture of lower lumbar vertebrae.

2. A spinal cord injury.

3. Compression of a lumbar disc.

4. History of spinal cord injury.

64. A male child with pectis excavatum and an associated scoliosis should be evaluated for:

1. Pulmonary dysfunction.

2. Cardiac compromise.

3. Marfan's syndrome.

4. Joint deformities.

Pharmacology

65. The nurse practitioner is seeing a middle-aged, severely arthritic female who has been on maintenance therapy of prednisone 10 mg/day for the past 6 weeks. She now presents as acutely ill with signs and symptoms of acute pneumonia. She complains of feeling fatigued and weak, she has a loss of appetite, and her blood pressure is lower than previous visit measurements. Treatment should include:

1. Immediately discontinue the prednisone.

2. Increase dosage to 60 mg/day and then taper back to 10 mg/day.

3. Gradually taper the prednisone from 10 mg/day to 1 mg/day.

4. Maintain dose of prednisone at 10 mg/day.

66. The primary drug of choice for a client with RA is:

1. NSAIDs.

2. Aspirin.

3. Methotrexate.

4. Hydrocortisone.

67. A client with rheumatoid arthritis is placed on prednisone 5 mg PO per day. In teaching the client about her medication, it would be important for the nurse practitioner to include what information?

1. When the symptoms of arthritis subside, she will be able to quit taking her medication.

2. It is important to take the medication as prescribed, even after the redness and swelling decrease.

3. Increased fluid intake is important to prevent renal damage by the steroids.

4. The medication should be taken about 30 minutes before eating.

68. A correct medication and dose for the treatment of an adult with an acute episode of gout is:

1. Indomethacin (Indocin) 25 mg PO prn.

2. Naproxen (Naprosyn) 100 mg PO bid.

3. Colchicine 0.6 mg qid.

4. Indomethacin (Indocin) 50 mg q8h for six to eight doses then decrease to 25 mg PM q8h until gout episode resolved.

69. If a client's 24-hour urine indicates that the client is secreting too much uric acid (a result of > 900 mg/day), the nurse practitioner would prescribe:

1. Aspirin 325 mg PO per day.

2. Tylenol 325 mg PO q4–6h prn.

3. Indomethacin (Indocin) 25 mg PO q8h and then increase at weekly intervals by 25 mg daily.

4. Allopurinol (Zyloprim) 100 mg PO × 1 week then increase the daily dose by 100 mg to a maximum of 300 mg/day.

70. Disease-modifying drugs for RA in adults include:

    1. Ibuprofen (Motrin, Advil), sulindac (Clinoril), and salicylates (aspirin, Disalcid).

    2. Corticosteroids (prednisone, methylprednisolone).

    3. Misoprostol (Cytotec).

    4. Hydroxychloroquine (Plaquenil), sulfasalazine (Azulfidine), methotrexate, and gold sodium thiomalate (Myochrysine).

71. Gold compounds are contraindicated in clients with all of the following **except**:

    1. Renal disease.

    2. Hepatic disease.

    3. Rheumatoid arthritis disease.

    4. Blood dyscrasia.

72. The most appropriate medication used to control pain for a client with osteoarthritis would be:

    1. Acetaminophen.

    2. Systemic corticosteroids.

    3. Gold salts.

    4. Misoprostol.

73. What is a serious side effect of ibuprofen in the elderly client?

    1. Rebound headaches.

    2. Impairment of renal function.

    3. Neuropathy.

    4. Liver failure.

74. A client has been on methotrexate (Rheumatrex) for 6 weeks. This was the medication of choice for her severe refractory rheumatoid arthritis. What parameters should the nurse practitioner monitor?

    1. Monthly platelet count, CBC, and differential.

    2. Urinalysis, blood sugar, and electrocardiogram (ECG) every 2 weeks.

    3. Monthly CBC, urinalysis, and electrolytes.

    4. Coagulation studies, electrolytes, and CBC every week.

75. A middle-age male client presents with a complaint of waking up yesterday morning with his big toe swollen and painful. The client reports he has never had anything like this before and has not had any previous health problems. Physical exam finds his big toe to be red, hot, and tender in the joint with inflammation extending into the surrounding tissue. His temperature is 99.8°F and WBCs are mildly elevated. Needle aspiration of joint fluid reveals urate crystals. The best treatment choice the nurse practitioner could recommend for this client is:

    1. Bed rest, very-low-calorie diet, and increase fluid intake.

    2. Initiate pharmacologic therapy with allopurinal (Zyloprim) 200 mg PO qd and educate client on the need to remain on this medication for maintenance therapy once symptoms resolve.

    3. Start on naproxen (Naprosyn) 500 mg PO tid and instruct client to continue full-dose until symptoms resolve and then taper and discontinue over 72 hours.

    4. Administer an injection of intra-articular corticosteroid therapy to the affected joint.

10 Answers & Rationales

Physical Examination & Diagnostic Tests

1. **(2)** The goniometer is used to determine the degree of joint flexion and extension. It provides a means of measuring degree of angle flexion and extension.

2. **(3)** Apley's sign, locking of the knee or the sound of clicks and pain, may indicate a loose body, such as torn cartilage. This test is performed to detect a torn meniscus. The drawer sign tests the collateral ligaments with the client in a sitting and lying position, not prone. The McMurray's test is a test for medial meniscus injury. In this test, the knee is fully flexed and the tibia is externally rotated. Varus pressure is applied to the knee while it is extended. To test for medial meniscus tear, the test is performed while applying valgus pressure to the knee.

3. **(4)** Phalen's maneuver, when present, is suggestive of carpal tunnel syndrome. Tinel's sign is also a test for carpal tunnel syndrome, but is performed by lightly percussing over the median nerve on the palmar side of the wrist; and abnormal result would be tingling or shock-like sensations across the palm, thumb, and first two fingers. The drawer sign and McMurray's tests are used to assess the knee.

4. **(3)** The balloon sign occurs in instances when considerable fluid is in the suprapatellar pouch; ballottement of the patella may be possible. The bulge sign is for testing fluid in the knee joint and is elicited with the knee extended by applying pressure to the medial aspect of the knee and watching for a bulge or fluid wave. A patellar tap suggests fluid in the knee as the patella clicks against the femur. The drawer sign tests the collateral ligaments with the client in a sitting and lying position. Kernig's sign, a sign of meningeal irritation, is the inability to extend the lower leg when that leg is flexed at the hip, or there may be resistance or pain during elicitation of the sign.

5. **(1)** Pain with gentle deviation of a fist in which the thumb is tucked under the other four fingers to the ulnar side is a positive Finkelstein's sign and an indication of De Quervain's disease, which is swelling and tenderness over the volar portion of the "snuff box" resulting from chronic tenosynovitis. Treatment is usually a thumb splint, NSAIDs, and possible steroid injection into the area. A positive Tinel's sign (tapping gently over the carpal tunnel, causing tingling in the thumb, index finger, and middle and lateral half of the ring finger) and a positive Phalen's sign (holding hands that are flexed at 90 degrees back-to-back with this same distribution of tingling) are indicative of carpel tunnel syndrome. A Lachman's sign is an indication of the stability of the cruciate ligament of the knee.

6. **(3)** The musculoskeletal system is examined by a visual inspection and palpation of bones, joints, and surrounding muscular tissue. Percussion is generally not done, and auscultation is not appropriate to the system being examined.

7. **(3)** Clients with PMR have a rapid, dramatic clinical response to corticosteroid therapy. The serum protein electrophoresis is used to rule out myeloma. The ESR is elevated in a number of diseases and is not specific to PMR. The chest radiograph is used to diagnose diseases affecting the lungs and thorax.

8. **(3)** The wrist, MCP, and PIP joints along with other small joint of the hands and feet, are involved with RA. The great toe is most often involved with gout. The large joints of the hip, knee, and shoulder along with the distal interphalangeal (DIP) joint and the base of the thumb are involved with degenerative joint disease (i.e., osteoarthritis).

9. **(2)** It would not be necessary to obtain a CBC. The HgbA$_{1c}$ would be ordered to evaluate the actual control of diabetes. The EMG is most often performed to evaluate both nerve conduction and needle electrode examination. Many toxins and inflammatory processes are involved with polyneuropathy, hence the sedimentation rate would be a helpful diagnostic tool.

10. **(4)** A thorough history is very important in assessing any client with injury, but in the event of a back injury, the mechanism of injury will provide the greatest clue as to the extent of injury and the proper path to take in diagnosis and treatment.

11. **(2)** Carpel tunnel syndrome, a compression of the median nerve at the wrist is commonly caused by repetitive finger motion and results in a positive Tinel's sign and Phalen's maneuver. Tinel's sign is considered positive when tapping over the nerve with a reflex hammer causes tingling in the distribution of the nerve. Phalen's maneuver is performed by fully flexing the wrist passively and noting tingling in the thumb or fingers.

12. **(2)** The clinical assessments point to a chronic inflammatory process such as RA.

The dizziness, fatigue, lightheadedness, and weakness may be a problem with anemia. The anemia of chronic disease is either a micro- or normocytic anemia. The value that differentiates the anemia of chronic disease from other anemias is the serum ferritin (iron stores). The value will be either normal or high. The MCV of 104 indicates a macrocytic anemia, which would not include the anemia of chronic disease. The low serum ferritin would not be considered a possibility with this disorder. The uric acid level would be elevated in gout. The WBC count does not address the signs of anemia.

13. **(2)** Gentle inversion of the affected ankle in an ankle injury is compared with the unaffected ankle in the talar tilt test. Anterior ankle stability is tested in the anterior drawer test, in which the tibia is grasped by the examiner's one hand while the heel is firmly grasped and backward pressure is applied to the tibia with the examiner's other hand. In passive range of motion, the examiner inverts, everts, dorsiflexes, and plantar flexes the foot and ankle. The client puts the foot and ankle through complete range of motion in active range of motion.

14. **(2)** Varus pressure on a slightly flexed knee tests for lateral collateral ligament stability. Valgus pressure tests for medial collateral ligament stability. Cruciate ligaments are tested with the anterior drawer test. The McMurray's test is a test for medial meniscus injury. In this test, the knee is fully flexed and the tibia is externally rotated. Varus pressure is applied to the knee while it is extended. To test for medial meniscus tear, the test is performed while applying valgus pressure to the knee.

15. **(1)** The child should remove her shirt (leave on bra or swimsuit top) and bend at the waist. The nurse should examine for uneven hips and shoulders.

16. **(4)** Typical findings include Ortolani's (hip click) sign, limited abduction, shortening of the extremity on the affected side, and asymmetric gluteal folds. The lax hamstrings allow for full extension of the hip when the knee is fully flexed.

Disorders

17. **(1)** Osgood-Schlatter disease (tibial tubercle apophysitis) is characterized by a painful, self-limiting tibial tubercle swelling that leads to knee pain, especially during periods of rapid growth. Extension of the knee against resistance or application of pressure over the tibial tubercle aggravates the pain. Pain worsens with activity and lessens with rest.

18. **(3)** Impingement syndrome is usually caused by rotator cuff tendinitis, which occurs when internal/external rotation is impaired. Frozen shoulder can occur after a rotator cuff injury, especially if a sling is used for a prolonged period of time. Thoracic outlet syndrome would note a decrease or loss of the radial pulse when the client abducts the arm and holds a deep breath, while simultaneously hyperextending the neck and turning the chin toward the raised arm.

19. **(3)** These are common symptoms of chondromalacia patella. With anterior cruciate tears, the client generally cannot bear weight on the extremity without it buckling or giving way. With a dislocated patella, there would be considerable effusion (loss of normal knee hollow on sides of patella) and possible patellofemoral compartment.

20. **(1)** With a complete rotator cuff tear (rupture of the supraspinatus tendon), the client would have difficulty abducting the arm and impaired internal/external rotation. Touching the hand to the opposite shoulder is adduction.

21. **(3)** Growing pains usually occur at night and resolve by morning. The pain is deep and does not involve the joints. Osgood-Schlatter disease is due to degeneration of the tibial tubercle due to overuse and a rapid growth spurt. Pain and swelling occur over the tibial tubercle. Symptoms are exacerbated by activities that involve the quadriceps muscle. Another form of overuse syndrome is patellofemoral stress syndrome. Pain of a dull, aching quality is present in the knee, sometimes with clicking. Long periods of sitting or activities that involve knee flexion as well as compression of the patella in the groove cause increased pain.

In shin splints, inflammation of muscles along the medial shaft of the tibia is due to overuse and causes aching pain. Rest improves the pain. Improper warm-up exercises or a lot of exercise by an unconditioned person, especially in unsuitable shoes, can lead to this pain.

22. **(4)** Also, anemia is common in PMR, along with an elevated ESR. There is a common complaint of morning stiffness; rheumatoid factor is negative. Option #1 is characteristic of SLE. Option #2 is characteristic of osteoarthritis. Option #3 is characteristic of ankylosing spondylitis.

23. **(3)** Diagnostic studies are of little value and benefit, except to rule out other causes, such as PMR or hypothyroidism. Treatment is symptomatic; the usual drugs are amitriptyline (Elavil), NSAIDs, cyclobenzaprine (Flexeril), temazepam (Restoril), and triazolam (Halcion). Daily, slow, low-impact aerobics, preferably in the late afternoon or early evening, is encouraged. Heat and massage are helpful, but not on the "trigger points."

24. **(3)** The chronic inflammatory disorder of RA has synovial hypertrophy from chronic synovitis and pannus formation that results in progressive destruction of the cartilage, ligament, tendons, and bone. Ankylosing spondylitis usually involves the large peripheral joints (e.g., sacroiliac), and is characterized by extreme kyphosis. There is no inflammation with OA. SLE has a distribution of symptoms similar to that of RA, but no pannus formation.

25. **(3)** Moist heat or cold, whichever relieves the pain more effectively, is appropriate to use on acutely affected joints. Physical therapy is recommended after the acute involvement of the joint; care must be taken to decrease repetitive movements. Immobilization is avoided, as it tends to increase the stiffness of the joint. The ESR is not an appropriate indicator of activity of osteoarthritis.

26. **(3)** Option #1 describes the malar or "butterfly" rash of SLE. The arthritis symptoms and other complications (meningitis and myocarditis) occur later in the disease process, especially if the client is not treated with antibiotics (usually tetracycline, doxycycline, or amoxicillin).

27. **(4)** Deformities (bony protuberances) of the DIP are called Heberden's nodes and are cardinal signs of osteoarthritis. The DIP joints are seldom involved with RA. Gouty arthritis most often affects the great toe. Joints are warm, red, tender, and swollen with septic arthritis.

28. **(3)** The unaffected leg goes up the step first then the crutches and affected leg follow. This allows for stability and weight-bearing on the unaffected leg, with the crutches supporting the affected leg.

29. **(2)** Cellulitis usually presents with warm, erythematous, painful areas of the skin. Symptoms of erythema, edema, and pain of the first metatarsophalangeal joint are a common presentation for gout. Symptoms that can be present in RA are similar: red, swollen, painful joint(s). The inflammation of RA is usually symmetric but can present as erythematous, swollen joints. Systemic symptoms may also be present. Osteoporosis most often occurs in postmenopausal women due to bone loss that occurs with the decline of the estrogen in the blood. Bone thinning leads to fractures, not inflammation of joints or skin. Osteoarthritis presents as pain and stiffness with decreased range of motion, stiffness in the morning for a few minutes, and occasionally joint effusions. Point tenderness in 11 of 18 sites with digital palpation is present in fibromyalgia. Joint swelling and erythema are not present. In septic arthritis, joint pain, inflammation, and erythema would be accompanied by systemic symptoms of fever and chills. It would be considered in the differential for this client.

30. **(1)** Lyme arthritis, rheumatic heart disease, ankylosing spondylitis, psoriatic arthritis, RA, Reiter's syndrome, osteoarthritis, gonococcal arthritis, SLE, and PMR commonly occur as polyarthritic diseases. Most often gout, septic arthritis, and pseudogout occur as monoarthritis.

31. **(4)** A client that sustained a meniscal tear can usually recall a twisting injury of the knee followed by pain and effusion over the joint line. A strong force or injury that causes external rotation or hyperextension of the knee is a common mechanism of injury for collateral or cruciate ligament injuries. A test for stability of the knee joint involves applying medial and lateral pressure to the knee during full extension and flexion of 30 degrees.

32. **(4)** As the soft tissue swells, pain onset is usually about 12–36 hours after injury.

33. **(2)** Herniated intervertebral disc pain typically shoots to the lower leg and foot. Lumbosacral strain causes pain in the back, buttock, and sometimes thigh. Osteomyelitis must be preceded by an event that permits an infectious agent to enter the bone. Osteoporosis occurs most commonly in postmenopausal women.

34. **(4)** At the time a patellar subluxation occurs, a traumatic event causes the knee to "give out" and the patella is laterally displaced. Severe pain and an effusion result. Subsequent to the injury, the client will notice a locking sensation in the knee with pivoting or turning. Patellofemoral stress syndrome is a form of overuse syndrome. Pain of a dull, aching quality is present in the knee, sometimes with clicking. Long periods of sitting or activities that involve knee flexion as well as compression of the patella in the groove cause increased pain. Growing pains usually occur at night and resolve by morning. The pain is deep and does not involve the joints. In shin splints, inflammation of muscles along the medial shaft of the tibia due to overuse causes aching pain. Rest improves the pain. Improper warm-up exercises or a lot of exercise by an unconditioned person, especially in unsuitable shoes, can lead to this pain.

35. **(1)** In quadriceps setting, with the foot dorsiflexed, the thigh is pressed down against the floor and held for 5 seconds. The straight leg raise involves lifting an extended leg while sitting on the floor and leaning back on the elbows with the opposite leg flexed to 90 degrees. A terminal arc extension requires that the client lie on the floor supine with extended legs flexed to 20 degrees over a rolled up towel. The client then extends one leg and holds for 5 seconds. The exercise is repeated with the opposite leg. All of the above exercises can be used to stretch and strengthen the quadriceps muscles in those suffering from

patellofemoral stress syndrome. Resistive exercises with an elastic band are general exercises that can be done with the extremities.

36. **(3)** Gout generally affects men over 30 and is associated with obesity, lead intoxication, starvation, and use of some medications, including salicylates, diuretics, pyrazinamide, and alcohol.

37. **(4)** A third-degree strain is a complete tear of the ligament resulting in marked edema, ecchymosis, pain, and an unstable joint.

38. **(3)** Morning stiffness or activity and the length of time it takes for maximal improvement is one of the American Rheumatism Association Classification criteria for RA and is a useful, measurable tool for effects of treatment. The other questions are good indicators of quality of activities of daily living but do not give a full, overall, measurable picture of the client's joint discomfort.

39. **(1)** This client meets the classification criteria for fibromyalgia based on history of widespread pain and pain in 11 of 18 tender points. Myofascial syndrome symptoms are more focal and there is no associated fatigue or sleep disorder. Rheumatoid disease would have abnormal serologic studies. Depression may cause musculoskeletal pain and fatigue but would not have reproducible tender points.

40. **(2)** This is a subtherapeutic amount of calcium and vitamin D. The other choices are recommendations for prevention of osteoporosis.

41. **(4)** Most whiplash injuries are associated with a cervical neck strain due to a motor vehicle accident. These injuries take a considerable time to heal, usually five times longer than a strain involving another part of the body.

42. **(2)** This client's symptoms are indicative of septic arthritis, which is a medical emergency; if not treated promptly, the joint may be destroyed. Examination of the joint fluid is the single most important diagnostic test. The other choices may provide some symptomatic relief, but the first goal of

treatment is to determine if the joint is septic.

43. **(3)** When developing a differential diagnosis, the history and physical exam will help narrow the differentiation. Other procedures are important in completing the evaluation, but the most important information is the pattern of joints affected and whether it is inflammatory or noninflammatory disease.

44. **(2)** Corticosteroids have limited value in treating AS, and long term-effects are associated with many serious side effects. Important treatment includes regular exercise to strengthen supporting muscles and use of NSAIDs for pain. Approximately one third of clients have recurrent attacks of acute iritis.

45. **(3)** Osgood-Schlatter disease is common in late childhood and adolescence. The likelihood increases in clients who are involved in strenuous activity, especially that involving the quadriceps muscle. The usual treatment is NSAIDs and rest.

46. **(1)** Trauma, alcoholic binge, and physical stress have all been implicated in the occurrence of acute gout. Gout occurs primarily in adult men. Decreased circulation, ecchymosis, and bone deformity are not likely with acute gout.

47. **(2)** The calcium intake is important in minimizing the development of osteoporosis. Both of these foods contain calcium. The other distractors are not focused on the calcium intake.

48. **(4)** Signs and symptoms of osteoarthritis include asymmetrical joint pain worse with movement and relieved by rest. Stiffness is of short duration (<15 minutes) after inactivity, or in the morning. Pain may be described as aching and poorly localized. Options #1, #2, and #3 are indicative of RA.

49. **(3)** Low back pain is the number one cause of disability and accounts for 25% of disabling work-related injuries.

50. **(2)** Most do not have disease persistent into adulthood. JRA symptoms present very similar to adult arthritis. Most disease activity diminishes with age; although some do have some residual joint damage, it is not this high a percentage. Aspirin is the treatment of choice and cytotoxic drugs are reserved only for clients that have failed other therapy.

51. **(1)** The RICE principle is used for initial treatment: **R**est, **I**ce, **C**ompression, and **E**levation. All other treatments mentioned may be appropriate, but not as the primary treatment.

52. **(1)** Although all of the above symptoms may be associated with cauda equina syndrome, urinary retention is the most important clue to the immediate need for surgery.

53. **(2)** Anular tears are the first step toward herniation, and early recognition can help to avoid the need for surgical repair of a subsequent herniation.

54. **(4)** Fibromyalgia is a poorly understood condition that can prolong the normal treatment course of an injury considerably and is very difficult to treat. Osteoarthritis may follow an injury, as can reflex sympathetic dystrophy or tendinitis, but they do not have specified tender points.

55. **(2)** This example demonstrates five of the risk factors for osteoporosis, which include female, Caucasian or Asian, over age 45, low body weight, postmenopausal, sedentary lifestyle, low calcium intake, and smoker.

56. **(1)** Her occupation and symptoms are both suggestive of carpal tunnel syndrome. Initial treatment would involve night splinting, ice, and anti-inflammatory medication.

57. **(3)** PMR is an inflammatory disorder of the proximal muscles presenting as described. Polyarteritis nodosa is an inflammatory disorder affecting the small arteries. It presents with muscle weakness, myalgias, headache, and subcutaneous nodules along the arteries in the extremities. Wegener's disease presents with mild anemia, dyspnea, cough, chest pain, hemoptysis, and abnormal urinalysis.

58. **(3)** Up to 40% of clients with temporal arteritis have a previous history of PMR. Presenting complaints include headache, low-grade fever, aching and stiffness of PMR, fatigue, malaise, and anorexia.

59. **(2)** Development of iridocyclitis may be insidious and asymptomatic, and if left untreated may cause blindness. Although children may develop any of the other listed diseases, there is no correlation with JRA.

60. **(3)** A positive McMurray's test (palpable click and pain when rotating the foot laterally and extending the leg) along with the symptoms is indicative of a medial meniscus tear. The drawer test evaluates for anterior cruciate ligament tears (i.e., knee flexed with foot on table; sit on foot and grasp both sides of tibia at the knee; pull tibia forward; abnormal if movement of tibia away from the joint).

61. **(4)** Toxic synovitis and increased femoral anteversion, while causing pain, are not bone threatening. Legg-Calvé-Perthes disease results in necrosis of the proximal femoral epiphysis; however, there is later revascularization. Avascular necrosis results in death of the femoral head with revascularization.

62. **(3)** In Adam's position (forward bending, arms loose at side, thumbs hooked together), true scoliosis (structural) is demonstrated (by an elevated rib hump) whereas the functional type related to other conditions is not apparent. Persistent functional scoliosis can eventually become structural.

63. **(3)** The client is presenting with the classic symptoms of nerve root compression secondary to pressure from a protruding lumbar disc. The sciatic stretch test (straight leg raise) maneuver will increase the radiation of pain down the hip.

64. **(3)** Pectus excavatum can affect cardiopulmonary function, but when associated with scoliosis, the child should be evaluated for Marfan's syndrome.

Pharmacology

65. **(2)** Clients on chronic steroid therapy should be evaluated for adrenal insufficiency during an acute illness, which increases stress. Signs and symptoms indicate subtle clinical manifestations of adrenal insufficiency. Recommended treatment is to empirically treat with stress-dose corticosteroid during acute illness. Stopping the medication or maintaining it at same dose may precipitate acute adrenal insufficiency.

66. **(2)** Aspirin is the first choice. NSAIDs can be used, but the anti-inflammatory and antipyretic effects of aspirin, plus low cost, make it the drug of choice. Methotrexate is used for severe cases that do not respond to either aspirin or NSAIDs. Steroids may be given, but are not the drug of choice.

67. **(2)** The client needs to understand the importance of maintaining her dose of the steroids. When symptoms decrease, the medication is effective. It is not influenced by fluids and it should be taken with food.

68. **(3)** This is the only effective dose listed for the treatment of an acute episode of gout. The other doses are incorrect and insufficient as dosed.

69. **(4)** Allopurinol works to keep the serum uric acid level lower. The goal of therapy is a serum uric acid level of <6.5 mg/dl. The other medications listed do not help to lower serum uric acid levels, and aspirin can precipitate a gout attack.

70. **(4)** These drugs modify the disease when NSAIDs (ibuprofen, sulindac, salicylates) have not worked. Corticosteroids can be used until the disease-modifying agents begin to work. Misoprostol (Cytotec) is used to prevent ulcer development related to long-term medication use.

71. **(3)** Gold is indicated for treatment of RA and is contraindicated in the presence of the other listed diseases.

72. **(1)** Acetaminophen or NSAIDs are generally used for pain relief for clients with osteoarthritis. Systemic corticosteroids are not indicated in osteoarthritis. Gold salts may be one of several pharmacologic approaches to the treatment of RA. Misoprostol is used to minimize the development of NSAID-induced gastric ulcers.

73. **(2)** Renal function may already be reduced in the elderly, and ibuprofen can further impair renal function, which in turn can result in nephrosis, cirrhosis, and congestive heart failure.

74. **(1)** This client should be monitored for blood dyscrasias on a monthly basis. Women of child-bearing age should avoid pregnancy.

75. **(3)** NSAIDs are recommended treatment for an acute gout attack in clients able to take NSAID therapy. Allopurinol (Zyloprim) is contraindicated in an acute attack and can even precipitate an attack in the early stages of treatment. Low-calorie diets increase risks of gouty attacks. Joint injection would not be first-line choice of treatment. However, in refractory cases in clients unable to take oral medication, it may be an option.

11 Neurology

Physical Examination & Diagnostic Tests

1. To evaluate the neurologic system for appropriate sensory system functioning in the geriatric client, stereognosis is determined. This is done by having the client:

   1. Rapidly touch the index finger and then the nose.

   2. Distinguish between a coin and a key by touch.

   3. Stand with heels together and eyes closed.

   4. Close eyes and identify familiar odors.

2. To determine cerebellar functioning in the geriatric client, the nurse practitioner evaluates:

   1. Ability of the client to balance on one foot, then the other.

   2. Ability to discriminate between two familiar objects by sensation.

   3. Ability to recall names of three U.S. presidents.

   4. Range of motion and ability to move extremities.

3. What is considered a "soft" (or equivocal) neurologic sign?

   1. Positive Babinski's reflex in an adult.

   2. Mirroring hand movements of the extremities.

   3. Brudzinski's sign.

   4. Kernig's sign.

4. A client is having problems controlling her seizures and is referred to have electroencephalography (EEG) performed. Prior to the test, the nurse practitioner explains to the client that:

   1. This test will cause some discomfort and she will be given a sedative before the test.

   2. It will be important for her to take her regular dose of fluoxetine (Prozac) and phenytoin (Dilantin) prior to the test.

   3. The procedure is painless and she will not be in any discomfort or experience electrical shock during the procedure.

   4. After the test, she will be on bed rest for 8 hours and will be given full liquids for 12 hours.

5. Which cranial nerve is being tested when the nurse practitioner asks the client to raise his eyebrows, smile, frown, or puff out his cheeks?

1. Hypoglossal nerve.

2. Acoustic nerve.

3. Glossopharyngeal nerve.

4. Facial nerve.

6. The nurse practitioner notes in a healthy individual an absent knee jerk reflex. What might the nurse practitioner ask the client to do?

1. Lift both arms above the head and count to 5 slowly as the reflex is tested.

2. Raise both legs slowly and then lower and immediately test for the reflex.

3. Clench both hands together and pull while the reflex is tested.

4. Close eyes and hold breath while examiner tests for the reflex.

7. The nurse practitioner gently flexes a client's neck in the direction of the chin touching the chest. If there is pain and resistance to the flexion and the hips and knees flex at the same time, the nurse practitioner accurately describes this finding as:

1. Phalen's sign.

2. Romberg's sign.

3. Kernig's sign.

4. Brudzinski's sign.

8. The nurse practitioner understands that dysdiadochokinesia refers to:

1. Trouble with speech.

2. Memory impairment.

3. Trouble with attempts at rapidly alternating movements.

4. A neurologic triad of symptoms with gait, memory, and speech.

Disorders

9. The nurse practitioner understands that the most common form of facial paralysis in the adult client is:

1. Facial nerve fasciitis.

2. Trigeminal neuralgia.

3. Bell's palsy.

4. Herpes zoster.

10. A client has a history of injury at thoracic level 5 (T5) and his condition has stabilized. The nurse practitioner understands that, with this level of injury, the client is most likely not going to be able to:

1. Perform coordinated movements with his hands, such as writing.

2. Achieve lower body strength and coordination for walking.

3. Have upper body strength adequate enough to drive a car.

4. Maintain upper body coordination required to feed himself.

11. An older client, who as a young child recovered very quickly after extensive initial impairment due to poliomyelitis, is diagnosed with postpolio syndrome. The most common symptom is:

1. Gastrointestinal upset, headache, and malaise.

2. New onset of weakness, fatigue, and pain.

3. Sudden onset of lower limb paralysis following an acute infection.

4. Headache, fever, and elevated blood pressure and pulse.

12. A client has Parkinson's disease. The nurse practitioner is discussing safety measures for the home environment. It would be important for the nurse practitioner to include what information?

1. Sleep on a firm mattress that is high off the floor to facilitate getting into and out of bed.

2. Pour hot liquids with the cup or container placed on the table to avoid spilling.

3. Place a sheepskin pad on the bed to decrease the development of decubiti.

4. Perform passive and active range of motion twice daily to prevent contracture.

13. A client is admitted to a rural clinic after a diving accident. The nurse practitioner suspects a spinal cord injury at cervical level 5 (C5). While awaiting emergency transport services, the nurse practitioner assesses for the development of complications by:

1. Checking for voluntary movement of extremities and sensation below the level of injury.

2. Assessing breath sounds and evaluating movement of diaphragm with respirations.

3. Maintaining cervical flexion to facilitate airway until cervical traction is initiated.

4. Beginning neurologic checks with careful documentation of location of pain sensations.

14. Many clients who suffer from recurrent headaches have similar symptoms with each episode. Which is a sign that a headache may be from a more serious cause?

1. It occurs on the right side.

2. Rhinorrhea occurs with the headache.

3. Headache that continuously becomes more and more painful.

4. The client is able to sleep through the pain of the headache.

15. Epidemic meningococcal meningitis occurs rarely. This control is due to:

1. Use of active immunization.

2. Lower community carrier rates.

3. Improved socioeconomic conditions.

4. Earlier detection and recognition of outbreaks.

16. The nurse practitioner understands that benign paroxysmal positional vertigo:

1. Is described as vertigo and nystagmus with positional change and occurs most commonly in the elderly.

2. Is more common in the young and occurs suddenly and in episodes that include vertigo, tinnitus, hearing loss, feeling of fullness in the ears, and nausea and vomiting.

3. Follows a viral syndrome (upper respiratory or gastrointestinal), with exacerbation of the vertigo with position change without hearing loss or tinnitus.

4. Involves gradual hearing loss and tinnitus along with vertigo; eventually facial numbness and weakness develops.

17. All of the following are included in the differential diagnosis of a client with facial paralysis **except**:

1. Herpes zoster.

2. Bell's palsy.

3. Trigeminal neuralgia.

4. Otitis media.

18. What would be appropriate to include in the treatment plan for health promotion in a client with a diagnosis of multiple sclerosis?

1. Avoid aerobic exercise, due to muscle weakness.

2. Keep warm (especially extremities) to improve neurologic function.

3. Avoid antioxidants (vitamins C and E, beta-carotene), as they contribute to loss of myelin sheath.

4. Consume a low-fat, high-fiber diet, with daily cranberry juice and calcium supplement.

19. A client who has had a cerebrovascular accident is incontinent of urine. The family should be taught to:

    1. Restrict fluid intake.

    2. Insert a Foley catheter.

    3. Establish a scheduled voiding pattern.

    4. Reposition the client often to reduce the discomfort of urgency.

20. The best way to test the hearing of a client with Bell's palsy would be to:

    1. Stand out of sight of the client and ask the client to move or do something.

    2. Use a tuning fork to test for lateralization of sound.

    3. Stand in front of the client and whisper, "Raise your hand."

    4. Snap your fingers next to the client's ear and ask if the sound was heard.

21. The physical examination findings on a 50-year-old female client who wears a left lower leg brace are: weight 100 lb, height 65 inches, and vital signs within normal limits. In assisting this client who has developed postpolio symptoms, the nurse practitioner suggests the client:

    1. Gain weight to prevent further disability.

    2. Exercise all muscle groups vigorously to prevent disuse syndrome.

    3. Avoid exposure to cold or chilling, as it may cause a loss of strength in the affected muscle.

    4. Reduce the amount of time using the brace for joint support to prevent further loss of strength.

22. In infants, especially preterm infants, seizures can present as:

    1. Coughing spells.

    2. Poor feeding.

    3. Awake apnea.

    4. Regurgitation.

23. Inflammation and swelling of the seventh cranial nerve with resultant unilateral facial muscle paralysis is called:

    1. Bell's palsy.

    2. Transient ischemic attack.

    3. Facial droop.

    4. Trigeminal neuralgia.

24. A skin change associated with carpal tunnel syndrome is:

    1. Rapidly appearing and disappearing wheals.

    2. Lichenification of skin of the flexor surface of the elbow.

    3. Vesicular lesion of the hand.

    4. Dry skin on the thumb and index and middle fingers.

25. Which is a pathophysiologic reason for a headache?

    1. Vascular constriction of the middle meningeal artery.

    2. Muscle strain.

    3. Dysregulation of the ascending brainstem serotonergic system.

    4. Inflammation of the scalp.

26. A symptom that can occur in a client who has experienced a transient ischemic attack in the anterior cerebral circulation is:

    1. Bilateral vision disturbance and/or diplopia.

    2. Dysarthria (speech disturbance).

    3. Disorders of behavior and cognition.

    4. Motor and sensory problems on both sides of the body at once.

27. Many visits to emergency departments by adults are prompted by headaches. One symptom that may help the nurse practitioner differentiate a headache that is life threatening is:

    1. It is preceded by an "aura."

    2. It occurs mainly behind one eye and tends to be grouped.

3. The onset is sudden and is accompanied by nuchal rigidity.

4. The headache occurs mainly on awakening.

28. An adult client presents with a complaint of facial paralysis that started suddenly. In making a diagnosis, the nurse practitioner considers the following symptoms of Bell's palsy.

    1. Concurrent paralysis of the opposite arm and leg.

    2. Pain in the ear that accompanied or preceded the paralysis.

    3. Loss of bowel control.

    4. Loss of hearing on the opposite side.

29. A student nurse practitioner studying for the nurse practitioner certification examination begins to have numbness and tingling in her hands and face. Convinced she is having a stroke from brain overload, she calls a fellow student to come to her aid. What should this friend offer her?

    1. A ride to the emergency department.

    2. A phone call to the local magnetic resonance imaging (MRI) center.

    3. A paper bag.

    4. A different study source.

30. The nurse practitioner is evaluating an elderly client's tremor. Which assessment would assist in differentiating an essential tremor from a parkinsonian tremor?

    1. The handwriting is not affected.

    2. The tremor occurs with purposeful movements.

    3. The tremor occurs at rest.

    4. The tremor gets worse with β-blockers or alcohol.

31. Which assessment may be evaluated in a client with Parkinson's disease?

    1. Macrographia.

    2. Micrographia.

3. Exaggeration of rapid successive movements.

4. Increased swinging of arms while walking.

32. A 3-week-old infant has been diagnosed with bacterial meningitis. The nurse practitioner is aware that the most common causative organism is:

    1. *Streptococcus pyogenes*.

    2. *Escherichia coli*.

    3. *Neisseria meningitidis*.

    4. Group B *Streptococcus*.

33. A client recently diagnosed with multiple sclerosis asks the nurse practitioner about the disease process. The nurse practitioner knows that:

    1. 90% of all clients have a quickly progressive form of the disease.

    2. 90% of all clients, after the first onset of symptoms, have relapses and remissions.

    3. 10% of all clients will respond to corticosteroids.

    4. 10% of all clients have problems with optic neuritis and sensory loss.

34. The nurse practitioner is caring for a 10-year-old child with meningitis. To assess for the presence of nuchal rigidity, the nurse practitioner would:

    1. Have the child bend forward at the waist and observe the line of the spine.

    2. Place her hand on the child's forehead and ask the child to press her hand with his head.

    3. With the child relaxes, attempt to move the child's head side to side.

    4. Place her hand on the back of the child's head and assist the child to put his chin on his chest.

35. A young adolescent is accompanied to the clinic by her mother who states the school reports that the girl stares off into space a lot and does not seem to pay attention during these brief periods, which typically last 1–3 minutes. The neurologic exam is within normal limits. The nurse practitioner suspects:

    1. Grand mal seizure.

    2. Complex partial seizure.

    3. Absence seizure.

    4. Simple partial seizure.

36. A child is admitted to the rural clinic following a car accident in which she sustained a closed head injury and a fractured femur. The child is very lethargic and follows commands very slowly, and her pupils are equal and reactive. The child is to be transferred to a hospital by air ambulance. In evaluating significant changes in her condition, the nurse practitioner would note:

    1. Urine output is below 500 ml in 24 hours.

    2. Complaints of a headache in the frontal area.

    3. Able to move lower extremities to command.

    4. Vital signs are blood pressure (BP) 130/50, pulse 70.

37. A parent, whose son was recently diagnosed with Tourette's syndrome asks the nurse practitioner about the condition. The nurse practitioner understands that:

    1. Tourette's syndrome is commonly treated with antianxiety agents, such as diazepam (Valium).

    2. Tics occur many times throughout the day and they change over time.

    3. Children rarely will have attention deficit hyperactivity disorder (ADHD) in conjunction with Tourette's syndrome.

    4. Tics are commonly neuromuscular, such as facial grimacing, tongue protruding, neck twitching; rarely are the tics vocal.

38. A 30-year-old female client has had several episodes of incontinence, weakness, visual loss, and some ataxia. Physical exam reveals slight swelling of the optic disc on funduscopic exam, difficulty in walking heel-to-toe, lower extremity weakness, 2+ deep tendon reflexes. The nurse practitioner suspects:

    1. Multiple sclerosis.

    2. Parkinson's disease.

    3. Amyotrophic lateral sclerosis.

    4. Postpolio syndrome.

39. A 3-year-old child presents to the nurse practitioner with a history of hospitalization at 18 months for bacterial meningitis. The nurse practitioner would want to be sure to include:

    1. Vision testing.

    2. Hearing testing.

    3. Lumbar puncture.

    4. Electrocardiogram (ECG).

40. Which is considered a likely cause of seizures in adolescents and young adults?

    1. Congenital abnormalities and metabolic disturbances.

    2. Metabolic disorders, central nervous system (CNS) infection, and fever.

    3. Idiopathic seizures, trauma, and substance abuse.

    4. Trauma, malignant tumor, and cerebral vascular accident.

41. A client has a history of recurrent headache for the past 3 years, occurring one or two times per month and lasting 12–18 hours, for which she take acetaminophen. The client has been using acetaminophen 6 gm in the past 12-hour period and has had no relief, and presents to the clinic. The nurse practitioner would:

    1. Refer the client to a neurologist for headache work-up.

    2. Consider analgesic rebound relative to the dose of acetaminophen taken.

3. Order naproxen (Anaprox) for prophylactic treatment of the headaches.

4. Order an EEG and MRI to rule out pathology.

42. A child presents with a history of a purpuric rash with a centrifugal distribution and a fever. The nurse practitioner who examines this child should be highly suspicious of:

1. Rubella.

2. Lyme disease.

3. Meningococcemia.

4. Roseola.

43. A client presents to the emergency room with the "worst headache of my life"; the most common diagnosis and most important to rule out is:

1. Brain tumor.

2. Migraine.

3. Onset of newly diagnosed seizure disorder.

4. Subarachnoid hemorrhage.

44. A client with a recent history of a left hemisphere stroke returns to the clinic for a checkup. What symptoms would the nurse practitioner anticipate the client to exhibit?

1. Left-sided weakness.

2. Bilateral weakness or lower extremities.

3. Difficulty with speech.

4. Left visual field deficit.

45. The nurse practitioner is evaluating a group of geriatric clients for risk factors of an embolic stroke. Which condition would be least likely to precipitate this type of stroke?

1. Mitral valve disease.

2. Atrial fibrillation.

3. Endocarditis.

4. Diabetes mellitus.

46. A client returns to the clinic for a follow-up visit. She has a history of simple, partial seizures. When questioning the client regarding the recurrence of seizures, the nurse practitioner would identify the recurrence of this seizure activity if the client reported:

1. Short episodes where she loses consciousness, but does not fall.

2. No loss of consciousness but jerking and tingling of her right leg, then right hand.

3. Auditory hallucinations, unconsciousness, and urinary incontinence.

4. Short period of unconsciousness, followed by period of confusion.

47. An elderly lady comes to the clinic complaining of having difficulty when she tries to do her needlework. She walks straight, although somewhat slowly, and no rigidity is noted on movement. She states the shaking in her hands stops when she holds her hands in her lap. The nurse practitioner makes a tentative diagnosis of:

1. Parkinson's disease.

2. Transient ischemic attack.

3. Benign essential tremor.

4. Simple partial seizure activity.

48. The mother of a 5-year-old boy brings him to the clinic with complaints that he is "acting funny." She states there are short periods of time when he does not respond to her, he does not fall, then he suddenly responds and acts as if nothing has happened. The nurse would initially evaluate the child further for the presence of:

1. Petit mal or absence seizures.

2. Attention deficit disorder.

3. Horner's syndrome.

4. Avoidance disorder of childhood.

49. A client with a history of myasthenia gravis presents with ptosis, facial weakness, dysphagia, and generalized weakness. What is important for the nurse practitioner to establish initially?

    1. When did the symptoms first begin, and have they increased in severity?

    2. What medications is the client on and when did he last take them?

    3. What activity was the client participating in when the symptoms began?

    4. Has the client experienced any seizure activity with the increase in symptoms?

50. A client presents with miosis and ptosis with anhidrosis of the ipsilateral face and neck. The initial diagnosis would be:

    1. Horner's syndrome.

    2. Damage to cranial nerves III and IV.

    3. Meniere's syndrome.

    4. Mycotic aneurysm.

51. The nurse practitioner is reviewing the records of a client who is recovering from a stroke (brain accident). The records indicate the client is experiencing homonymous hemianopia. This is interpreted as:

    1. Partial loss of visual acuity in the peripheral area of the visual field.

    2. Diplopia in the eye contralateral to the cerebral lesion.

    3. Nystagmus in both eyes, but movements are dissimilar.

    4. Loss of vision in both eyes in either the right or left halves of the visual field.

Pharmacology

52. An elderly client is diagnosed with herpes zoster. To reduce the occurrence of postherpetic neuralgia, the nurse practitioner orders which medication?

    1. Prednisone (Deltasone).

    2. Acyclovir (Zovirax).

    3. Ketorolac (Toradol).

    4. Carbamazepine (Tegretol).

53. A client is on antiepileptic medication. The nurse practitioner understands that antiepileptic medication:

    1. Must be taken indefinitely.

    2. Is usually discontinued after 4 years of no seizure activity, following an EEG test to confirm lack of seizure activity.

    3. Is usually given in combination with other antiepileptics or sedatives to reduce the seizure threshold.

    4. Must be given to all clients who experience a seizure.

54. The medication management of clients with peripheral vestibulopathy includes:

    1. Meclizine (Antivert) 100 mg PO qid.

    2. Dimenhydrinate (Dramamine) 5 mg PO tid to qid.

    3. Scopolamine transdermal disc (Transderm-Scōp) 1 disc applied behind the ear and left in place for 3 days.

    4. Prochlorperazine (Compazine) 25–50 mg PO q4h prn.

55. A medication and dose that can be used for abortive therapy for an adult client with symptoms of a migraine headache are:

    1. Sumatriptan (Imitrex) 6 mg IM.

    2. Ergotamine (Ergostat) 2 mg SL.

    3. Ketorolac (Toradol) 100 mg IM.

    4. Amitriptyline (Elavil) 100 mg PO.

56. During a physical exam of a child diagnosed with chronic recurrent seizures who is receiving antiepileptic medication, the nurse practitioner notes hyperplasia of the gums. The nurse understands that hyperplasia of the gums is:

    1. An unusual side effect of phenobarbital.

    2. A common side effect of phenytoin.

    3. A common occurrence with chronic recurrent seizures.

    4. Due to poor oral hygiene.

57. The family of a Parkinson's client brings him to the clinic because his tremors and difficulty walking have increased. The physician increases the client's trihexyphenidyl (Artane) from 3 mg/day to 5 mg/day in divided doses. What is important for the nurse practitioner to teach the family regarding the increase in the dose of this medication?

1. There may be an increase in the fluctuations of his symptoms.

2. There will be an increased tendency for urinary retention.

3. Initially an increase in confusion is not uncommon.

4. Closely observe the client for dizziness when he stands up.

11 ⟩ Answers & Rationales

Physical Examination & Diagnostic Tests

1. **(2)** Stereognosis is the ability to determine familiar objects by shape rather than visual identification. Option #1 determines fine motor and coordination, Option #3 determines proprioception (balance, posture), and Option #4 determines the functioning of the first cranial nerve (i.e., olfactory).

2. **(1)** The cerebellar area controls gross motor movements and balance, as well as fine motor movements of the upper and lower extremities. Discriminatory sensation tests the sensory system, and a remote memory test is a mental status examination involving the cerebral cortex.

3. **(2)** Soft neurologic signs involve slight deviations of the CNS that are present occasionally or inconsistently. Examples are short attention span, clumsiness, frequent falling (disturbances of gait), hyperkinesis, left-handed but right-footed, language disturbances, anisocoria, and mirroring movements of the extremities (when one hand performs a movement, the other is also in motion). The other three options indicate a CNS problem that occurs consistently (Brudzinski's and Kernig's signs indicate meningeal irritation; a positive Babinski's reflex in an adult may indicate an upper motor lesion in the corticospinal tract).

4. **(3)** The procedure is painless and there is no danger of electrical shock. All anticonvulsants, antidepressants, stimulants (caffeine, tobacco), and alcohol should be stopped. There is no restriction on movement or diet after the procedure.

5. **(4)** The facial nerve is tested by facial movement, taste, sensation, and corneal reflex. The hypoglossal nerve is tested by the client sticking out his tongue. The acoustic nerve is tested by a hearing test. The glossopharyngeal nerve is tested by taste, gag reflex, and giving the client a drink and asking him to swallow.

6. **(3)** Augmentation of the knee jerk reflex can be obtained by having the client isometrically tense muscles not directly involved with the reflex arc being tested. This is called Jendrassik's maneuver.

7. **(4)** This describes Brudzinski's sign. Phalen's sign is elicited in carpal tunnel syndrome. Romberg's test is done to assess gross swaying by asking the client to stand with feet together and eyes closed for 5 seconds. Kernig's sign (inability to extend the lower leg when the leg is flexed at the hip or when there is resistance or pain during the process) along with Brudzinski's sign indicate meningeal irritation and should be further evaluated.

8. **(3)** Dysdiadochokinesia is trouble with attempts at rapidly alternating movements (i.e., finger to nose).

Disorders

9. **(3)** The most common form of facial paralysis is Bell's palsy, which is a disorder affecting the facial nerve and is characterized by muscle flaccidity of the affected side of the face. Trigeminal neuralgia is a disorder of cranial nerve V characterized by an abrupt onset of pain in the lower and upper jaw, cheek, and lips. Herpes zoster affects the dermatomes and does not cause a paralysis, but rather pain and possible postherpetic neuralgia.

10. **(2)** T5 injuries do not affect the coordination or capacity of the upper body, arms, and hands; the lower body is paralyzed. The client should be able to do all of the activities listed except walk.

11. **(2)** The cardinal signs of postpolio syndrome include onset of new weakness, fatigue, and pain along with hot or cold intolerance, and swallowing, speech, breathing, and/or sleep disturbances.

12. **(2)** Pouring liquids is frequently a complicated task for this client due to his tremors. If the cup or container in which the client is pouring the liquid is placed on the table, there is less chance of spilling the contents.

13. **(2)** At this level of injury (C5), the intercostal muscles and diaphragm can be affected and the client with have respiratory compromise. Airway maintenance and avoiding flexion of the neck are critical.

14. **(3)** If a headache becomes more and more severe, if there is new onset of severe headache in a client over 35 years old, if the headache's character or progression is different from other headaches, or if there is vomiting but no nausea, there could be a new and serious cause for the headache. The side on which the headache occurs, accompanying rhinorrhea, and sleeping through a headache may or may not be significant, depending on other symptoms.

15. **(3)** Undoubtedly, improved sanitary and socioeconomic conditions have led to the marked reduction in the number of cases of epidemic meningitis. There is no research to support increased cases in communities with higher carrier numbers.

16. **(1)** Benign paroxysmal positional vertigo usually occurs in older clients. Younger persons who experience a sudden episode of vertigo, tinnitus, hearing loss, sensation of fullness, and nausea and vomiting typically have Meniere's disease. Peripheral vestibulopathy usually follows upper respiratory or gastrointestinal viral illness and involves nearly incapacitating vertigo that increases with positional changes, but not hearing loss or tinnitus. Suspect an acoustic neuroma if gradual hearing loss, tinnitus, and vertigo develop before the facial numbness and weakness develop.

17. **(3)** The differential diagnosis for facial paralysis includes numerous problems: bacterial infections of the ears, Lyme disease, herpes zoster, mumps, temporal bone fracture, acoustic neuroma, other types of tumors, and demyelinating diseases. Trigeminal neuralgia is associated with intense facial pain, not paralysis.

18. **(4)** In addition to the factors listed, keeping cool, not warm, is associated with improvement of neurologic function. A regular exercise program is encouraged along with daily intake of a multivitamin, antioxidants, and low-dose aspirin (81 mg); maintaining ideal body weight, having rest periods or naps daily, and becoming informed about the disease process are important aspects of promoting health.

19. **(3)** Re-establishing regularity will assist in maintaining bladder control. A catheter exposes the client to infection. Fluids should not be restricted.

20. **(1)** Bell's palsy involves a sensorineural hearing loss. In contrast to the client being able to read lips, he must be able to hear the direction of sound without any visual prompting. The tuning fork assists in differentiating between air or bone conduction of sound.

21. **(3)** In addition to encouraging the client to have regular health maintenance visits, the client should be advised to avoid gaining weight and exercising to the point of muscle pain. Cold temperatures can cause a loss of muscle strength in the affected muscle groups and should be avoided. Assistive or orthotic devices (canes, walkers, braces, etc.) should be used, along with periodic evaluation of muscle strength and function.

22. **(3)** While it is important to investigate all episodes of apnea in infants, premature infants may not exhibit the typical tonic-clonic type seizures but may have awake apnea.

23. **(1)** The symptoms describe Bell's palsy, which is believed to be caused by a virus. This sudden onset of unilateral facial paralysis usually resolves within a couple of weeks, but can endure for months. A few clients can have residual problems. Transient ischemic attacks last <24 hours. Facial droop occurs with Bell's palsy due to paralysis of the muscles innervated by the facial nerve (seventh cranial nerve). Trigeminal neuralgia is sudden pain along the fifth cranial nerve.

24. **(4)** These changes are typical of carpal tunnel syndrome. Rapidly appearing and disappearing wheals are known as urticaria and could have one of many causes, including allergic response to a substance that was ingested. A vesicular lesion of the hand could be caused by one of many etiologies, including a burn, local allergic reaction, and friction.

25. **(3)** Stimulation of pain-sensitive structures, vessel and meningeal inflammation, vasodilation, severe muscle contraction in the head and neck area, and dysregulation of the ascending brainstem serotonergic system are causes for headaches.

26. **(3)** A wide variety of changes can occur in behavior and cognition after a transient ischemic attack. Bilateral vision disturbance, diplopia, dysarthria (speech disturbance), and motor/sensory problems on both sides of the body are problems associated with a transient ischemic attack in the posterior cerebral circulation.

27. **(3)** Classic migraine headaches are accompanied by auras. Cluster headaches occur behind one eye and are grouped. Headaches associated with hypertension occur mainly on awakening. A sudden onset and nuchal rigidity may indicate a subarachnoid hemorrhage.

28. **(2)** Bell's palsy is typically preceded or accompanied by pain in the ear on the paralyzed side. The paralysis is confined to the face and there is no bowel involvement.

29. **(3)** Clients who are under stress have periods of hyperventilation in which they "blow off" more carbon dioxide than necessary. They experience numbness and tingling in their hands and faces and can experience syncope. Breathing into a paper bag increases the carbon dioxide level and relieves the symptoms of respiratory alkalosis.

30. **(2)** The differentiating feature between the two tremors is that the essential tremor occurs with purposeful movements. Handwriting may be affected with both tremors. The tremor with Parkinson's disease occurs at rest. Essential tremors improve with β-blockers as well as alcohol.

31. **(2)** Micrographia is a classic manifestation of Parkinson's disease. There is an impairment of rapid successive movements and a loss in automatic movements such as swinging the arms while walking.

32. **(4)** The most common cause of bacterial meningitis in the first month of life is the Group B *Streptococcus. Streptococcus pneumoniae* and *Neisseria meningitides* are usually associated with meningitis after the age of 1 month in areas where the conjugate Hib vaccines are used.

33. **(2)** Multiple sclerosis is characterized by exacerbations and remissions of the symptoms. Only 10% have a progressive form of the disease from onset. Many clients (35–40%) have problems of optic neuritis, sensory loss, and weakness and do respond to corticosteroids.

34. **(4)** Nuchal rigidity is a stiff neck; the child cannot move his head forward and cannot bring his chin in contact with his chest.

Movement of the head from side to side does not elicit nuchal rigidity.

35. **(3)** This accurately fits the description of a petit mal or absence seizure, which is a type of generalized seizure that begins in childhood and usually ends in early adulthood (30s). There is usually impairment of consciousness, automatic symptoms, and mild tonic/clonic symptoms. Classically, "the staring off into space," is the reporting symptom.

36. **(4)** Increase in the pulse pressure and decrease in pulse rate are indications of increasing cerebral edema and intracranial pressure and would necessitate immediate intervention. A child's urine output should be between 20 and 30 ml/hr.

37. **(2)** Tourette's syndrome is a hereditary, chronic neuromuscular disorder consisting of various motor and vocal tics. Tics are sudden, involuntary, brief, repetitive, motor movements that often begin in childhood and change over time. Neuroleptic drugs, such as haloperidol (Haldol), are the medications of choice. ADHD frequently occurs concomitantly with Tourette's syndrome.

38. **(1)** Involvement of more than one area of the CNS, age 15–60 years, two or more separate episodes of symptoms involving different sites, or a gradual progression over at least 6 months meets the criteria for multiple sclerosis.

39. **(2)** It would be most important to do a formal hearing acuity test on a child with a history of bacterial meningitis due to the use of ototoxic medications used to treat the disease. A vision test should be done on all children but is not specific for a child with a history of meningitis. A lumbar puncture or ECG would not be appropriate.

40. **(3)** The most likely causes of seizures in adolescents and young adults are idiopathic disease, trauma, and substance abuse. Congenital abnormalities are the likely cause of seizures in newborns. In children <6 years old, metabolic causes, CNS infection, and fever can cause seizures. Trauma, malignant tumor, and CVA are likely causes for seizures in the elderly.

41. **(2)** The recommended dose for acetaminophen is no more than 4 gm/day. This client may be experiencing analgesic rebound headache. Appropriate prophylactic medications for migraine include β-blockers (propanolol), tricyclic antidepressants (amitriptyline), selective serotonin reuptake inhibitors (fluoxetine), monoamine oxidase inhibitors (phenelzine), and calcium channel blockers (verapamil). It is not necessary to order expensive tests for clients with migraine or tension headache. Usually, a careful, thorough history is sufficient.

42. **(3)** The most common finding in children with meningococcemia (71%) is fever and a purpuric rash. The rash of rubella, Lyme disease, and roseola is finer and none of these problems is life threatening, as is meningococcemia, making it a "do not miss" diagnosis.

43. **(4)** This is a common complaint of the client with subarachnoid hemorrhage headache. This client should be immediately referred to a neurologic surgeon.

44. **(3)** The speech center (Broca's area) is most often located in the left hemisphere. The client would experience weakness of the right side of the body and a right-sided visual deficit as well.

45. **(4)** Options #1, #2, and #3 all precipitate the development of an embolus that can result in an embolic stroke (brain accident). Diabetes will precipitate occlusive disease of the cerebral arteries and the possible development of a thrombotic stroke, not an embolic stroke.

46. **(2)** A simple partial seizure is characterized by unilateral paresthesia, numbness and tingling, and spastic movement of the extremities (old term is Jacksonian seizure). There is no loss of consciousness or incontinence of bowel or bladder.

47. **(3)** The characteristics of a benign tremor are a fine to coarse rhythmic tremor of the hands and feet that increases with activity, and may be absent at rest. Frequently, the voice is also involved. An ingestion of a small amount of alcohol may decrease symptoms.

48. **(1)** The description is that of a petit mal or absence seizure. The client should have a neurologic work-up to determine the cause of the seizures.

49. **(2)** It is important to determine if the client has stayed on his medication schedule. The symptoms may be the result of missed medication, or may also occur due to too much medication. This is especially true with pyridostigmine bromide (Mestinon). This should be addressed first. The symptoms may also be exacerbated by exercise and heat.

50. **(1)** The clinical presentation is classic of Horner's syndrome, especially the lack of sweating, or anhidrosis, on the ipsilateral, or same, side of the face and neck as the eye symptoms. The client needs to be referred for further neurologic work-up.

51. **(4)** Homonymous hemianopia is the loss of the vision in one half of the visual field. Either the right or left field of vision may be affected. It is most often caused by a lesion or pathology to the optic tract or the occipital lobe.

Pharmacology

52. **(1)** Elderly clients are particularly susceptible to postherpetic neuralgia, which is pain at the site that may last for months or years. Discomfort is alleviated by pain medication. Systemic corticosteroids may reduce the occurrence of postherpetic neuralgia. Usually, 60 mg prednisone qd for 2 weeks with a rapid taper is prescribed. Acyclovir is used for immunocompromised clients.

53. **(2)** Although most medication is discontinued after 4 years of no seizure activity, this should be confirmed by an EEG. Not all seizure clients require medication; referral to and monitoring by a neurologist are appropriate.

54. **(3)** Scopolamine patches are placed behind the ear and provide medication for 3 days. Meclizine (Antivert) is dosed 12.5–25 mg PO tid to qid. The correct dose for dimenhydrinate (Dramamine) is 50 mg tid or qid. Compazine is dosed 5–10 mg q4h prn.

55. **(2)** The correct dose is ergotamine (Ergostat) 2 mg SL. Sumatriptan (Imitrex) is given SC or 100 mg PO. Ketorolac (Toradol) is dosed 30–60 mg IM. Amitriptyline (Elavil) is not used for abortive therapy.

56. **(2)** Hyperplasia of the gums is a common side effect of phenytoin (Dilantin). The child should have regular dental prophylactic hygiene to deal with the problem.

57. **(2)** Trihexyphenidyl (Artane) is an anticholinergic medication. Geriatric men frequently have problems with benign prostatic hypertrophy and are more likely to develop a problem with urinary retention when on Artane.

Gastrointestinal & Liver

Physical Examination & Diagnostic Tests

1. The nurse practitioner is preparing to examine the abdomen of a client. What is the correct sequence in which to conduct the examination?

    1. Inspection, palpation, percussion, auscultation.

    2. Palpation, percussion, auscultation, inspection.

    3. Percussion, palpation, auscultation, inspection.

    4. Inspection, auscultation, percussion, palpation.

2. When obtaining a history from a client with abdominal pain, the following areas are to be examined:

    1. The quality, quantity, and location of the pain.

    2. The location, the way in which the pain developed (gradually over hours or suddenly), whether the pain has changed since onset, and associated symptoms.

    3. If the pain is referred to other sites, what aggravates of alleviates the pain, and the client's past medical history and medication history.

    4. All of the above.

3. To test for a positive obturator sign in a client with abdominal pain, the nurse practitioner:

    1. Passively rotates the right hip from the 90-degree hip/knee flexion position.

    2. Asks the client to take a deep breath while applying pressure in the area of the gallbladder.

    3. Percusses over the costovertebral angles.

    4. Positions the supine client with hips flexed and auscultates for bowel sounds, then palpates the abdomen, beginning with superficial palpation of nontender areas.

4. Serologic features* of acute hepatitis B are:

   1. HBsAg, HBeAg, and a high titer of immunoglobulin M (IgM) anti-HBc.

   2. HBeAg- and HBsAg-positive.

   3. HBeAg- and HBsAg-negative.

   4. IgM anti-HBc- (high titer) HBsAg-negative.

5. The nurse practitioner is performing a physical examination on a middle-aged man. The history reveals the client's father died of colon cancer. What diagnostics are used to screen this client?

   1. Barium enema and upper gastrointestinal (GI) series.

   2. Carcinoembryonic antigen (CEA) titer.

   3. Proctoscopy and biopsy.

   4. Colonoscopy and Hemoccult.

6. The anti-HCV test indicates the client has:

   1. Acute hepatitis C.

   2. Chronic hepatitis C.

   3. Resolved hepatitis C.

   4. Acute, chronic, or resolved hepatitis C.

7. The diagnosis of early acute pancreatitis will be considered by the nurse practitioner based on physical findings and the following laboratory result:

   1. A white blood cell (WBC) count of 10,300/mm^3.

   2. A serum amylase of 75 U/L.

   3. A serum amylase of 300 U/L.

   4. A serum lipase of 75 U/L.

8. A middle-aged woman who is overweight has right upper quadrant pain that radiates to her right subscapular area and is severe and persistent. She is also experiencing anorexia, nausea, and a fever. For her last meal, she ate a double quarter-pound hamburger with cheese, French fries, and a vanilla shake. Based on this information, the nurse practitioner examines the abdomen and percusses for costovertebral angle tenderness. The abdomen is tender in the right upper quadrant and, if there is a positive:

   1. Obturator sign, the client has appendicitis.

   2. Costovertebral angle tenderness, the client has a urinary tract infection.

   3. Murphy's sign, the client has cholecystitis.

   4. McBurney's sign, the client has a strangulated hernia.

9. A client complains of extreme pain in his abdomen and points to the right lower quadrant. In examining the acute abdomen, the nurse practitioner would:

   1. Immediately order a WBC, and abdominal x-ray.

   2. Percuss the abdomen in all quadrants followed by auscultation and gentle palpation.

   3. Palpate the right side of the abdomen first, paying close attention for guarding in the area of pain.

   4. Palpate the left side of the abdomen then gently palpate the right side noting guarding and tenderness.

Disorders

10. Diarrhea is often associated with:

    1. Infectious gastroenteritis, inflammatory bowel disease, diverticulitis.

    2. Diseases of the colon or rectum.

    3. Fever and abdominal pain in sexually transmitted diseases.

    4. Dysuria and flank pain in urinary tract infections.

11. Esophageal pain may radiate to the:

    1. Infrascapular area.

    2. Right shoulder.

    3. Neck and left arm.

    4. Periumbilical area.

---

*HBsAg, hepatitis B surface antigen; HBeAg, hepatitis B e antigen; anti-HBc, antibody to hepatitis B core antigen.

12. The most important goal of assessing a client with abdominal pain is to:

    1. Palpate the area of pain right away.

    2. Rule out emergent conditions.

    3. Determine the exact etiology of the pain on the first visit for every client.

    4. Determine what tests to order.

13. The nurse practitioner suspects peritonitis in a client, the best action is to:

    1. Percuss over the costovertebral angle and watch for signs of pain.

    2. Perform a rectal exam and test the stool for blood.

    3. Auscultate the abdomen for decreased bowel sounds.

    4. Palpate for a tense, hard abdomen and check for a positive obturator sign.

14. Which of the following suggests an emergent condition?

    1. Pain in an adolescent that is rated as 5 on a scale of 1–10 and is relieved by having a bowel movement.

    2. Pain that is progressive, localized, and steady for more than 6 hours and accompanied by rebound tenderness and guarding.

    3. Pain in an adolescent girl that is sudden in onset and localized in the lower right or left quadrant and lasts 14–36 hours.

    4. Pain that follows the onset of vomiting and diarrhea.

15. Under what circumstances should peptic ulcer disease (PUD) **not** be treated empirically before diagnostic studies are done? When the client's ulcer pain:

    1. Awakens him or her from sleep early in the morning.

    2. Can be relieved by food, antacids, or vomiting.

    3. Is worsened by food ingestion.

    4. Is atypical or occurs with anemia, blood in the stool, or weight loss.

16. A careful history of a client with a chief complaint of diarrhea reveals that this adult has recurrent abdominal pain and diarrhea that alternates with constipation. The most likely diagnosis is:

    1. Drug-induced diarrhea.

    2. Inflammatory bowel disease.

    3. Giardiasis.

    4. Irritable bowel syndrome (IBS).

17. Clients with dysphagia due to motility disorders:

    1. Usually have more difficulty swallowing solids than liquids.

    2. Can have a stricture due to esophagitis following a long history of reflux disorder.

    3. Usually complain of cold liquids causing pain.

    4. Can have marked weight loss.

18. The pathogenesis of gastroesophageal reflux disease (GERD) is:

    1. Frequent and excessive retrograde movement of stomach contents into the esophagus due to an abnormal lower esophageal sphincter (LES) function.

    2. A hiatal hernia that leads to the esophageal irritation and inflammation.

    3. Reflux of the gastric contents after meals when a client is in the upright position often after a period of vigorous exercise.

    4. Initiated by erosion of the gastrointestinal mucosa into the LES, causing weakening of LES pressure and a burning sensation in the stomach.

19. A client comes to emergent care concerned about pain and swelling in his groin. He tells the nurse practitioner that his doctor told him that he has an incarcerated hernia. The examination of the client reveals a hernia that:

    1. Easily moves back and forth across the abdominal wall.

    2. Protrudes from the groin area and cannot be reduced into the abdomen.

    3. Is very painful to palpation with significant abdominal swelling.

    4. Decreases in size when the client increases intra-abdominal pressure.

20. Which of the following findings would indicate a need for endoscopy in clients with PUD?

    1. All new cases of dyspepsia.

    2. Symptoms persisting after 6–8 weeks of therapy.

    3. All clients with dyspepsia who smoke and use alcohol.

    4. Good response to empiric treatment after 7–10 days.

21. The nurse practitioner's understanding of which principle will be helpful in educating clients with GERD?

    1. A hiatal hernia is always a coexisting and major contributing factor.

    2. The lower esophageal sphincter (LES) has become a poor antireflux barrier.

    3. The amount of acid reflux is dependent on a familial tendency for GERD.

    4. Overeating and use of caffeine and alcohol cause GERD.

22. Inflammatory toxigenic gastrointestinal illness is characterized by:

    1. Fecal leukocytes, secretory diarrhea, site: colon.

    2. No fecal leukocytes, watery diarrhea, site: distal small bowel.

    3. Fecal leukocytes, site: colon, secretory diarrhea.

    4. Fecal leukocytes, watery diarrhea, site: colon.

23. Clinical features of IBS include which of the following?

    1. IBS affects men more then women.

    2. IBS affects children more than those in early adulthood.

    3. IBS affects women more than men.

    4. IBS predominantly affects elderly clients more than those in early adulthood.

24. The nurse practitioner understands that hepatitis B can be transmitted in blood and blood products. Another common mode of transmission of hepatitis B is:

    1. Respiratory contact.

    2. Contaminated fluid.

    3. Fecal–oral route.

    4. Perinatal exposure.

25. A young adult client presents to the nurse practitioner's office with a chief complaint of intermittent heartburn, which became worse 2 months ago from job stress. The discomfort is worse after eating and at night and is relieved temporarily by antacids. The client also states that several times in the last 14 days he has regurgitated very bitter tasting material into the mouth. The physical exam by the nurse practitioner is unremarkable. The nurse practitioner's most likely diagnosis is:

    1. Viral esophagitis.

    2. Irritable bowel syndrome.

    3. Gastroesophageal reflux disease.

    4. Carcinoma of the esophagus.

26. All of the following should be referred to an internist for management due to the high rate of chronic hepatitis **except**:

    1. Hepatitis A.

    2. Hepatitis B.

    3. Hepatitis C.

    4. Hepatitis D.

27. An indirect inguinal hernia:

    1. Is a portion of the bowel or omentum that protrudes directly through the floor of the inguinal canal and exits through the external inguinal ring.

2. Occurs mainly in middle and later years.

3. Is due to a weakness in the abdominal structure.

4. Passes through the internal abdominal ring, traverses the spermatic cord through the inguinal canal, and exits at the external inguinal ring.

28. Which is true about enterobiasis?

   1. The parasite is in the soil and enters the body through the feet. It can cause anemia.

   2. The parasite causes pruritus around the anus because the gravid females exit through the anus at night and lay eggs on the skin. The human is the only host of this parasite.

   3. The eggs of this parasite enter the body by ingestion of dirt (pica) or dirt on unwashed vegetables that contain the eggs, or through water containing eggs.

   4. This parasite is a protozoan. The source is usually contaminated water but it is spread from person to person by oral–fecal contamination.

29. The therapeutic energy diet modification in GERD consists of which type of diet?

   1. Low energy.

   2. Energy controlled.

   3. High energy.

   4. Small feedings.

30. Nonpharmacologic management of GERD includes which of the following:

   1. Weight reduction and sleep with head of bed elevated 4–6 inches with blocks.

   2. Lying down and resting after meals, and weight reduction.

   3. Drinking large amounts of fluids with meals and avoiding alcohol.

   4. Avoiding mint, orange juice, and high-energy diet.

31. An organism associated with etiology of PUD is:

   1. *Streptococcus pneumoniae.*

   2. *Helicobacter pylori.*

   3. *Moraxella catarrhalis.*

   4. *Staphylococcus aureus.*

32. The most common cause of cirrhosis is:

   1. Hepatitis A.

   2. Hepatitis B.

   3. Hepatitis D.

   4. Alcoholic hepatitis.

33. Prolapse of a vascular anal cushion through the anal canal with resultant entrapment by the internal anal sphincter describes a:

   1. Prolapse of the rectal mucosa.

   2. Hemorrhoid.

   3. Tumor.

   4. Hernia.

34. An acute febrile illness with jaundice, anorexia, malaise, and an incubation period of 45–160 days; having a chronic and an acute form; and transmitted by parenteral, sexual, and perinatal routes describes:

   1. Hepatitis A.

   2. Hepatitis B.

   3. Hepatitis C.

   4. Hepatitis D.

35. A client presents to the nurse practitioner's office with a history of cholelithiasis. Which client complaining of increased pain would require immediate admission to the hospital for possible prompt intervention?

   1. A client who is human immunodeficiency virus positive (HIV+).

   2. A 75-year-old diabetic.

   3. A client who is 5 weeks pregnant.

   4. A client who is vomiting and has a slight fever.

36. An older adult male presents to the nurse practitioner for evaluation of "heartburn." The client states that he has been taking antacids and an oral histamine (H_2) blocker. The client states that, after eating, he feels like there is a knot in his stomach. He also gives a history of being a cigar smoker. What differential diagnosis must the nurse practitioner consider first?

    1. Gastric ulcer.

    2. Acid reflux.

    3. Esophageal tumor.

    4. Lung tumor.

37. An older adult male presents to the nurse practitioner complaining of weakness and vomiting. The client gives a history of "several" drinks per day for the past 12 years. The nurse practitioner observes that the client's lips appear to have dark blood on them. What emergent condition does the nurse practitioner suspect?

    1. Seizure disorder.

    2. Cerebral hemorrhage.

    3. Pancreatitis.

    4. Esophageal varices.

38. A usually benign diagnosis that can result in small bowel obstruction and infarction and that requires immediate referral to a surgeon is:

    1. Gastric ulcer.

    2. Endometriosis.

    3. Hernia.

    4. Ectopic pregnancy.

39. A young adult female presents to the nurse practitioner for evaluation of 2 days of increasing crampy, abdominal pain. She states that she also has some mild nausea and anorexia, and a low-grade fever. The client states that the pain is periumbilical. Her STAT complete blood count (CBC) reveals a slightly elevated white count but is otherwise normal. The nurse practitioner's next step for the care of this client is:

    1. Referral to a gynecologist for evaluation of a possible ectopic pregnancy.

    2. Referral to surgeon for evaluation of possible appendicitis.

    3. Observe the client overnight and reassess the next day.

    4. Place the client on a clear liquid diet and have her watch for increasing symptoms.

40. A previously benign condition that can cause a client severe rectal pain and be the cause of an emergency visit to the nurse practitioner is:

    1. Hookworms.

    2. Pinworms.

    3. Thrombosed hemorrhoid.

    4. Cystitis.

41. An elderly client presents with fever, leukocytosis, lower left quadrant pain, and diarrhea alternating with constipation. The nurse practitioner would make the diagnosis of:

    1. Appendicitis.

    2. Diverticulitis.

    3. Irritable bowel syndrome.

    4. Pancreatitis.

42. Which clients would be the lowest risk for developing diverticular disease?

    1. Vegetarians.

    2. Type A personality.

    3. The elderly.

    4. Fad dieters.

43. The nurse practitioner knows that the following symptom is characteristic of left-sided colon cancer:

    1. Anemia.

    2. Tenesmus.

    3. Bright red rectal bleeding.

    4. Change in bowel habits.

44. The nurse practitioner knows that a history of pancolonic ulcerative colitis requires careful surveillance because of an increased risk of:

    1. Colon cancer.

    2. Anemia.

    3. Depression.

    4. Perforation.

45. Which is true of PUD in the elderly?

    1. Smoking does not increase the risk of PUD.

    2. Duodenal ulcers are more common in the elderly.

    3. Perforation is a rare complication.

    4. Weight loss and anorexia are often the only symptoms.

46. Which is true of early cancer of the esophagus in the elderly client?

    1. Alcoholism and smoking increase the risk for cancer of the esophagus.

    2. It is usually an adenocarcinoma.

    3. Dysphagia for liquids, cough, and hoarseness are early symptoms.

    4. A boring-type midchest pain indicates mediastinal involvement and requires immediate surgery.

47. A client has a history of colon polyps. The nurse practitioner knows:

    1. Polyps of the cecum are most likely to be malignant.

    2. Polyps <1 cm are more suspicious for malignancy.

    3. Villous polyps are rarely malignant.

    4. Sessile polyps are more likely to be malignant than pedunculated.

48. The nurse is interpreting the notation of "string sign" on an upper GI series performed on an infant. This is associated with a diagnosis of:

    1. Intussusception.

    2. Aganglionic congenital megacolon.

    3. Pyloric stenosis.

    4. Esophageal atresia.

49. The nurse practitioner identifies which of these conditions as most conducive to the development of metabolic aklalosis in a child?

    1. Severe anxiety resulting in hyperventilation.

    2. Excessive vomiting related to gastroenteritis.

    3. Depressed respirations from excessive narcotics ingestion.

    4. Decreased renal function with glomeruli damage.

50. The nurse practitioner in the emergency room examines a child who has severe diarrhea and vomiting resulting in dehydration. One of the orders is to start an IV of 500 ml normal saline with 10 mEq of potassium to run at 23 ml/hr. The child is NPO. What would be a priority action prior to initiating the IV fluid?

    1. Weigh the child.

    2. Obtain serum electrolyte values.

    3. Make sure the child is voiding adequately.

    4. Determine amount of previous fluid loss.

51. A young child is brought to the clinic by her mother complaining of abrupt onset of vomiting followed by over ten liquid stools with mucus for the past 48 hours. The temperature is 100°F orally. The stool smear by the nurse practitioner is negative for WBC. The most likely etiologic pathogen for this young child's gastroenteritis is:

    1. Rotavirus.

    2. *Shigella dysenteriae*.

    3. *Campylobacter jejuni*.

    4. *Salmonella*.

52. The symptoms of abdominal discomfort associated with meals, diarrhea or constipation, anorexia, weight loss, failure to grow, and failure to develop sexually are most associated with:

    1. Ulcerative colitis.

    2. Irritable bowel syndrome.

    3. Carcinoma of the colon.

    4. Crohn's disease.

53. What is the most consistent finding in clients with acute appendicitis?

    1. An elevated WBC count.

    2. High fever.

    3. Periumbilical dull pain.

    4. Nausea and vomiting.

54. What question by the nurse practitioner would be appropriate to ask the parents of an infant who is suspected of having intussusception?

    1. "Does the infant have clay-colored stools?"

    2. "Does the infant have projectile vomiting?"

    3. "Does the infant have constant abdominal pain?"

    4. "Does the infant have red currant jelly stools?"

55. The major symptom of reflux in infants is:

    1. Vomiting or regurgitation, especially after feeding.

    2. Poor weight gain in infants.

    3. Hyperirritability and refusal of feeding.

    4. Fever and diarrhea.

56. Medical therapy for young infants with vomiting or regurgitation of GERD consists of the following:

    1. Small feedings and burping after each feeding.

    2. Placing the infant prone after feedings.

    3. Placing the infant supine in the infant seat after feedings.

    4. Thickening the feedings.

57. A baby is born to a mother who is HBsAg-positive. Which is true regarding the management of the baby?

    1. No prophylaxis against hepatitis B needs to be given to the baby.

    2. This baby should have one dose of hepatitis B immunoglobulin administered.

    3. This baby should have one dose of hepatitis B vaccine administered by the nurse practitioner.

    4. This baby should have one dose of hepatitis B immunoglobulin and a complete three-dose immunization of hepatitis B vaccine administered.

58. What physical findings would lead the nurse practitioner to suspect Hirschsprung's disease in a 6-month-old infant?

    1. Rectal bleeding, diarrhea, and prolonged jaundice at birth.

    2. History of constipation and current abdominal distention.

    3. Irritability, vomiting, and dehydration.

    4. History of colic, bloody diarrhea, and nausea.

59. A common cause of acute abdominal pain in children <5 years old is:

    1. Appendicitis.

    2. Intussusception.

    3. Incarcerated hernias.

    4. Gastroenteritis.

60. The nurse practitioner understands that common causes of recurrent abdominal pain in children are:

    1. Intussusception, gastroenteritis, peptic ulcer disease, and right lower lobe pneumonia.

2. Psychogenic pain, mittelschmerz, trauma, and urinary tract infections.

3. Parasitic infestation, musculoskeletal pain, dysmenorrhea, and chronic stool retention.

4. Incarcerated hernias, appendicitis, inflammatory bowel disease, and ectopic pregnancy.

61. An adolescent client is brought to the nurse practitioner by his mother for evaluation after a dirt-bike accident. The client states that the bike flipped over and struck him on the abdomen. There is a hematoma noted just below the left anterior rib area. In this case, the nurse practitioner must be particularly aware of the possibility of:

1. Ruptured bowel due to blunt trauma.

2. Bladder trauma.

3. Hypovolemia due to ruptured spleen.

4. Dysrhythmias.

62. A 2-year-old Asian-American child comes to the clinic with her parents and infant brother. The chief complaint is abdominal pain and flatulence and diarrhea after eating. Until 3 months ago, she had continued to be breast-fed twice a day. The nurse practitioner would suspect:

1. Irritable bowel syndrome.

2. Hirschsprung's disease.

3. Lactose intolerance.

4. Food allergy.

63. A 10-year-old girl comes to the clinic with complaints of nausea, vomiting, and right upper quadrant pain during vigorous play; she is also more tired than usual. Serologic test for IgM antibodies are ordered to rule out:

1. Cholecystitis.

2. Hepatitis A.

3. Infectious mononucleosis.

4. Hepatitis B.

64. A 3-year-old presents to the clinic with diffuse abdominal pain, irritability, and a low-grade fever. The mother states the toddler has not had a bowel movement since the previous morning. Physical exam reveals umbilical tenderness, guarding, and hypoactive bowel sounds. The nurse practitioner's next step is to:

1. Refer to physician/surgeon for further evaluation.

2. Assess for rebound tenderness and do a rectal exam.

3. Prescribe a pediatric Fleets.

4. Assess dietary intake for past 24 hours.

65. A 2-year-old child is seen for a foreign body in the GI tract. The nurse practitioner pays particular attention to the size of the object, knowing that passing the ligament of Treitz is difficult with objects larger than:

1. 5 cm.

2. 8 cm.

3. 10 cm.

4. 12 cm.

66. A 2-month-old infant presents with coughing that results in emesis that occurs when laid supine after eating. The infant has lost 1.3 lb since birth, with a birth weight of 7.5 lb. The nurse practitioner focuses her assessment toward the possibility of:

1. Suck-swallow incoordination.

2. Gastroesophageal reflux.

3. Tracheoesophageal fistula.

4. Infantile colic.

Pharmacology

67. An adult client has been treated on and off for PUD for the past 12 years. He has always responded quickly to cimetidine (Tagamet) and antacids. He continues to smoke. He presents to the nurse practitioner's office with severe epigastric pain, weakness, and lightheaded feelings. The stool guaiac is positive and his hemoglobin is 11.2 gm/dl. His weight has decreased slowly over the past 6 months for unknown reasons. Based on this information, what should the nurse practitioner do next?

    1. Refill his medications.

    2. Give medications and refer to smoking cessation clinic.

    3. Discontinue cimetidine and start omeprazole (Prilosec).

    4. Consult with physician.

68. The nurse practitioner is examining a 30-year-old obese man who is complaining of indigestion and heartburn with a strong acid taste in the mouth about an hour after meals. The history is negative for chronic illnesses. A diagnosis of GERD is made. The best way to treat this client is:

    1. Lie down after meals, eat five smaller meals per day.

    2. Probanthine 15 mg tid 30 minutes prior to eating.

    3. Decrease weight, ranitidine (Zantac) 150 mg bid.

    4. Omeprazole (Prilosec) 40 mg once a day, antacids.

69. Which of the following would be prescribed as initial treatment for uncomplicated PUD?

    1. Cimetidine (Tagamet) 400 mg bid.

    2. Doxepin (Sinequan) 25 mg qhs.

    3. Omeprazole (Prilosec) 20 mg qd.

    4. Pirenzepine 50 mg tid.

70. Which drug would be most useful for the nurse practitioner to prescribe for a client to prevent ulcers due to nonsteroidal anti-inflammatory drugs (NSAIDs)?

    1. Misoprostol (Cytotec).

    2. Cimetidine (Tagamet).

    3. Doxepin (Sinequan).

    4. Pirenzepine.

71. After percutaneous or permucosal exposure to an HBsAg-positive source:

    1. In an unvaccinated person, begin the hepatitis B series.

    2. In a known hepatitis B responder with an adequate response, no treatment is necessary.

    3. In a known hepatitis B responder with inadequate anti-hepatitis B surface antigen, give hepatitis B immune globulin (HBIG) and initiate a new hepatitis B vaccine series.

    4. In an unknown hepatitis B responder who completed the entire hepatitis B vaccine series, give a hepatitis B booster.

72. *Helicobacter pylori* has been found to be a causative factor in many cases of PUD. Successful treatment requires therapy with which regimen?

    1. Combination of H_2-blockers, antacids, and omeprazole (Prilosec).

    2. Combination of Pepto-Bismol, amoxicillin (Amoxil), and metronidazole (Flagyl).

    3. Combination of lifestyle changes, Pepto-Bismol, and cimetidine (Tagmet).

    4. Combination of H_2 blocker, amoxicillin (Amoxil), and antacid.

73. A primary therapy for clients with mild ulcerative colitis is:

    1. Metronidazole (Flagyl).

    2. Sulfasalazine (Azulfidine).

    3. Amoxicillin (Amoxil).

    4. Cephalexin (Keflex).

74. The stepwise approach to management of GERD is:

1. Lifestyle changes and antacids as needed and cimetidine (Tagamet) 800 mg qhs.

2. Lifestyle changes and antacids as needed followed by lifestyle changes plus ranitidine (Zantac) 150 mg bid.

3. Lifestyle changes and antacids as needed followed by lifestyle changes plus omeprazole (Prilosec) 20 mg qd.

4. Cisapride (Propulsid) 10 mg taken 15 minutes before meals and at bedtime; Lifestyle changes can be added if this therapy is not effective.

75. After exposure to household or sexual contacts with hepatitis A, the nurse practitioner would:

1. Give immunoglobulin 0.02 mg/kg as soon as possible but no later than 2 weeks after exposure.

2. Give one dose of HBIG and immunoglobulin 0.02 mg/kg as soon as possible.

3. Give immunoglobulin 0.02 mg/kg and two doses of HBIG.

4. Understand that no injections are needed.

76. Shigellosis is treated by:

1. No medication intervention, careful toileting and bathroom sanitation, and keeping the perineal area clean.

2. Symptomatic treatment and antidiarrheal agents.

3. Symptomatic treatment and trimethoprim-sulfamethoxazole (Septra) dosed for age and weight bid × 5 days.

4. Boiling water and quinacrine (Atabrine) 100 mg PO tid × 5 days.

77. Pharmacologic management of nausea and vomiting includes:

1. Emetrol 15–30 ml PO in adults.

2. Promethazine (Phenergan) 25 mg for children over 6 years old and adults.

3. Hydroxyzine hydrochloride (Vistaril) 1 mg IM for adults and children 12 years old and older.

4. Trimethobenzamide (Tigan) 10 mg PO prn for adults.

78. The two major factors that lead to disruption of the gastrointestinal mucosa with subsequent development of an ulceration are:

1. Alcohol consumption and NSAIDs.

2. NSAIDs.

3. NSAIDs and *Helicobacter pylori*.

4. *Helicobacter pylori* and smoking.

79. A young woman presents with a history of recent unprotected sexual activity with a partner now diagnosed with hepatitis B. She is currently asymptomatic and she does not recall having a vaccine in the past. The best action for the nurse practitioner is:

1. Draw a hepatitis B e antibody test (anti-HBe).

2. Administer one dose of HBIG.

3. Administer two doses of HBIG and initiate vaccination.

4. Administer one dose of HBIG and initiate vaccination.

80. What condition is a contraindication for the administration of the hepatitis B vaccine?

1. Pregnancy.

2. Lactating mothers.

3. Severe hypersensitivity.

4. Age >60 years.

81. A 78-year-old client is diagnosed with enterocolitis and the physician prescribes vancomycin (Vancocin) 125 mg PO qid. The nurse practitioner will follow the progress of the client. What areas will be monitored with regard to the medication tolerance?

    1. CBC, platelet count, clotting studies.

    2. Serum creatinine, blood urea nitrogen (BUN), hearing changes.

    3. Serum electrolytes, urinalysis, ataxia.

    4. Changes in bowel habits, diarrhea, electrocardiographic changes.

82. A client with PUD is treated with a regimen that includes bismuth subsalicylate (Pepto-Bismol), tetracycline, and metronidazole (Flagyl). The client calls the nurse practitioner to report that his stools are unusually dark. He is not experiencing any gastric discomfort, orthostatic hypotension, or increased lethargy. The nurse practitioner's interpretation of this information is:

    1. He is probably bleeding and should come in immediately.

    2. He ate something to affect the color of his stool.

    3. His stools are dark secondary to the Pepto-Bismol.

    4. The stool discoloration is due to the metronidazole (Flagyl).

83. A 3-year-old child is seen in the clinic for chronic, relapsing diarrhea. A stool for ova and parasites is obtained and is positive for *Giardia*. The most appropriate pharmacologic intervention would be:

    1. Ampicillin (Omnipen).

    2. Erythromycin (E-Mycin).

    3. Metronidazole (Flagyl).

    4. Tetracycline (Achromycin).

Answers & Rationales

Physical Examination & Diagnostic Tests

1. **(4)** Inspection and auscultation should be conducted first in order to prevent undue guarding. If the examination is painful initially, the client is going to be very uncomfortable with allowing the examiner to continue.

2. **(4)** All of the information is important in sorting out the cause of abdominal pain. The location and character may help identify the origin of the pain. Abrupt onset of pain usually has a different etiology than pain that develops over hours. Whether or not the pain has changed since onset can help in determining if a larger area of the abdomen is becoming involved or if the pain is subsiding. Both visceral and parietal pain can be referred to remote sites along shared nerve pathways. Aggravating and alleviating factors can provide clues as to the origin of the pain. Fever, chills, vomiting, diarrhea, constipation, and urogenital-associated symptoms are important in determining the cause of the abdominal pain. Past medical history and medication history can give clues to known conditions and to medications that may be causing the symptoms or are being used for conditions that can cause abdominal pain. For example, a client taking ranitidine (Zantac) may fail to mention a history of GERD.

3. **(1)** If abdominal pain results from passive internal rotation of the right hip from the 90-degree hip/knee flexion position, the client has a positive obturator sign, which is suggestive of appendicitis. In a positive Murphy's sign (Option #2), pain and a brief inspiratory arrest result when a client takes a deep breath while the examiner applies pressure over the gallbladder. This is suggestive of cholecystitis. Percussion over the costovertebral angles that elicits pain is a positive costovertebral angle tenderness suggestive of pyelonephritis. Positioning of the client in a supine position with hips flexed and then auscultating and palpating the abdomen, beginning with light palpation in nontender areas, is the sequence for examining the abdomen.

4. **(1)** HBsAg is found in active or chronic hepatitis B disease. HBeAg indicates active replication of the virus. IgM anti-HBsAg indicates chronic disease. Positive HBsAg indicates chronic disease. And negative HBsAg indicates prior exposure.

5. **(4)** These are standard diagnostics used for screening a client with a high risk of colon cancer. CEA is used more to determine recurrence of cancer; barium enema, upper GI, and proctoscopy do not provide sufficiently reliable information for detecting the malignancy.

6. **(4)** This is the surface marker for hepatitis C. At present there is no way to differentiate the diffuse forms of hepatitis C, as the viremia level is well below the threshold of most assays.

7. **(3)** Options #2 and #3 are almost identical. (*Note: use the testing strategy; both are wrong or one is the correct answer.*) In acute pancreatitis the serum amylase increases within 3–6 hours of onset. The serum lipase elevates after the increase in amylase. (Normal levels of serum amylase in adults are 50–180 U/L; those of serum lipase are 55–417 U/L.)

8. **(3)** The history, right upper quadrant pain that radiates to the right subscapular area, and positive Murphy's sign are all commonly associated with cholecystitis. A positive obturator sign at McBurney's point is a sign associated with appendicitis. Clients with strangulated hernias have colicky abdominal pain, nausea, vomiting, abdominal distention, and hyperperistalsis. Those with reducible hernias are asymptomatic or have only mild pain.

9. **(4)** Always palpate the nontender areas first, before going to the area of pain and tenderness. Option #2 is not described in the correct order of assessing an abdomen, which is inspection, auscultation, percussion, and palpation. Although Option #1 may be done, it does not answer what the question is asking.

Disorders

10. **(1)** Diarrhea is a common symptom in infectious gastroenteritis, inflammatory bowel disease, diverticulitis, and early intestinal obstruction. Diseases of the colon or rectum are often associated with constipation that clearly precedes the onset of abdominal pain. With sexually transmitted diseases, abdominal pain can often occur with vaginal discharge or bleeding and sometimes irregular menses. Dysuria, flank pain, hematuria, and urinary frequency are common signs and symptoms of upper or lower urinary tract infections or ureteral calculi.

11. **(3)** Esophageal pain may radiate to the neck and left arm. Gallbladder pain can radiate to the infrascapular area, diaphragm pain to the right shoulder, and the pain of appendicitis to the periumbilical area.

12. **(2)** The most important goal in evaluating a client who presents with abdominal pain is to rule out emergent conditions. Palpation is done after auscultation. Begin in an area away from the site of the pain. It is important to rule out emergent causes and ideal to make an exact diagnosis every time. However, due to the sometimes complicated nature of abdominal pain, it is not always possible to do this. Ordering appropriate laboratory tests is important but is not the most important goal.

13. **(4)** A tense, hard abdomen; verbal refusal or severe pain when asked to jump; or a positive obturator sign are positive peritoneal signs. Costovertebral angle tenderness is a sign of a renal disorder. Stool for occult blood is not a test for peritonitis. Decreased bowel sounds could be present in appendicitis or bowel obstruction but are not a peritoneal sign.

14. **(2)** Localized pain that steadily increases for 6 or more hours with rebound tenderness and guarding could be caused by an emergent condition, such as appendicitis or ruptured ectopic pregnancy. Pain in an adolescent girl that is relieved by having a bowel movement could be constipation; pain that is sudden in onset and is in the right lower quadrant, lasting 14–36 hours, could be mittelschmerz, if the girl is midway through her menstrual cycle. Pain that follows the onset of vomiting and diarrhea usually occurs in gastroenteritis.

15. **(4)** Atypical pain or pain that occurs with hematochezia, anemia, or weight loss could be caused by a disorder other than peptic ulcer, such as gastric cancer. Or the client's ulcer could be bleeding. Pain that awakens a client early in the morning from sleep or is relieved or worsened by food ingestion is typical of peptic ulcer pain.

16. **(4)** IBS presents with abdominal pain and/or altered bowel habits. These symptoms can be aggravated by psychological stresses. Symptoms disappear while sleeping. Bacterial or viral gastroenteritis presents as abdominal pain with diarrhea and vomiting of abrupt onset. Drug-induced diarrhea follows initiation of drug therapy, and in this situation, there is no mention of previous drug therapy. In inflammatory bowel disease, nocturnal diarrhea and

abdominal pain are often accompanied by rectal fistula, fever, and/or skin lesions. Diarrhea occurring with giardiasis is malodorous. Weight loss occurs over a period of weeks.

17. **(3)** Cold liquids causing pain, dysphagia for both liquids and solids, and repeated swallowing or performance of a rapid Valsalva maneuver that helps food or liquid pass into the stomach are experiences reported by clients with dysphagia caused by a motility disorder. Those with dysphagia due to obstruction have more difficulty swallowing solids than liquids, can have a stricture due to esophagitis resulting from longstanding esophageal reflux, and may report marked weight loss if a tumor is present.

18. **(1)** Esophageal inflammation caused by excessive reflux that overpowers the normal mucosal defense mechanism leads to symptoms of reflux. People with and without a hiatal hernia can experience gastroesophageal reflux. Physiologic or normal reflux occurs in most people after eating when they are in an upright position, especially during vigorous exercise, but its low frequency and small volume do not lead to symptoms. Symptoms of PUD are initiated by erosion of the gastrointestinal mucosa.

19. **(2)** The most common hernia is an inguinal hernia, protruding at the inguinal canal. Incarcerated means the hernia cannot be reduced or returned to the abdominal cavity. A reducible hernia easily moves across the abdominal wall. There should be no abdominal swelling and, if the hernia is particularly painful and associated with nausea and vomiting, then incarceration should be considered.

20. **(2)** All cases of recurrent, not new, dyspepsia indicate a need for endoscopy. Endoscopy is reserved for those clients with no response to empiric therapy after 7–10 days and symptoms persisting after 8 weeks of therapy. Dyspepsia can be characterized by fullness, belching, and regurgitation and can include PUD and gastroesophageal reflux. Smoking should be discontinued and alcohol intake should be decreased to a moderate level in PUD and GERD, but endoscopy is not indicated for these clients.

21. **(2)** The factor contributing most to reflux is an abnormal LES, the antireflux barrier. Hiatal hernia is not believed to play an important factor in the etiology of reflux. Reflux occurs postprandially in the upright position and may be exacerbated by meals, but overeating is not a direct cause. Alcohol and excessive use of caffeine may affect the LES pressure.

22. **(3)** The etiologic agents that produce inflammation and cause diarrhea are characterized by positive fecal leukocytes. Viral diarrhea is free of pus, thus no fecal leukocytes would be found on the smear. Noninflammatory diarrhea is usually caused by rotavirus. Toxigenic bacteria cause diarrhea by elaborating toxins that have been released after bacterial growth in the intestine. These poisonous substances result in secretory diarrhea.

23. **(3)** The female-to-male ratio for IBS is 4:1. It is a disease of young or middle-aged adults, frequently appearing at age 20–25.

24. **(4)** A common means of hepatitis B transmission is from mother to baby, perinatally. Other mechanisms of transmission are by infected body fluids, sexual contact, and parenterally. Hepatitis E virus is spread in contaminated water. Hepatitis A's mode of transmission is fecal–oral and person–person.

25. **(3)** The client is presenting with the most reliable symptoms of GERD. GERD is most often related to inappropriate relaxation of the LES, which allows reflux of gastric acid and pepsin into the distal esophagus. Common presentations of IBS are differentiated by cramping, abdominal pain, or altered bowel habits predominating. Clients with esophagitis complain of the acute onset of chest pain, dysphagia, and odynophagia. Bleeding is associated with carcinoma.

26. **(1)** Hepatitis A and E do not have a chronic stage, and generally resolve without any long-term effects.

27. **(4)** Because indirect hernias are due to a congenital defect in which the processus vaginalis remains patent, they occur more often in younger persons. A portion of the bowel and/or the omentum comes through the internal abdominal ring, traverses the spermatic cord through the inguinal canal, and exits at the external inguinal ring. In a direct hernia, the omentum or bowel protrudes directly through the floor of the inguinal canal and exits through the external inguinal ring. Because it is due to a weakness in the abdominal structures, it occurs more often in middle and later years of life.

28. **(2)** These parasites reside in the intestine. Females lay eggs on the skin outside the anus resulting in extreme pruritus. The only host is humans. Hookworm larvae reside in the soil, enter the body through the feet, and can cause anemia. When dirt containing roundworm eggs is ingested due to pica or on unwashed vegetables or contaminated water is consumed, an intestinal infestation occurs. Giardiasis results from ingestion of the protozoan *Giardia lamblia* through contaminated water or via oral–fecal transmission.

29. **(4)** The small-feedings diet used for GERD results in decreased gastric volume and decreased likelihood of continued reflux. Low-energy diets are used in obesity for weight loss. Energy-controlled diets are used for clients with diabetes mellitus for increased glucose tolerance. High-energy diets are used for clients with anorexia for increased weight and fat.

30. **(1)** A high-energy diet is used for clients with anorexia. Management of GERD includes reduce weight, avoid lying down after meals, avoid large meals, avoid exercise after meals, and elevate the head of the bed. Certain foods and drinks, such as alcohol, mint, and orange juice, should be avoided, as they may cause symptoms of heartburn.

31. **(2)** *Helicobacter pylori* has been implicated in the etiology of ulcer disease. The other organisms listed are implicated in other types of infections, such as acute otitis media and skin infections.

32. **(4)** Alcohol is the most important cause of cirrhosis in the United States. Especially in men, one six-pack of beer or four to six glasses of wine daily significantly increases the risk for long-term hepatic injury leading to cirrhosis. The corresponding amount for women is about half that. Hepatitis A is a self-limited infection without a known chronic state. Hepatitis B and D acute infections do not directly result in a high incidence of cirrhosis.

33. **(2)** A hemorrhoid results when a vascular anal cushion prolapses through the anal canal and is entrapped by the internal anal sphincter. In a rectal mucosa prolapse, the wall of the rectum prolapses. A tumor is not a vascular anal cushion.

34. **(2)** These characteristics describe hepatitis B. Hepatitis A has similar symptoms but can be transmitted by the oral–fecal or oral–genital route and has an incubation period of 15–50 days and no chronic form. Hepatitis C infection rarely causes jaundice. It is transmitted parenterally and has an incubation period of 14–140 days and a chronic form. Hepatitis D coexists with hepatitis B, is transmitted parenterally, and can also become chronic. Hepatitis E is characterized by oral–fecal transmission associated with contaminated food and water, and has an incubation period of 14–60 days and no chronic disease state.

35. **(2)** Although most clients need eventual intervention, those who are elderly and diabetic are at increased risk and should be hospitalized for prompt diagnosis, intravenous fluids, pain control, and surgical consultation.

36. **(3)** A typical description of a "knot" is given by clients who have esophageal tumors. The symptom of heartburn caused by either gastric ulcer or acid reflux should be controlled with a H_2 blocker.

37. **(4)** Clients with a history of heavy alcohol intake are at increased risk for cirrhosis and portal hypertension, which may result in variceal bleeding. These clients often present clinically with bleeding, hypotension, and eventual shock.

38. **(3)** A strangulated hernia is irreducible and the blood supply to the trapped bowel is

compromised, resulting in bowel infarction. Ulcers, endometriosis, and ectopic pregnancy can cause abdominal pain and can be surgical emergencies, but they do not cause bowel obstruction.

39. **(2)** Increasing crampy abdominal pain that starts as periumbilical pain, anorexia, and fever are classic symptoms of appendicitis. The client should be evaluated by a surgeon to decrease the risk of rupture of the appendix. Although ectopic pregnancy should always be a consideration in young females with abdominal pain, the characteristics of the pain and other symptoms are not typical of an ectopic pregnancy.

40. **(3)** Thrombosed hemorrhoids can cause severe pain for clients and should be quickly decompressed. Although they are irritating and cause itching, pinworms do not cause rectal pain. Hookworms penetrate the soles of the feet, and cystitis usually causes lower abdominal, not rectal, pain.

41. **(2)** Diverticular disease presents with change in bowel habits (diarrhea alternating with constipation or both) and blood in the stool; if diverticulitis develops, flatus, low-grade fever, and leukocytosis may be present. The majority of clients with diverticulosis may have no symptoms; some may have abdominal pain in the left lower quadrant. Appendicitis may present with pain in the right lower quadrant and may not be severe until perforation occurs. Other signs, including nausea and vomiting, leukocytosis, and fever, may or may not be present. IBS may present with aching or cramping periumbilical or lower abdominal pain often precipitated by meals and relieved by defecation. Pain may radiate to the left chest or arm. There may be alternating episodes of diarrhea and constipation. Pancreatitis may present with epigastric pain or tenderness that lasts for hours and may radiate to the back, fever, nausea and vomiting, mental confusion, and jaundice.

42. **(1)** A high-fiber diet is the treatment for this disease, and vegetarians eat increased amounts of fruits, vegetables, grains, and cereals. Options #2, #3, and #4 are at higher risk.

43. **(4)** Colorectal cancer occurs most commonly in individuals over age 50. A change in bowel habit, with reduced caliber of stool and blood mixed with the stool, are characteristic of left-sided colon cancer, which is the most common site. Anemia is found with right-sided lesions. Bright red rectal bleeding and tenesmus are characteristic of rectal cancer.

44. **(1)** Colon cancer risk in pancolonic ulcerative colitis increases by 2% per year after the tenth year of diagnosis.

45. **(4)** PUD in the elderly often does not cause the usual pain and indigestion associated with the disease in younger individuals. Smoking does increase the risk and, without the pain, perforation is common. Gastric ulcers are more commonly seen in the elderly.

46. **(1)** Cancer of the esophagus is found mostly in elderly men. Alcoholism and smoking are the primary risk factors for cancer of the esophagus. The cell type is usually squamous cell. Dysphagia for liquids, cough, and hoarseness as well as boring midchest pain indicate late disease, which does not usually respond to any treatment, including surgery.

47. **(4)** Flexible sigmoidoscopy and colonoscopy are screening tools for colorectal cancer recommended after age 50. They are useful for identifying adenomatous polyps, which are considered premalignant. Sessile or flat polyps are more suspicious for malignancy. Polyps of the cecum and polyps <1 cm are less likely to be malignant, and villous polyps are often malignant.

48. **(3)** The string sign is indicative of a narrow pyloric channel and is associated with pyloric stenosis. Intussusception would be evaluated by a barium enema. Hirschprung's disease can be diagnosed by doing a Wagenstein-Rice series (air rises in the inflated colon).

49. **(2)** Excessive vomiting with loss of acid is a common problem with metabolic alkalosis. Respiratory problems do not precipitate primary metabolic acid-base imbalance, and renal disease most often causes metabolic acidosis.

50. **(3)** It is critical that a child be voiding prior to starting an IV solution with potassium. The problem with renal compromise is always a possibility, and adequate output should be established prior to initiating fluid.

51. **(1)** Rotavirus is the most frequent cause of gastroenteritis in children ages 6 months to 2 years. The Norwalk virus is more predominant in school-age children. Up to 58% of diarrhea in children is due to viral causes. Viral causes result in vomiting and then diarrhea. The stool smear is negative for WBC in viral causes, and positive in bacterial causes (Options #2, #3, and #4). In viral diarrhea the fever is mild, and diarrhea is watery and nonbloody.

52. **(4)** Clinical features of Crohn's disease include severe weight loss, abdominal pain, growth failure, and weight loss. In IBS abdominal pain predominates. Altered bowel habits with either diarrhea or constipation are also seen. Clinical findings associated with carcinoma of the colon include mild, occult blood loss with intermittent episodes of acute bleeding. Ulcerative colitis clinical features include diarrhea, rectal bleeding, and moderate weight loss.

53. **(3)** Appendicitis usually begins as dull periumbilical pain accompanied by anorexia and nausea, but not necessarily vomiting. Within a few hours there may be low-grade fever. Most laboratory tests are normal. A WBC count of more than 15,000/mm^3 is often noted but neither confirms nor excludes the diagnosis of appendicitis.

54. **(4)** Red currant jelly stools are seen in intussusception and are caused by a mixture of stool, mucus, and blood. Clay-colored stools are seen with hepatitis. Projectile vomiting is associated with pyloric stenosis. Infants with intussusception usually have periods of severe pain followed by intervals in which they appear comfortable.

55. **(1)** The major symptom of reflux is vomiting or regurgitation. It may occur during sleep, and frequently after feeding. Poor weight gain, hyperirritability, and refusal of feeding may be signs in some infants, but are not the major symptoms. Fever or diarrhea may be present in clients with acute otitis media, gastroenteritis, or urinary tract infections.

56. **(1)** The optimal therapy for GERD should include frequent small feedings, burping after each feeding, and placing the baby prone, on an inclined surface at 30 degrees. The prone position is not advocated, as it allows gravity to pronate reflux. The supine position leads to more reflux as compared with prone. Proof of the effectiveness of thickening feedings has not been demonstrated.

57. **(4)** For an infant born to an HBsAg-positive mother the recommendations are: the baby should have one dose of hepatitis B immunoglobulin (by 12 hours after birth) and a complete three-dose immunization of hepatitis B vaccine administered. The vaccine will stimulate the newborn's active immunity.

58. **(2)** Classic signs and symptoms of Hirschsprung's disease in later infancy include alternating diarrhea and constipation and abdominal distention. The stools are offensive and ribbon-like, the abdomen is enlarged, and the veins are prominent.

59. **(4)** Gastroenteritis is the most common cause of abdominal pain in all age groups. The incidence of appendicitis increases after the age of 5. Intussusception and incarcerated hernias are not common events and certainly occur less often than gastroenteritis.

60. **(3)** Parasitic infestations cause recurrent episodes of abdominal pain often with diarrhea, nausea, and vomiting, depending on the type of infestation. Musculoskeletal pain is usually sharp and recurs with various activities or body movements that trigger the pain. Dysmenorrhea accompanies or precedes menses. Chronic stool retention occurs in a child with a history of ineffective toilet training. There is often a family history of constipation. All of the other conditions present with acute symptoms, except for psychogenic pain that is recurrent and is a diagnosis of exclusion and mittelschmerz, which may occur monthly.

61. **(3)** The location of the injury indicates the possibility of a ruptured spleen. While bowel and bladder problems are possible with blunt trauma to the abdomen, the upper abdominal location makes a spleen injury more likely.

62. **(3)** Lactose intolerance is common among Asian clients. The primary symptoms are bloating, flatulence, abdominal cramps, and diarrhea 2 hours after lactose-containing food consumption.

63. **(2)** Right upper quadrant pain during exercise along with malaise, nausea, and vomiting are early signs of hepatitis A. Elevated IgM antibodies indicate a recent/ current infection.

64. **(2)** Further physical examination is needed to rule out appendicitis (although rare, it can occur in young children); also needed would be further diagnostic testing and assessment for differential diagnosis of lactose intolerance, urinary tract infection, or extra-abdominal causes.

65. **(1)** Objects 3–4 cm or larger have difficulty passing the ligament of Treitz and other points of narrowing such as the cardioesophageal juncture.

66. **(2)** Increased abdominal pressure after eating with the infant in a supine position can result in passage of gastric contents into the esophagus which, frequently during sleep, can be aspirated resulting in the forceful coughing and resultant emesis. Suck-swallow incoordination can cause the same problems regardless of position, as will a tracheoesophageal fistula.

Pharmacology

67. **(4)** For clients with reoccurring symptoms after a course of treatment for PUD, consult the physician. The client is having symptoms of active bleeding, and endoscopy may be indicated at this point. The physician should be consulted regarding the next step. Omeprazole (Prilosec), a proton pump inhibitor that inhibits acid secretion, is useful for hypergastrinemia, and may be useful in PUD clients not controlled by H_2 antagonists in the absence of active bleeding.

68. **(3)** H_2 blockers, changes in diet, and weight reduction are the first line of treatment for GERD. The client should be advised to sit up after meals and sleep with his head elevated. Anticholinergics (Pro-Banthine) may increase the problem by lowering the LES pressure. Omeprazole is not recommended for the first phase of treatment.

69. **(1)** Goals of PUD treatment include relief of pain, healing of ulcer, and cost effectiveness. The H_2 receptor antagonists heal 90% of duodenal ulcers and 70% of gastric ulcers. The proton pump inhibitors such as omeprazole are recommended for ulcers unresponsive to the receptor antagonists after 8–12 weeks with full dosing and GERD. The anticholinergic drugs, doxepin (Sinequan) and pirenzepine, are useful when used with the H_2 receptors but are limited by side effects and used only in Canada and Europe at this time.

70. **(1)** The prostaglandins, such as misoprostol (Cytotec), are used to decrease recurrent ulcerations in client who require NSAIDs. They have not, however, been shown to increase ulcer healing. Cimetidine (Tagamet) has been shown to increase healing. Doxepin (Sinequan) and pirenzepine are not prescribed in the United States as of this date.

71. **(2)** If a person exposed to a client known to be positive for hepatitis B has sufficient immunity to hepatitis B, no treatment is necessary. If this same person had not been vaccinated, in addition to initiation of the hepatitis B vaccine series, HBIG 0.06 ml/kg IM is also administered. If an exposed person has had an inadequate immune response to the hepatitis B vaccine series, a hepatitis B booster is to be given. There is no need to repeat the series. If the response to the hepatitis B vaccine series is unknown, test the exposed person's HBsAg level and decide what intervention, if any, is needed.

72. **(2)** Therapy for clients with refractory ulcers due to *H. pylori* are most successfully treated with the triple-drug therapy of Pepto-Bismol, amoxicillin or tetracycline, and metronidazole (Flagyl). Less effective but well-tolerated regimens consist of omeprazole (Prilosec) and amoxicillin.

73. **(2)** Sulfasalazine (Azulfidine) therapy for clients with mild ulcerative colitis results in symptomatic improvement in 50–75% of cases. If no response is seen after 2–4 weeks, the addition of prednisone is recommended. This drug prevents relapse of ulcerative colitis once remission is induced. The other drugs listed are not recommended as first-line treatment.

74. **(2)** Since 25% of clients are effectively treated with lifestyle changes, therapy should begin with use of these measures. If these are not completely effective, an H_2 receptor antagonist can be added. Twice-daily dosing is recommended. Omeprazole (Prilosec) is recommended only for refractory cases. Cisapride (Propulsid) can be effective, but lifestyle changes and antacid tablets as needed is the recommended starting point for therapy.

75. **(1)** To minimize the risk of a contact developing hepatitis A, immunoglobulin 0.02 ml/kg should be given as soon as possible after exposure. It has not been shown to be effective if administered more than 2 weeks after exposure.

76. **(3)** Treatment with sulfamethoxazole and trimethoprim shortens the course and prevents further spread of the organism. Prevention of dehydration that can result from the diarrhea is accomplished through symptomatic treatment (clear liquids for 24–48 hours, no dairy products, electrolyte-rich sports drinks, advance diet as tolerated). Antidiarrheal medications are not recommended because intestinal motility is important in recovery. Option #4 would be appropriate treatment for nonpregnant adults who have giardiasis.

77. **(1)** The Emetrol dose for adults is 15–30 ml. Phenergan 25 mg can be given to children over 12 years old (not 6 years old)

and adults. The older child and adult dose for hydroxyzine hydrochloride (Vistaril) is 25–100 mg. Trimethobenzamide (Tigan) is dosed at 200 mg, not 10 mg.

78. **(3)** NSAIDs are more often associated with mucosal disruptions causing gastric ulcers. *Helicobacter pylori* is associated with mucosal disruption that leads to PUD. Alcohol and smoking are not causes of gastrointestinal mucosal disruption.

79. **(4)** For unvaccinated clients with exposure to hepatitis B, administer one dose of HBIG and initiate the vaccine. If the client thinks he/she may have been vaccinated but does not know if there was a response, the nurse practitioner may have a prevaccination antibody testing done. The HBe antibody is drawn to determine the potential for transmission; it generally appears about 3 months after the onset of the infection.

80. **(3)** The only contraindication to the hepatitis B vaccine is a prior anaphylaxis or severe hypersensitivity to the vaccine or components of the vaccine.

81. **(2)** This medication causes problems with nephro- and ototoxicity (eighth cranial nerve). Laboratory tests to monitor renal function should be done on a regular basis. The client should be frequently evaluated for any hearing loss. The geriatric client is particularly susceptible to the complications and toxicity.

82. **(3)** This is a common observation for a client on Pepto-Bismol. He may also experience a problem with discoloration of his tongue.

83. **(3)** The drug of choice for treating *Giardia* is metronidazole 5 mg/kg (up to 250 mg) tid × 5 days (80–90% effective). This drug is well tolerated in children. Metronidazole does have a disulfiram-like effect and should not be used in children or adolescents receiving ethanol-containing medications. All of the other drugs are ineffective for *Giardia*. Tetracycline should never be prescribed to children under age 8 for any reason.

13

Hematology

Physical Examination & Diagnostic Tests

1. On physical examination a palpable, firm, nontender supraclavicular lymph node is noted on the left side of the body. This information is consistent with a diagnosis of:

   1. Bacterial infection draining from the internal jugular chain.

   2. Thoracic or abdominal malignancy.

   3. Inflammation of the tonsils and adenoids.

   4. Non-Hodgkin's lymphoma.

2. The nurse practitioner describes a "shotty" lymph node as:

   1. Tender, mobile, and >5 mm.

   2. Small and pellet-like.

   3. Discrete and cystic.

   4. Irregular, soft, and fixed to surrounding tissue.

3. A macrocytic, normochromic anemia is diagnosed in an elderly man. The next test(s) that should be ordered is(are):

   1. Serum iron and total iron-binding capacity (TIBC) levels.

   2. Bone marrow biopsy.

   3. Colonoscopy.

   4. Vitamin B_{12} and red blood cell (RBC)–folate levels.

4. The nurse practitioner would suspect disseminated intravascular coagulation (DIC) if the client's laboratory results indicated:

   1. Increased prothrombin time, decreased platelet count, decreased fibrinogen.

   2. Decreased prothrombin time, increased hematocrit, increased fibrinogen.

   3. Increased platelet count, decreased hematocrit, increased prothrombin time.

   4. Increased platelet count, increased hematocrit, decreased prothrombin time.

5. In examining lymph nodes, the nurse practitioner understands:

   1. Children are more likely to develop generalized lymphadenopathy than adults in response to a mild infection.

   2. Older adults frequently have enlarged, nontender supraclavicular and epitrochlear lymph nodes due to aging.

   3. Lymphadenopathy in an adult indicates acute or chronic infection and rarely malignancy.

   4. Enlarged neck lymph nodes in children with no other physical findings are highly suspicious of Burkitt's lymphoma.

6. After confirming the diagnosis of iron deficiency anemia in an adult client based on standard laboratory values (complete blood count [CBC], peripheral smear, serum iron, TIBC, serum ferritin), what would be the next essential test for the nurse practitioner to order?

   1. Stool guaiac ×3.

   2. Prothrombin time (PT)/partial thromboplastin time (PTT).

   3. Liver function tests.

   4. Endoscopy.

7. Evaluation of an elderly male client reveals a macrocytic, normochromic anemia. Subsequent testing shows a folate level that is normal and a decreased vitamin B_{12} level. Further evaluation should include:

   1. Referral to a hematologist for a bone marrow biopsy.

   2. Schilling's test.

   3. Upper gastrointestinal (GI) series.

   4. No tests are indicated at this time.

8. The most sensitive test for the diagnosis of sickle cell anemia is:

   1. CBC with a peripheral smear.

   2. Bone marrow biopsy and aspiration.

   3. Hemoglobin electrophoresis.

   4. Hemoglobin and hematocrit.

9. A school-age child presents to the clinic. His mother reports a recent history of easy fatigability ("he can't keep up with his brother anymore"), unexplained bruising, and that he has been treated for an upper respiratory infection (URI) with multiple antibiotics over the past 6 months. Physical exam reveals scattered bruising in no apparent pattern, pallor, and cervical lymphadenopathy. The diagnostic work-up for this child should include:

   1. Chest x-ray and electrocardiogram (ECG).

   2. Liver function tests and an abdominal ultrasound.

   3. PT/PTT.

   4. CBC with differential, and platelet count.

10. In evaluating the laboratory findings on a child with iron deficiency anemia, the nurse practitioner expects:

    1. Mean corpuscular volume (MCV) 80 and low reticulocyte count.

    2. MCV 120 and hemoglobin 12 gm.

    3. MCV 99 and hematocrit 34%.

    4. MCV 96 and normal reticulocyte count.

11. The nurse practitioner explains a bone marrow aspiration procedure to a 4-year-old child. Which behavior of the child would reflect effective teaching?

    1. Appears calm as the nurse takes her for the procedure.

    2. Asks if she can have ice cream after the procedure.

    3. States that her blood is bad and the doctor will make it better.

    4. Points at her doll saying that they have to put a needle here to look at my blood.

12. An elderly male presents to the nurse practitioner's office with complaints of fatigue, dizziness, decreased activity tolerance, and occasional bounding heart rate. Physical examination reveals pallor (including mucous membranes), tachycardia, and general appearance of lethargy. The following tests are ordered: CBC with differential, peripheral smear, serum iron,

TIBC, and serum ferritin. These tests are ordered because there is a high index of suspicion of:

1. Sideroblastic anemia.

2. Pernicious anemia.

3. Folic acid deficiency anemia.

4. Iron deficiency anemia.

13. Anemia of chronic disease would reveal which of the following lab findings?

    1. Decreased iron, decreased TIBC, and decreased serum ferritin.

    2. Decreased iron, decreased TIBC, and increased serum ferritin.

    3. Decreased iron, increased TIBC, and decreased serum ferritin.

    4. Decreased iron, increased TIBC, and increased serum ferritin.

Disorders

14. Sickle cell anemia is caused by:

    1. Exposure to ionizing radiation.

    2. A genetically induced production of abnormal hemoglobin S.

    3. A deficiency of dietary folic acid.

    4. Long-term use of thiazide diuretics.

15. An adult client presents to the nurse practitioner with a history of erythrocytosis. One common complaint that could cause a serious complication for this client is:

    1. A laceration.

    2. Vomiting and diarrhea.

    3. Coughing.

    4. Dizziness.

16. A client has a folic acid deficiency anemia. The nurse practitioner teaches the client to eat foods rich in folic acid, such as:

    1. Green leafy vegetables, nuts, and liver.

    2. Carrots, salmon, and avocados.

    3. Cottage cheese, yogurt, and skim milk.

    4. Lima beans, brussels sprouts, and potatoes.

17. Which of the changes occur in the RBC indices for pernicious anemia?

    1. Microcytic, normochromic.

    2. Microcytic, hypochromic.

    3. Normocytic, normochromic.

    4. Macrocytic, normochromic.

18. Iron deficiency anemia is an example of:

    1. Macrocytic, normochromic anemia.

    2. Macrocytic, hypochromic anemia.

    3. Microcytic, hypochromic anemia.

    4. Normocytic, normochromic anemia.

19. A client with pernicious anemia may present with which signs and symptoms?

    1. Paresthesias, unsteady gait, lethargy and fatigue.

    2. Hepatomegaly, jaundice, and right upper quadrant pain.

    3. Hypertension, angina, and peripheral edema.

    4. Blurred vision, diplopia, and decreased visual acuity.

20. Anemia of chronic disease is a:

    1. Normochromic, normocytic anemia.

    2. Normochromic, microcytic anemia.

    3. Hypochromic, microcytic anemia.

    4. Hypochromic, macrocytic anemia.

21. A young adult presents to the clinic for a routine checkup. History is unremarkable, and on physical exam, an enlarged (2-cm) mobile, nontender and rubbery lymph node is palpated on the left posterior cervical chain. The nurse practitioner's next step is:

    1. Order a throat culture and monospot.

    2. Referral to a surgeon for a lymph node biopsy.

    3. Order a stat chest x-ray.

    4. No intervention is necessary at this time.

22. The nurse practitioner understands that "B" symptoms associated with non-Hodgkin's lymphoma (NHL) include:

    1. Bruising and bleeding.

    2. Peripheral edema, shortness of breath, and ascites.

    3. Fever, night sweats, and unexplained weight loss (>10% of body weight).

    4. Headache, fatigue, and weakness.

23. In teaching a client with anemia to include foods rich in iron in the diet, the nurse practitioner encourages the client to eat:

    1. Cheese, milk, and yogurt.

    2. Red beans, whole-grain bread, and bran cereal.

    3. Tomatoes, cabbage, and citrus fruits.

    4. Beef, spinach, and peanut butter.

24. Anemia of chronic disease is associated with:

    1. Malnutrition and B_{12} deficiency.

    2. Infections, inflammation, and neoplasms.

    3. Traumatic injuries and folate deficiency.

    4. Excessive menstrual flow, trauma, and heredity.

25. The nurse practitioner is concerned about the development of which complication in a young child with a diagnosis of iron deficiency anemia?

    1. Crohn's disease.

    2. Pernicious anemia.

    3. Impaired cognitive development.

    4. Hepatic and spleen dysfunction.

26. The nurse practitioner is counseling a client who has a child with sickle cell disease. The client asks, "If my child has sickle cell disease, does that mean that I am at an increased risk for developing the same problems?" The nurse practitioner's response would be based on what principle of sickle cell disease?

    1. The mother is at an increased risk, because the condition is inherited; she

    probably has the condition and has not had an active episode.

    2. There is no risk for the mother developing the condition, as males are the carriers of the trait.

    3. There is a 25% chance that the mother will be affected by the disease, especially at times of stress.

    4. The parents are both carriers of the trait, but they do not have the active disease; each child has a 25% chance of having the condition.

27. During a clinic visit, the nurse practitioner notes that an 11-month-old is pale. The physical examination reveals pulse 170, height 25th percentile, weight 95th percentile. The nurse practitioner questions the mother about the infant's diet. The mother states that the infant eats mostly pureed fruits and whole milk. The nurse practitioner expects which diagnostic finding?

    1. Normal hemoglobin.

    2. Elevated MCV.

    3. Low serum ferritin level.

    4. Macrocytic, hyperchromic anemia.

28. The nurse practitioner knows that an infant who is exclusively breast-fed is at risk for developing iron deficiency anemia at:

    1. 1 month of age.

    2. 2 months of age.

    3. 4 months of age.

    4. 6 months of age.

29. The nurse practitioner understands that most adult clients with Hodgkin's disease present with:

    1. Nausea, vomiting, and diarrhea.

    2. Night sweats, weight loss, and fever.

    3. Painless, movable mass in the neck, axilla, or groin.

    4. Hepatosplenomegaly with a painful mass in the mediastinum.

30. What is the most common leukemia found in the older adult and is typically asymptomatic and characterized by a median survival rate of approximately 10 years?

    1. Acute myelogenous.

    2. Chronic myelogenous.

    3. Acute lymphocytic.

    4. Chronic lymphocytic.

Pharmacology

31. The nurse practitioner determines that an adult male client has an iron deficiency anemia, and has ruled out gastrointestinal (GI) bleeding as the cause. The nurse practitioner:

    1. Refers the client to a hematologist.

    2. Refers the client to a GI specialist.

    3. Prescribes ferrous sulfate 300 mg PO tid, and has the client return in 1 month for a repeat CBC, serum iron, and TIBC.

    4. Have the client return in 6 months for additional stool guaiac testing.

32. Teaching clients regarding the treatment of vitamin B_{12} deficiency includes:

    1. The client will take vitamin B_{12} tablets given bid for 1 year.

    2. Oral folic acid supplements will be taken daily for the client's lifetime.

3. Monthly cyanocobalamin (vitamin B_{12}) injections will be given for the client's lifetime (after being given weekly for the first month).

4. Iron supplementation and monthly blood transfusions will be required until the deficiency is corrected.

33. Treatment of anemia of chronic disease should include:

    1. A folic acid supplement, 1 mg PO qd.

    2. Iron sulfate ($FeSO_4$) supplement, 300 mg PO tid.

    3. Treatment of the underlying condition.

    4. Weekly epoetin alfa (Epogen) injections.

34. A toddler has been diagnosed as having iron deficiency anemia and the nurse practitioner has prescribed elemental iron 6 mg/kg/day in three divided doses. Instructions to give the parents would include:

    1. Give the iron with food to increase the absorption of the medication.

    2. Give the medication through a straw to decrease the staining of the teeth.

    3. Avoid foods containing ascorbic acid because it will decrease the absorption of the medication.

    4. If a dose is missed, double up on the next two doses.

13   Answers & Rationales

Physical Examination & Diagnostic Tests

1. **(2)** A Virchow's node in the left supraclavicular region is of concern due to the high correlation with abdominal or thoracic malignancy. Infections and inflammatory conditions produce tender, inflamed lymph nodes.

2. **(2)** Shotty or small and pellet-like, lymph nodes that are movable, cool, nontender, discrete, and up to 3 mm in diameter are usually considered normal.

3. **(4)** It is important to determine which type of macrocytic anemia a client has, so that the appropriate therapy can be ordered. Therefore, the vitamin B_{12} and RBC-folate levels would be ordered. These tests would determine if the client has a pernicious anemia (the most common type) or a folate deficiency (also common in the elderly). Serum iron and TIBC would be ordered if an iron deficiency anemia was suspected (it is not in this case because this is a microcytic anemia). There is no indication for a colonoscopy. It would be premature to order a bone marrow biopsy at this point, without performing initial testing and thereby potentially overlooking an easily treated condition (i.e., pernicious anemia, folate deficiency anemia).

4. **(1)** DIC is a complication of infection, malignancy, and sometimes trauma. DIC is the inappropriate accelerated systemic activation of the coagulation cascade, resulting in simultaneous hemorrhage and thrombosis. The lab results would show increased prothrombin and a decrease in platelet and fibrinogen in response to the hemorrhage and clotting.

5. **(1)** Children often have generalized lymphadenopathy in response to mild infections of the skin or respiratory tract. Palpable lymph nodes are generally not present in healthy individuals; however, some individuals may have small, discrete, nontender nodes that are not clinically significant. Enlarged lymph nodes may indicate infection, inflammation, and malignancy in both child and adult. Painless, firm supraclavicular or cervical lymph node is a common sign of Hodgkin's disease in children, not Burkitt's lymphoma, where the child has other associated symptoms depending on the system affected.

6. **(1)** Stool guaiac would identify blood loss from the GI tract, the most common cause of iron deficiency anemia. The other tests should be done if the stool guaiacs are positive. Finding the cause of the iron deficiency is paramount, and the stool guaiac is an easy, noninvasive method of ruling out bleeding as the cause.

7. **(2)** A Schilling's test will determine the cause of the vitamin B_{12} deficiency. It will distinguish between inadequate intake, an intrinsic factor deficiency, or a malabsorption problem. This will allow the practitioner to prescribe the most appropriate therapy for the client. A bone

marrow biopsy and an upper GI series are not indicated at this time.

8. **(3)** Normal and abnormal hemoglobins can be detected by electrophoresis, which matches hemolyzed red cell material against standard bands for the various known hemoglobins, including hemoglobin S (the abnormal hemoglobin that is associated with sickle cell anemia). CBC with peripheral smear and hemoglobin/hematocrit would not yield enough information to diagnose sickle cell anemia. Bone marrow biopsy would not be necessary and would not indicate the presence of hemoglobin S.

9. **(4)** This clinical presentation would make the practitioner consider the diagnosis of leukemia, necessitating a work-up. A CBC with differential, along with platelet count (indicators of bone marrow function), is diagnostic for leukemia. Further testing may be necessary, but the work-up should always include a CBC.

10. **(1)** The findings associated with iron deficiency anemia include a low MCV (<90), decreased hemoglobin and hematocrit, and a low reticulocyte count. An elevated MCV is associated with macrocytic anemias (i.e., pernicious anemia).

11. **(4)** Dolls and puppets are effective teaching tools for the preschool child. Using the doll reflects the child's understanding of the procedure. Children will often withdraw and appear calm when they have feelings of anxiety.

12. **(4)** This client's clinical picture is a classic presentation for anemia. Further testing would be needed to determine the type of anemia involved. The most common cause in elderly males is GI bleeding, which would cause an iron deficiency anemia. The tests that were ordered would confirm or rule out this diagnosis; the peripheral smear is especially important in diagnosing the specific type of anemia. If the smear ruled out the diagnosis of iron deficiency anemia, it would lead the practitioner to other diagnoses (including the remaining choices) and appropriate laboratory tests required for confirmation.

13. **(2)** Normal to increased iron stores (serum ferritin) with concurrent low serum iron is the hallmark finding of anemia of chronic disease. The serum iron is decreased along with the TIBC. Options #1 and #4 contain incorrect information for the anemias. Option #3 contains the findings for iron deficiency anemia.

Disorders

14. **(2)** Sickle cell anemia is a genetic disorder characterized by the production of hemoglobin S, an anemia secondary to shortened erythrocyte survival, microvascular occlusion by sickle-shaped erythrocytes, and an increased susceptibility to certain infections. Exposure to ionizing radiation has been associated with the development of certain malignancies, especially leukemia. A deficiency of dietary folic acid does not cause sickle cell anemia, although folic acid is used in the treatment of these clients to help increase hematopoiesis and aid in recovery from aplastic events. Long-term use of thiazide diuretics has been implicated in the development of hemolytic or aplastic anemias, in very rare cases.

15. **(2)** Erythrocytosis (or polycythemia) can be worsened by dehydration from any cause. Coughing and dizziness will have no effect on the condition, and a laceration may actually improve the symptoms, due to the blood loss.

16. **(1)** Green leafy vegetables, nuts, and liver are excellent sources of folic acid. Also, cereals and breads are now fortified with folic acid. The other foods are not significant sources of folic acid.

17. **(4)** A macrocytic (MCV >100), normochromic anemia resulting from atrophic gastric mucosa not secreting intrinsic factor is the definition of pernicious anemia. These indices could also include folic acid deficiency anemia. Options #1 and #2 could include iron deficiency anemia or anemia of chronic disease. Option #3 could also include anemia of chronic disease.

18. **(3)** Iron deficiency anemia is a microcytic, hypochromic anemia. The red blood cells are smaller (microcytic) due to the decrease in hemoglobin production caused by inadequate amounts of iron. This also makes the cell appear pale (hypochromic). The other selections describe other types of anemia, which would be determined by the peripheral smear.

19. **(1)** A deficiency in vitamin B$_{12}$ can cause neurologic signs and symptoms including paresthesias, an unsteady gait, lethargy, and fatigue. These findings are specific to pernicious anemia, and so must always be assessed for in any client who presents with an anemia. The other signs and symptoms are not characteristic of pernicious anemia.

20. **(1)** Anemia of chronic disease is a chronic normochromic, normocytic anemia. There is normal production of hemoglobin, along with normal maturation of red blood cells.

21. **(2)** Lymphadenopathy as described, without evidence of infection, should always be referred to a surgeon for biopsy, because biopsy is the only definitive test to rule out a malignancy (a frequent cause of lymphadenopathy not caused by infectious processes). There are no signs or symptoms to suggest the need for a throat culture, monospot, or chest x-ray. Not intervening is not appropriate because the cause of lymphadenopathy needs to be determined.

22. **(3)** This constellation of symptoms (fever, night sweats, weight loss) is used in the staging of NHL, the presence of which is considered to be a poor prognostic indicator. The other symptoms may occur depending on the amount of disease involvement, but they are not considered "B" symptoms, also known as constitutional symptoms.

23. **(4)** Beef, spinach, and peanut butter are iron-rich foods. Options #1, #2, and #3 are examples of foods rich in calcium, fiber, and vitamin C, respectively.

24. **(2)** Anemia or chronic disease is associated with infections (e.g., tuberculosis), chronic inflammatory conditions (i.e., systemic lupus erythematosus [SLE], rheumatoid arthritis [RA]), and malignancies. Excessive blood loss from menstrual flow or traumatic injuries would more likely cause an iron deficiency anemia. Malnutrition can contribute to iron, vitamin B$_{12}$, and folate deficiencies.

25. **(3)** With an iron deficiency anemia, there is a reduced amount of hemoglobin, which carries the oxygen. Long-term oxygen deprivation can lead to impaired cognitive and motor development. Pernicious anemia is associated with lack of the intrinsic factor. Crohn's disease has a familial incidence and leads to problems associated with diarrhea. The liver and spleen are both involved with RBC production.

26. **(4)** Sickle cell disease is transmitted by two parents who have the sickle cell trait; however, they do not show symptoms of the disease. Each pregnancy carries a 25% chance of sickle cell disease and a 25% chance of the child carrying the trait.

27. **(3)** An iron deficiency anemia is commonly found in this age group, especially in infants who do not eat a balanced diet that includes foods rich in iron (i.e., iron-fortified cereals). This is a microcytic, hypochromic anemia with a decrease in serum iron (ferritin). The MCV would be decreased (<90).

28. **(4)** The normal, full-term infant is born with sufficient iron stores to prevent iron deficiency for the first 6 months of life.

29. **(3)** Most clients present with a painless, movable mass in the neck, axilla, or groin. Older clients may present with fatigue, weight loss, or persistent fever, and night sweats. Often, there is pain in diseased areas after consuming alcohol (an unexplained finding). Hepatosplenomegaly presents with advanced disease.

30. **(4)** Chronic lymphocytic leukemia (CLL) is found primarily in the middle and older adult; fewer than 10% of all clients are under the age of 50. Acute myelogenous leukemia (AML) incidence increases with age, and approximately 50% of clients are younger than 50 years of age. Chronic myelogenous leukemia (CML) occurs most often at a median age of 45. Acute lymphocytic leukemia (ALL) is most common in children and gradually increases in frequency in later life.

Pharmacology

31. **(3)** Treatment with iron orally for at least 6 months is necessary to correct both the anemia and the depleted body iron stores. The client should have the hemoglobin, hematocrit, iron, and TIBC rechecked after 1 month on iron supplementation. If there is not improvement in all parameters, most notably a rise in the hemoglobin by 1 gm/dl, the client should be referred to a hematologist. There is no need to refer to a GI specialist or repeat the guaiac, because there is no indication that this client's condition is caused by bleeding.

32. **(3)** If the deficiency is not due to inadequate intake, the client will require lifetime supplementation of vitamin B_{12}. It must be given in the form of an intramuscular or subcutaneous injection to ensure absorption. Oral folic acid, iron, and blood transfusions would not treat the cause of the deficiency, and therefore the resulting anemia would not be corrected.

33. **(3)** Treatment of the underlying condition leads to resolution of the anemia of chronic disease. Folic acid and iron supplements are indicated for folate and iron deficiency anemias, respectively. Epoetin alfa (Epogen) injections are indicated for those conditions that affect erythropoiesis, namely, chronic renal failure, chemotherapy-induced anemia, and acquired immunodeficiency syndrome.

34. **(2)** Iron medications can cause staining of the teeth, so it is a good practice to give the medication through a straw. It is best to give iron on an empty stomach (if tolerable) to increase absorption. Ascorbic acid increases absorption of iron. If a dose is missed, it is best to give the dose when it is remembered as long as it is not too close to the next dose. You would not increase the next two doses.

14

Urinary

Physical Examination & Diagnostic Tests

1. A urinalysis that suggests a urinary tract infection shows:

   1. Protein only.

   2. Alkaline pH and positive nitrite and leukocyte esterase.

   3. Hematuria and pyuria only.

   4. Red color without the presence of red blood cells (RBCs).

2. An intravenous urography and voiding cystourethrography assists in diagnosing:

   1. Congenital anomalies, stone formation, or foreign bodies.

   2. Renal size and the presence of stone.

   3. A problem in the urethra, prostate, or bladder.

   4. Visualization of the ureter and renal pelvis.

3. Physical exam on an adolescent reveals 2+ proteinuria. The next step in differential diagnosis would involve:

   1. Quantify protein excretion.

   2. Evaluate for orthostatic proteinuria.

   3. Reassure patient and follow-up in 6 months.

   4. Evaluate for nephritis.

4. According to the Agency for Health Care Policy and Research (AHCPR) Guideline Panel, the basic continence evaluation for the primary care provider includes:

   1. History, physical examination, measurement of postvoid residual volume, and urinalysis.

   2. Measurement of postvoid residual volume, blood urea nitrogen (BUN), serum creatinine, and urinalysis.

   3. History, physical examination, serum glucose, BUN, serum creatinine, and urinalysis.

   4. Urodynamic, endoscopic, and imaging tests; urinalysis and serum creatinine.

5. The nurse practitioner is evaluating serum blood studies on a client who is experiencing a slight increase in blood pressure (BP). She has no previous history of high blood pressure and no other chronic diseases. Which serum lab values would the practitioner be most concerned about?

   1. Serum creatinine 5.2 mg/dl.

   2. BUN 30 mg/dl.

   3. Serum potassium 4.5 mEq/L.

   4. Serum osmolarity 290 mOsm/kg.

6. When taking a history on voiding patterns in adults, the nurse practitioner knows:

   1. Adults normally void q2–3h in a 24-hour period (8–12 times a day).

   2. The first sensation to void occurs when the bladder fills to 200–300 ml.

   3. Normally, 15–20 minutes passes between the first urge to void and the functional capacity is reached.

   4. Adults typically reach functional (comfortable) capacity at 200–300 ml and may experience some leakage if voiding is delayed.

7. The nurse practitioner expects which findings on examination of an older client with dehydration?

   1. Tongue furrows and skin tenting on the forehead.

   2. Specific gravity of urine 1.004.

   3. Pulse rate 58 strong and regular; BP 100/62.

   4. Geographic tongue and reduced saliva pool.

Disorders

8. A young adult female client explains to the nurse practitioner that she has been having frequent and painful urination. The nurse practitioner orders a clean-catch urine for routine urinalysis and culture and sensitivity. The laboratory culture and sensitivity report is as follows: 10^5 *Escherichia coli* and 10^4 *Staphylococcus*

epidermidis per milliliter. The nurse practitioner would:

   1. Treat the *E. coli*.

   2. Order penicillin.

   3. Treat the *S. epidermidis*.

   4. Encourage citric fruit juices.

9. An elderly female client is incontinent of urine. What would the nurse practitioner advise the family caregiver to avoid using on the skin in the perineal area?

   1. Petrolatum.

   2. Moisture-barrier films.

   3. Mild soap and water.

   4. Zinc oxide ointment.

10. A young adult comes to the student health clinic complaining of severe abdominal discomfort and bloody urine. Priority in the diagnostic work-up should include:

    1. Intravenous pyelography to rule out a kidney stone.

    2. Straining all urine.

    3. Microscopic urine exam.

    4. A 24-hour urine culture.

11. Which plan would be most appropriate for an older client with functional incontinence?

    1. Evaluate need for pads.

    2. Limit fluid intake in the evenings.

    3. Perform Credé's maneuver.

    4. Provide a bedside commode.

12. A male client presents with recurrent urinary tract infections. What is the most likely cause?

    1. Balanitis.

    2. Epididymitis.

    3. Chronic bacterial prostatitis.

    4. Benign prostatic hypertrophy.

13. A possible cause of transient urinary incontinence, which can be reversed, is:

   1. Poor pelvic support causing hypermobility of the base of the bladder in females.

   2. Lower urinary tract problems, such as carcinoma.

   3. Cystocele or uterine prolapse in women.

   4. Ingestion of certain medications, such as sedatives, diuretics, anticholinergic agents, α-adrenergic agents.

14. Functional incontinence is:

   1. Leakage of urine during activities that increase abdominal pressure, such as coughing, sneezing, laughing, or other physical activities.

   2. Mainly caused by factors outside the urinary tract, such as dementia or immobility, that prohibit proper toileting habits.

   3. Characterized by the inability to delay urination, with an abrupt and strong desire to void.

   4. The occurrence of incontinence with overdistention of the bladder.

15. The two most common pathogens in community-acquired urinary tract infections are:

   1. *Klebsiella pneumoniae* and *Proteus mirabilis*.

   2. *Staphylococcus saprophyticus* and *Escherichia coli*.

   3. *Proteus mirabilis* and *Staphylococcus saprophyticus*.

   4. *Escherichia coli* and *Proteus mirabilis*.

16. The usual clinical presentation of an adult client with cystitis is:

   1. No symptoms noted.

   2. Acute onset of chills, fever, flank pain, headache, malaise, and costovertebral angle tenderness.

   3. Complaints of dysuria, urgency, frequency, nocturia, and suprapubic heaviness.

   4. Signs and symptoms of fever, irritability, decreased appetite, vomiting, diarrhea, constipation, dehydration, and jaundice.

17. In children, the presence of hypertension and a history of a sore throat may be an indication of:

   1. Congestive heart failure.

   2. Glomerulonephritis.

   3. Vasculitis.

   4. Cushing's syndrome.

18. Recurrent urinary tract infections in females are due to relapse or reinfection. The nurse practitioner understands that relapse:

   1. Is less common than reinfection and occurs within 2 weeks of the completion of drug therapy for the infection.

   2. Is responsible for most recurrent urinary tract infections in females.

   3. May occur due to residual urine after voiding due to a prolapsed uterus or bladder or a lack of estrogen.

   4. Can be treated with the same medication regimen as the original infection.

19. The nurse practitioner understands that the treatment of pyelonephritis:

   1. In females is suggestive of a structural problem.

   2. Requires hospitalization, parenteral antibiotic therapy, and an intravenous voiding pyelogram in males.

   3. In females requires hospitalization, parenteral antibiotic therapy, and an intravenous voiding pyelogram.

   4. Requires no follow-up.

20. When assessing a child with glomerulonephritis, what symptoms would the nurse practitioner anticipate to be present?

   1. Fever >102°F and bilateral flank pain.

   2. Periorbital edema and increase in blood pressure.

   3. Anorexia and complaints of dysuria.

   4. Oliguria with strong concentrated urine.

21. When instructing the parents regarding the course of poststreptococcal glomerulo-nephritis, the nurse practitioner lets them know to expect the bloody urine for at least how long after onset of diuresis?

    1. 1 week.

    2. 1–2 weeks.

    3. 2–3 weeks.

    4. 4–7 days.

22. Urinary incontinence associated with conditions such as Parkinson's disease, Alzheimer's disease, and stroke is termed:

    1. Stress incontinence.

    2. Urge incontinence.

    3. Frequency incontinence.

    4. Overflow incontinence.

23. A client has a renal stone that consists of uric acid. What is the best diet to order for this client to decrease the incidence of stone formation?

    1. Alkaline ash diet and low purine.

    2. High purine and an acid ash diet.

    3. Increased fluid intake and high doses of vitamin C.

    4. High complex carbohydrate and decreased protein.

24. A mother brings in her 3-year-old daughter stating she noticed a swelling in the child's abdominal area just below the rib cage on the left side. The nurse practitioner observes a bulging of the area and the child does not want to be touched due to abdominal tenderness. What is the best action for the nurse practitioner at this visit?

    1. Immediately contact a pediatrician for consultation.

    2. Schedule a referral with a pediatrician in the near future.

    3. Perform a urinalysis and draw blood for creatinine and potassium.

    4. Explain to the child it is necessary to examine the abdomen.

25. A male client presents with complaints of blood in his urine; it is painless and he has no difficulty with voiding. The nurse practitioner obtains a urinalysis to confirm the presence of blood, and there are no bacteria present. What is the priority diagnosis that must be ruled out on this client?

    1. Cancer of the prostate.

    2. Prerenal failure.

    3. Renal calculi.

    4. Cancer of the bladder.

26. The nurse practitioner is taking the history of a client who has been diagnosed with renal calculi. What information in the history would the nurse practitioner identify as a precipitating factor in the development of renal calculi?

    1. Increased incidence of urinary tract infections over the past 3 years.

    2. Drinking 6–8 oz of milk daily.

    3. History of fractured femur and prolonged bed rest.

    4. High intake of citrus fruit and high-fiber carbohydrates.

27. A client is diagnosed with renal failure and the origin of the problem is thought to be postrenal. What would the nurse practitioner identify as a possible precipitating cause of this client's renal failure?

    1. History of myocardial infarction (MI) with severe hypotensive episode.

    2. Advanced prostate hypertrophy with hematuria.

    3. Renal vascular changes secondary to long history of diabetes.

    4. Exposure to carbon tetrachloride on his job site.

28. A nurse practitioner recognizes what factors as contributing to the development of prerenal failure?

    1. History of an anaphylactic reaction that rendered the client unconscious.

2. Extended treatment of an infection with gentamicin (Garamycin).

3. Acute pyelonephritis and consequently glomerulonephritis.

4. Renal vascular changes that occur secondary to atherosclerotic disease.

29. The nurse practitioner is teaching a female client some guidelines regarding bladder health, which include all **except**:

    1. Drink at least six to eight glasses of water per day.

    2. Avoid doing Kegel's exercises.

    3. Avoid constipation.

    4. Consider estrogen replacement after menopause.

Pharmacology

30. A client is diagnosed with benign prostatic hypertrophy. Which medication should be recognized by the nurse practitioner as likely to aggravate this condition?

    1. Glyburide (DiaBeta).

    2. Oral buspirone (Buspar).

    3. Inhaled ipratropium (Atrovent).

    4. Ophthalmic timolol (Timoptic).

31. Which of the following agents can be useful for stress incontinence?

    1. Propantheline (Pro-Banthine) 7.5–30 mg, three to five times a day.

    2. Oxybutynin (Ditropan) 2.5–5 mg tid to qid.

    3. Doxypin (Sinequan) 10–25 mg qd/bid/tid initially to a maximum total daily dose of 25–100 mg.

    4. Conjugated estrogen (Premarin) 0.3–1.25 mg/day orally or vaginally, medroxyprogesterone (progestin) 2.5–10 mg/day either continuously or intermittently.

32. In order to decrease the production of uric acid stones, the nurse practitioner orders what medication?

    1. Allopurinol (Zyloprim).

    2. Potassium citrate (Urocit-K).

    3. Bethanechol (Urecholine).

    4. Phenazopyridine (Pyridium).

33. A 70-year-old woman is treated with oxybutynin (Ditropan) for her urinary frequency and urgency. The nurse practitioner would explain to the client she will probably experience:

    1. Increased sensitivity to sunlight.

    2. Dizziness when she stands up.

    3. A dry mouth and increased thirst.

    4. Increased bruising.

34. A 6-year-old girl is brought to the clinic by her mother. The child is complaining of burning on urination and the urine is cloudy. A dipstick test of the urine is positive for leukocyte esterase. The mother states the child had a fever with nausea and vomiting the last time she took Gantrisin (sulfisoxazole). The medication of choice for this client is:

    1. Nitrofurantoin (Macrodantin) 50 mg PO qid × 7 days.

    2. Trimethoprim-sulfamethoxazole (Septra DS) 1 tab PO bid × 10 days.

    3. Ciprofloxacin (Cipro) 200 mg PO bid × 10 days.

    4. Clarithromycin (Biaxin) 250 mg PO bid × 10 days.

35. All of the following medications can cause urinary incontinence in the older adult **except**:

    1. Hypnotics.

    2. Antibiotics.

    3. Sedatives.

    4. Antidepressants.

36. The nurse practitioner has selected nitrofurantoin (Macrodantin) for treatment of a chronic urinary tract infection in a female geriatric client. What parameter should be evaluated prior to the administration of this medication?

    1. Creatine clearance (should be >50 ml/min).

    2. Levels of serum alanine aminotransferase (ALT).

    3. Any current medications that include anticoagulant agents.

    4. History of allergic reactions to sulfa-based medications.

37. A 46-year-old man with a history of renal calculi presents with complaints of severe flank pain radiating to his groin area; he is also experiencing nausea and vomiting. His temperature is 99°F. What is the best initial order for the nurse practitioner to give at this time?

    1. Morphine sulfate 10 mg sc now.

    2. Ibuprofen (Advil) 600 mg PO now and q6h.

    3. Increase fluid intake and strain all urine.

    4. Trimethobenzamide (Tigan) 250 mg PO now.

38. The nurse practitioner is prescribing nitrofurantoin (Macrodantin) for a woman who is experiencing problems with urinary tract infections. What specific directions are given to this client regarding the administration of this medication?

    1. Medication should be taken with food, anticipate the urine to have brown discoloration.

    2. Do not take medication with milk products, take on empty stomach for better absorption.

    3. Take the medication four times a day until the symptoms have subsided for at least 24 hours.

    4. Acetaminophen (Tylenol) and/or ibuprofen (Advil) should not be taken with this medication.

39. A young woman presents with complaints of burning on urination, frequency, and urgency. Phenazopyridine (Pyridium) is prescribed by the nurse practitioner. What specific directions are given to the client regarding this medication?

    1. May discolor contact lens; if sclera begin to turn yellow, return to the office.

    2. Always take the medication on an empty stomach to increase absorption.

    3. Do not take any medication containing aspirin or salicylate.

    4. May interfere with effectiveness of mini pill for birth control.

14 Answers & Rationales

Physical Examination & Diagnostic Tests

1. **(2)** These are results indicating the presence of a urinary tract infection. Proteinuria alone suggests glomerulonephritis. Hematuria and pyuria without bacteria may indicate chlamydia, gonorrhea, viral infection or, less commonly, tuberculosis. If a dipstick test is negative for RBCs but the urine color is red, a substance that can change the color of the urine is likely the cause.

2. **(1)** In intravenous urography and voiding cystourethrography, congenital anomalies, stone formation, or foreign bodies can be identified. Renal size and the presence of stones can be seen in flat plate and upright films of the abdomen. In a cystoscopy, the urethra, prostate, and bladder can be visualized. A urethroscopy can visualize the ureter and renal pelvis.

3. **(2)** Twenty-five to 60% of proteinuria in children is orthostatic in nature and must be evaluated first.

4. **(1)** The 1996 AHCPR Guideline Panel encourages primary health care providers to initiate the basic evaluation of urinary incontinence by performing a history and physical examination, measurement of postvoid residual volume, and urinalysis. The other tests may be performed based on the findings from the initial evaluation.

5. **(1)** The primary concern here is the increase in the serum creatinine. All of the other serum lab values are within normal limits. This client should be referred for a work-up for chronic renal failure.

6. **(2)** Adults normally void four to six times in a 24-hour period (q4–6h). Most usually do not get up in the middle of the night, unless they have a medical problem (e.g., benign prostatic hypertrophy, urge incontinence). The feeling of the bladder filling occurs around 90–150 ml, with first urge occurring at 200–300 ml. Normally, 1–2 hours pass between the first urge to void and the functional capacity is reached. Adults typically reach functional (comfortable) capacity at 300–600 ml and should *never* experience leakage if voiding is delayed.

7. **(1)** The classic sign of dehydration in the older adult is lack of skin turgor along with skin tenting on the forehead, concentrated urine (specific gravity >1.025), oliguria, sunken eyes, lack of axillary moisture, orthostatic blood pressure changes, tachycardia, dry mucous membranes of the mouth and nose, and absent or small saliva pool. It is important to examine the mouth, as it reveals reliable assessment data in the older adult suspected of having dehydration. A geographic tongue (patchy papillary loss giving rise to a map-like appearance) should not be confused with tongue furrows and tongue coating.

Disorders

8. **(1)** *E. coli* is the most common organism causing urinary tract infections in the young adult female, and counts of 10^5 are diagnostic and should be treated with trimethoprim-sulfamethoxazole (Bactrim DS) or any suitable, sensitive anti-infective agent. *S. epidermidis* is more often a contaminant due to inappropriate clean-catch specimen collection technique.

9. **(2)** Although moisture-barrier films may protect the skin from urine, they often contain alcohol and can further burn and irritate denuded skin. Cleansing with a mild soap and water helps prevent infections. Petrolatum and zinc oxide, which are types of moisture-barrier ointments, are used to prevent or treat irritant dermatitis.

10. **(3)** The nurse practitioner suspects a urinary tract infection and needs to confirm with a microscopic urinalysis exam to identify presence of white blood cells and bacteria.

11. **(4)** Functional incontinence is an inability to toilet appropriately due to impaired mobility. Providing physical assistance and guidance, such as with wheelchairs, bedside commodes, appropriate clothing that can be removed easily, and accessible facilities, is effective with this type of incontinence. Evaluating the need for pads is effective with stress incontinence. Limiting fluid intake in the evenings to reduce nocturnal incontinence is appropriate for urge incontinence. Performing the Credé's maneuver is appropriate for overflow incontinence.

12. **(3)** Chronic bacterial prostatitis is the most likely cause, as it is difficult to treat due to the bacteria being harbored in the prostatic calculi and in corpora amylacea. A 3- to 4-month treatment with trimethoprim-sulfamethoxazole or a quinolone may be necessary to prevent urinary symptoms.

13. **(4)** Sedative-hypnotics, diuretics, anticholinergic agents, α-adrenergic agents, and calcium channel blockers can cause transient reversible urinary incontinence. Poor pelvic support is a possible cause of stress incontinence. Urge incontinence, or the inability to delay urination with a sudden and powerful urge to void, is a possible result of lower tract problems. A prolapsed uterus or bladder can cause overflow incontinence with overdistention of the bladder.

14. **(2)** Functional incontinence results from a client's inability to toilet appropriately. Stress incontinence is leakage from the bladder during activities that increase intra-abdominal pressure and, therefore, increase the pressure on the bladder, forcing some urine out. An inability to delay urination, with a strong, abrupt urge to void, is urge incontinence and is due to bladder hyperactivity or a hypersensitive bladder. The client often has little warning before urine passes out of the bladder. Incontinence with overdistention of the bladder is called overflow incontinence and is due to an underactive detrusor or one that will not contract, or to bladder outlet or urethral obstruction. It is characterized by frequent urination in small amounts.

15. **(2)** *Escherichia coli* is the pathogen in 80–90% of community-acquired infections. Gram-positive *Staphylococcus saprophyticus* is the second most common pathogen. *Klebsiella pneumoniae* and *Proteus mirabilis* are also possible common pathogens. In hospital settings, *Escherichia coli* is less prevalent.

16. **(3)** Cystitis in adults usually presents with dysuria, urgency, frequency, nocturia, and suprapubic heaviness. Acute onset of chills, fever, flank pain, headache, malaise, and costovertebral angle tenderness are common in pyelonephritis in adults. Infants with cystitis may exhibit fever, irritability, decreased appetite, vomiting, diarrhea, constipation, dehydration, and jaundice.

17. **(2)** Acute hypertension in children and adolescents almost always is due to an identifiable secondary cause such as glomerulonephritis due to strep infections.

18. **(1)** Relapse is an uncommon cause of recurrent urinary tract infections in women and occurs within 2 weeks of completion of antibiotic therapy. It may need to be treated for 2–12 weeks. Reinfection is the cause of most urinary tract infections in women and may be due to residual urine resulting from

a prolapsed uterus or bladder or to lack of estrogen in perimenopausal women. If the client has two or fewer urinary tract infections in a year, the single-dose or 3-day regimen of antibiotic therapy may be used.

19. **(2)** Pyelonephritis in men is suggestive of a structural abnormality and is usually an indication for hospitalization, parenteral antibiotics, and an intraveneous voiding pyelogram. Pyelonephritis in women is usually a result of invasion of the urinary tract by bacteria that have ascended the urethra from the introitus of the urethra. If bacteremia is suspected, women need to be hospitalized, also. Suggested follow-up is by telephone contact within 12−24 hours of initiation of antibiotic therapy and at 2 weeks and 3 months for posttreatment urine cultures.

20. **(2)** The facial edema and increased blood pressure are common. Generally, the child does not have a high fever and the urine is not concentrated, but it may be decreased in amount.

21. **(2)** There can be gross hematuria for 1−2 weeks after the diuresis and microscopic hematuria for up to 2 years. If parents know what to expect they will know what is abnormal and when to notify a health care professional.

22. **(2)** Urge incontinence is associated with conditions that involve the central nervous system, causing detrusor motor and/or sensory instability.

23. **(1)** With an acid stone, the rule of thumb is to promote a diet that will render the urine more alkaline, that is, an alkaline ash diet. A high-purine diet contributes to the development of the renal stones, so the client needs decreased purine. Foods that are high in purines include liver, spinach, chicken, and dried peas. Milk is allowed on an alkaline ash diet. An increased fluid intake is recommended in all stones but does not particularly correlate with vitamin C intake. High carbohydrates do not contribute to the stone formation.

24. **(1)** The pediatrician should be contacted immediately; this is frequently the first sign of a Wilms' tumor, which is very fragile and possibly malignant. The child should not be referred due to the chance they will not be seen immediately. A urinalysis and blood test can be done, but often these tests are negative, so the child should be seen by a pediatrician immediately regardless of the test results. The abdomen should not be examined due to the fragility of the tumor.

25. **(4)** Painless hematuria is the most common symptom in the client with bladder cancer. This often occurs early, and it may be the only symptom the client will exhibit. There is no evidence of renal failure, renal calculi are characterized by flank pain, and cancer of the prostate will often present with the other symptoms of benign prostatic hypertrophy.

26. **(3)** A sedentary lifestyle or episodes of immobilization can predispose a client to the development of stones. Urinary infections usually do not precipitate problems with stones; however, the presence of stones will predispose the client to urinary tract infections; 6 to 8 oz of milk daily is not excessive, and the increased intake of citrus and high-fiber carbohydrates is good.

27. **(2)** Postrenal failure is the development of a complication that presents an obstructive problem distal to the kidney. The hypotensive episode is prerenal, and the vascular changes due to diabetes and the exposure to nephrotoxic chemicals are intrarenal.

28. **(1)** The precipitating factor in prerenal failure is most often an incident that precipitated renal ischemia, i.e., a shock situation. Nephrotoxic medications, pyelonephritis, and renal vascular changes are all causes of intrarenal failure.

29. **(2)** Kegel's (pelvic floor) exercises keep the bladder support strong. Weak pelvic floor muscles contribute to urinary incontinence, especially with activity. In addition, the teaching should include avoiding bladder irritants, such as caffeine, alcohol, and spicy foods.

Pharmacology

30. **(3)** Benign prostatic hypertrophy is a common cause of urinary retention in older men. Atrovent is an atropine-like bronchodilator that is used to treat chronic bronchitis, and its anticholinergic agent may aggravate urinary retention. Neither glyburide nor buspirone has an effect on the urinary system, and timolol does not have a systemic effect.

31. **(4)** Combination hormone replacement therapy can be useful for management of stress incontinence. Propantheline and oxybutynin may be useful in urge incontinence; research is limited on the use of these drugs for urge incontinence.

32. **(1)** To decrease the formation of uric acid stones, a urinary alkylating agent such as allopurinol (Zyloprim) is frequently used.

33. **(3)** The medication produces anticholinergic side effects. Dry mouth is very common. The other reactions listed are not consistent with oxybutynin.

34. **(1)** The clinical presentation is that of a urinary tract infection. The dipstick is positive for bacteria. Since the child may have had a reaction to a sulfa drug (Gantrisin), it would be best to avoid sulfa drugs at this time. The next best medication for a urinary tract infection in children is nitrofurantoin (Macrodantin). Ciprofloxacin is not recommended for children under 18 years old, and clarithromycin is not a first-line drug of choice for urinary tract infections.

35. **(2)** Sedatives and hypnotics lead to sedation and muscle relaxation. Antidepressants have anticholinergic effects and lead to sedation. Antibiotics have not been implicated in the development of incontinence in the older adult.

36. **(1)** If there is any impairment of renal function, the antibacterial concentration in the urine is inadequate and there is increased risk of toxicity. With normal doses there should be no serum or tissue accumulation of the medication. Liver function studies may be indicated if the client experiences adverse reactions to the medication. Anticoagulants and sulfa-based medications have not been reported as producing any significant drug interactions.

37. **(1)** The severe pain of renal calculi should be addressed prior to other treatments or diagnostics. The ibuprofen may be used for beginning pain, but severe pain needs to be treated with morphine or meperidine (Demerol). Tigan can be used, but only after the pain relief has been initiated.

38. **(1)** The most common side effect is gastrointestinal upset. This can be decreased if the medication is taken with food or milk. The discoloration of the urine is a very common occurrence. The medication should be taken for at least 3 days after sterile urine is obtained.

39. **(1)** Yellow discoloration of the sclera may indicate poor renal excretion. Pyridium should be administered with food, and there is no drug interaction with aspirin or with birth control pills.

Male Reproductive

Physical Examination & Diagnostic Tests

1. Which organ is **not** palpable on physical examination of a male client?

   1. Vas deferens.

   2. Testes.

   3. Epididymis.

   4. Cowper's glands.

2. A review of a lab report with an elevated serum gonadotropin would raise suspicion of which disorder?

   1. Seminal vesiculitis.

   2. Vas deferens disease.

   3. Testicular disease.

   4. Benign prostatic hypertrophy (BPH).

3. Which of the following structures can be palpated during an external examination of a male client?

   1. Epididymis.

   2. Cowper's ducts.

   3. Seminal vesicles.

   4. Ejaculatory ducts.

4. What would be most helpful in diagnosing gynecomastia?

   1. History and physical examination.

   2. Liver function test.

   3. Thyroid function test.

   4. Mammogram.

5. The correct position in which to place a healthy, adult male client to examine the rectum and prostate is:

   1. Left lateral Sims' position with right knee flexed and left leg extended.

   2. Supine position with hips and legs flexed and feet positioned on the examining table.

   3. Modified knee-chest position with client prone and knees flexed under hips.

   4. Leaning over the examination table with chest and shoulders resting on the table.

6. Which test is a tumor marker used to diagnose advanced prostatic cancer?

    1. α-Fetoprotein (AFP).

    2. Prostate-specific antigen (PSA).

    3. Prostatic acid phosphatase (PAP).

    4. Human chorionic gonadotropin (hCG).

7. Which statement is correct about the PSA test?

    1. It can be elevated in clients with BPH.

    2. It is not elevated in clients with prostatitis.

    3. Prostatic massage will not elevate levels.

    4. It does not increase in reoccurrence of prostate cancer.

8. Which procedure is used in screening males (age 40) for prostate cancer, but is not diagnostic?

    1. Prostate-specific antigen test.

    2. Digital-rectal exam (DRE).

    3. Urinalysis and complete blood count (CBC).

    4. Prostate-specific antigen test and digital-rectal exam.

9. When examining the scrotum of an adult Hispanic male, a normal finding is:

    1. Symmetrical scrotal sac with two movable testes.

    2. Smooth, rubbery, sac-like surface that is sensitive to gentle compression.

    3. Asymmetrical sac with the left side lower than the right side.

    4. A reddened color that is darker than body skin with sebaceous cysts.

Disorders

10. What finding is indicative of testicular torsion?

    1. Scrotal swelling with tenderness that occurs only after age 40.

    2. Sudden onset of pain with a firm, tender mass in the scrotum.

    3. Positive Prehn's sign.

    4. Cremasteric reflex.

11. On a routine physical examination the client expresses concern over the observation that one side of his scrotum is larger than the other. He states it has been getting larger for the past few months, the scrotum is smaller in the morning and gets larger through the day. He has felt a heaviness in the scrotum, denies any acute pain but does confirm some discomfort in his lower back. He denies any history of trauma to the scrotal area. On examination the nurse practitioner confirms the enlargement, and on further examination determines the scrotum will transilluminate and manual manipulation of the scrotum does not cause pain. The initial diagnosis for this client is:

    1. Hydrocele.

    2. Orchitis.

    3. Epididymitis.

    4. Traumatic injury.

12. Which statement is correct concerning circumcision?

    1. Circumcision is helpful in preventing phimosis.

    2. Circumcision is a cause of paraphimosis.

    3. Balanoposthitis is the direct result of circumcision in older men.

    4. Circumcision increases the incidence of cancer of the penis.

13. Acute epididymitis is characterized by:

    1. Absence of dysuria.

    2. Nonenlarged scrotum.

    3. Tenderness over the epididymis.

    4. Lack of abdominal pain.

14. Which one of the following is correct about hypogonadism?

    1. Usually presents with impotence.

    2. May cause an increased libido.

3. Is not associated with gynecomastia.

4. Does not contribute to infertility.

15. Which of the following is a true statement about impotence?

   1. Impotence can be caused by antihypertensives.

   2. Impotence is caused by infections only.

   3. Impotence is not the result of multicausal factors.

   4. Impotence is not the result of vascular problems.

16. Circumcision can prevent which of the following?

   1. Paraphimosis.

   2. Epididymitis.

   3. Sexually transmitted diseases.

   4. Prostatitis.

17. Which statement is true about the prostate?

   1. Secretes fluid that is acid.

   2. Secretes fluid that is alkaline.

   3. Secretes androgens.

   4. Produces sperm.

18. An elderly man presents to the clinic with complaints of difficulty voiding and hematuria. The rectal examination reveals a very firm prostate about 5 cm in diameter, asymmetrical, with firm nodules. The PSA level is 14. The next action is to:

   1. Medicate with finasteride (Proscar), 5 mg PO daily and re-evaluate in 3 months.

   2. Advise client to avoid caffeine, alcohol, and over-the-counter decongestants.

   3. Obtain a urinalysis to determine presence of infection and amount of hematuria.

   4. Refer to urologist for biopsy and diagnostic evaluation for prostatic cancer.

19. A 15-year-old male presents with complaints of severe scrotal pain for the past 2 hours. The scrotum is swollen and extremely tender; palpation of the epididmis is not

possible. The nurse practitioner recognizes the immediate treatment is:

   1. Narcotic analgesics and bed rest.

   2. Warm packs and scrotal support.

   3. Antibiotics, ice packs, and analgesics.

   4. Referral to surgeon for exploration.

20. A 20-year-old male client presents with scrotal pain. A suspected diagnosis that requires immediate referral is:

   1. Testicular torsion.

   2. Hydrocele.

   3. Epididymitis.

   4. Inguinal hernia.

21. An adult male client is being evaluated for dysuria, fever, and perineal pain. The physical exam by the nurse practitioner reveals a distended bladder. Further physical exam should **not** include:

   1. A urine culture.

   2. Prostate massage.

   3. Cultures for gonorrhea and chlamydia.

   4. A blood urea nitrogen (BUN) and creatinine.

22. An older adult male presents with a history of burning on urination and difficulty urinating that has been increasing over the past few days. A stat urinalysis reveals the presence of leukocytes and bacteria. The primary diagnosis considered by the nurse practitioner is:

   1. Bladder cancer.

   2. Testicular torsion.

   3. Benign prostatic hyperplasia.

   4. Renal failure.

23. The client with localized prostate cancer will exhibit which symptoms?

   1. Hesitancy, frequency, and dysuria.

   2. Fatigue, severe constipation, and dysuria.

   3. Hematuria, nocturia, and weight loss.

   4. Myalgia, confusion, and lethargy.

24. A young male client presents with a complaint of a feeling of fullness in the scrotum. Physical examination reveals a round, soft, nontender, nonadherent bluish discolored testicular mass resembling a "bag of worms"; there is no variation in size with respiration or Valsalva maneuver. The mass transilluminates and is located anterior to the testes. The most likely diagnosis is:

    1. Varicocele.

    2. Hernia.

    3. Tumor.

    4. Spermatocele.

25. An uncircumcised male client presents with a complaint of not being able to retract the foreskin over the glans penis. The most likely diagnosis is:

    1. Lateral phimosis.

    2. Phimosis.

    3. Peyronie's disease.

    4. Paraphimosis.

26. A middle-aged male client complains of a tight band causing a lateral curvature of the penis during erection and painful intercourse. The most likely diagnosis is:

    1. Phimosis.

    2. Lateral phimosis.

    3. Lateral paraphimosis.

    4. Peyronie's disease.

27. A middle-aged uncircumcised client presents with red pinpoint pustules and papules on the prepuce and glans. The most likely diagnosis is:

    1. Peyronie's disease.

    2. Balanitis.

    3. Phimosis.

    4. Paraphimosis.

28. A male client is diagnosed with balanitis; the most likely cause is:

    1. Candidiasis.

    2. Herpes genitalis.

    3. Lichen planus.

    4. Psoriasis.

29. A male client presents with a complaint of sexual dysfunction. The nurse practitioner understands that sexual dysfunction is impairment of:

    1. Erection only.

    2. Emission only.

    3. Ejaculation only.

    4. Erection or emission or ejaculation.

30. A client presents with a complaint of dysuria, enlarged scrotal tenderness over the epididymis, and abdominal pain. The most likely diagnosis is:

    1. Testicular torsion.

    2. Vas deferens inflammation.

    3. Epididymitis.

    4. Balanitis.

31. The nurse practitioner knows that erectile dysfunction is:

    1. Primarily psychological in origin.

    2. Primarily associated with the 70+ older male.

    3. Is the persistent inability to achieve and maintain an erection adequate for sexual intercourse.

    4. Is the physiological dysfunction when smooth muscle contracts causing a lack of adequate amount of blood in the penis to render a rigid, larger penis.

32. Priapism is classified as which type of sexual dysfunction?

    1. Erection.

    2. Emission.

    3. Ejaculation.

    4. None of the above.

33. In response to a male client's question concerning a possible cause of prostate cancer, which is correct?

    1. Syphilis.

2. Gonorrhea.

3. Cryptorchidism.

4. Balanitis.

34. A male client complains of impotence. Which one may be a contributing factor?

   1. Antihypertensives.

   2. Intercourse.

   3. Smoking.

   4. Masturbation.

35. A young male presents for a sports physical examination. In addition to examining for hernias, it would be appropriate for the nurse practitioner to do which of the following, especially if not previously performed?

   1. Teach testicular self-exam.

   2. Perform a PSA test.

   3. Examine for prostate cancer.

   4. Perform a PSA test and a DRE.

36. An older male presents with gynecomastia. The most likely cause is:

   1. Cirrhosis.

   2. Diabetes mellitus.

   3. Hypergonadism.

   4. Peptic ulcer disease.

37. Concerning the male breast, which is a correct statement?

   1. Gynecomastia is the result of low estrogen and normal levels of testosterone.

   2. Most breast cancers in men are estrogen-receptor positive.

   3. Breast cancer in males is very common.

   4. Gynecomastia is a nonhormonal or tissue alteration.

38. Which is true of prostate cancer?

   1. Rarely diagnosed in men >50 years of age.

2. Soft, indiscrete, symmetrical nodules of the prostate.

3. Rarely have obstructive symptoms.

4. Asymmetrical, discrete, hard nodules of the prostate.

39. Which symptoms would be a concern about a possible diagnosis of prostate cancer in a male over 50 years of age?

   1. Hesitancy, dribbling, and urgency.

   2. Decreased force of urinary stream.

   3. Pain and feeling of a full bladder.

   4. Rapid onset of obstructive symptoms of urinary output.

40. Which statement is correct concerning testicular cancer?

   1. There is a very common problem in men over 50 years.

   2. This problem is directly related to testicular trauma.

   3. Testicular cancer presents suddenly with pain.

   4. Testicular cancer is primarily found in young men.

41. Which statement is correct about acute bacterial prostatitis?

   1. Characterized by recurrent urinary tract infections.

   2. Ascending infection of urinary tract.

   3. Always occurs in men under 30.

   4. Usual treatment is a 12-week course of antibiotics.

42. Which finding is indicative of orchitis?

   1. Extremely painful scrotum.

   2. No history of parotitis.

   3. No evidence of systemic viral infection.

   4. Decreased serum amylase.

43. A client has nongonococcal urethritis (NGU). The nurse practitioner understands that:

    1. No related problems occur if it is untreated.

    2. It is often asymptomatic.

    3. It is easily differentiated from gonococcal urethritis on physical examination.

    4. There is a very purulent discharge with a foul odor.

44. What organism is the most common cause of NGU in men?

    1. *Chlamydia trachomatis.*

    2. *Neisseria gonorrhoeae.*

    3. *Escherichia coli.*

    4. *Streptococcus faecalis.*

45. Cryptorchidism is defined as:

    1. Testicular underdevelopment.

    2. Imbalance of estrogen-androgen ratio.

    3. Undescended testicles.

    4. Absence of spermatogenesis.

46. Which test is a useful tumor marker for testicular cancer?

    1. Alpha fetoprotein (AFP).

    2. Prostate-specific antigen.

    3. Prostatic acid phosphatase.

    4. Alkaline phosphatase (ALP).

47. The causative agent of orchitis is:

    1. Arbovirus.

    2. Echovirus.

    3. Mumps.

    4. Rubeola.

48. What are common symptoms of BPH?

    1. Dribbling, hesitancy, loss of stream volume and force, and recurrent urinary tract infections.

    2. Dysuria, urgency, frequency, nocturia, and suprapubic heaviness or discomfort.

    3. Obstructive symptoms, such as a weak urinary stream, abdominal straining to void, hesitancy, incomplete bladder emptying, and terminal dribbling.

    4. Acute onset of fever, chills, flank pain, headache, malaise, costovertebral angle tenderness, and possibly hematuria.

49. A 14-year-old boy comes into the clinic from school with complaints of severe scrotal pain radiating inguinally that began suddenly. He is experiencing no difficulty voiding, and has some nausea but no vomiting. Examination reveals scrotal edema and erythema, the scrotum on the affected side is slightly higher than the unaffected side, and the cremasteric reflex is negative. The nurse practitioner determines the best treatment for this client is:

    1. Bed rest with ice pack and scrotal elevation.

    2. Warm scrotal pack and return to clinic the next day.

    3. Immediate referral to a urologist.

    4. Schedule for an ultrasound in the morning.

50. A 25-year-old client with a history of sickle cell disease complains of a sudden problem with erections that are not sexually oriented. He is currently experiencing a painful erection and he is unable to void. The nurse practitioner determines the treatment of choice is:

    1. Meperidine (Demerol) and bed rest.

    2. Immediate referral to a urologist.

    3. Increased hydration for sickle cell crisis.

    4. Determination of PSA level.

51. The nurse practitioner is speaking with a group of male teenagers. They are most concerned about symptoms associated with gonorrhea. The nurse practitioner discusses with them that:

    1. There may be reddish lesions on the palms of the hands and soles of the feet.

    2. Men may observe a rash over the body of the penis.

3. Urinary dribbling may occur due to the irritation of the urinary tract.

4. Painful urination occurs due to the inflammation of the urethra.

Pharmacology

52. A client has been on doxazosin (Cardura) 2 mg PO daily for 3 weeks for treatment of his BPH. He returns to the clinic and is complaining of feeling dizzy when he stands up. The nurse practitioner:

   1. Determines his blood pressure with him lying down, standing, and sitting.

   2. Orders a urinalysis to determine hematuria and presence of bacteria.

   3. Reviews with the client his symptoms over the past 3 weeks.

   4. Performs a rectal exam to determine if the prostate is smaller than previously noted.

53. In planning the treatment for a client with balanitis, the nurse practitioner orders:

   1. Rest, ice, and elevation.

   2. Massage.

   3. Antifungals.

   4. Emergency circumcision.

54. A 28-year-old male presents with complaints of fever, low back pain, perineal pain, and intense pain on voiding. Rectal exam reveals a tender, swollen, firm, warm prostate. Based on the client's symptoms, the treatment of choice is:

   1. Trimethoprim-sulfamethoxazole (TMP-SMX; Septra DS) 1 tab bid, × 30 days.

   2. Tetracycline (Achromycin) 250 mg qid × 10 days.

   3. Amoxicillin (Amoxil) 500 mg tid × 14 days.

   4. Erythromycin (Ilosone) 250 mg q6h × 24 days.

55. A 70-year-old man complains of scrotal pain with dysuria and frequency that has been increasing over the past 2 weeks. Physical examination reveals extreme tenderness and swelling of the scrotum, there is a urethral discharge, and the testes are normal in size and position. A urinalysis reveals pyuria. Based on the client's symptoms, the treatment of choice for this client is:

   1. Nitrofurantoin (Macrodantin) 100 mg PO qid × 14 days.

   2. Trimethoprim-sulfamethoxazole (Septra DS) 1 tab PO bid × 10 days.

   3. Doxazosin (Cardura) 1 mg PO qd × 10 days.

   4. Oxbutynin (Ditropan) 5 mg PO tid × 10 days.

56. Finasteride (Proscar) is prescribed for a 50-year-old man who is experiencing a problem with urination secondary to an enlarged prostate. The nurse practitioner would teach this client that while on this medication it is important for him to:

   1. Increase his fluid intake.

   2. Restrain from sexual activity.

   3. Use contraceptives.

   4. Increase intake of folic acid.

57. A 75-year-old client is diagnosed with chronic bacterial prostatitis and the nurse practitioner selects TMP-SMX (Septra DS) as the treatment. How should the TMP-SMX be prescribed for this client?

   1. 2 tablets bid × 10 weeks.

   2. 1 tablet tid × 3 days then two tablets × 10 days.

   3. 2 tablets qid × 2 days, then one tablet bid × 14 days.

   4. 1 tablet bid for 30 days.

15 ▶ Answers & Rationales

Physical Examination & Diagnostic Tests

1. **(4)** Cowper's glands (bulbourethral glands) are located near the prostate and beside the urethra near the base of the penis. These glands are part of the internal and nonpalpable genitalia that consists of glands and ducts. The testes, vas deferens, and epididymis are part of the external genitalia.

2. **(3)** Gonadotropin is elevated in testicular disease, whereas PSA is elevated in disease of the prostate, such as BPH.

3. **(1)** The epididymis is part of the external genitalia, whereas the ducts and glands are part of the internal genitalia. The epididymis is palpated on the posterolateral surface of each testis and is a comma-shaped structure. The seminal vesicles (pair of glands) lie behind the urinary bladder in front of the rectum. These vesicles join the ampulla of the vas deferens to form the ejaculatory duct.

4. **(1)** A complete history and physical will usually provide the cause of gynecomastia without further testing, since it can be caused by medication, starving and refeeding, or lack of androgen production (atrophying testes), which changes the estrogen-androgen ratio.

5. **(4)** For client comfort and ease of examination, the healthy, ambulatory adult client is asked to lean over the examination table with his chest and upper body resting on the table. Although Option #1 is correct,

it is the position used for examining a client who is confined to bed.

6. **(3)** PAP is an enzyme marker. An increased value is the result of increased metabolism and catabolism of cancer cells of the prostate; in three fourths of clients the cancer arises in the posterior lobe of the prostate. This marker is also used to monitor therapy with antineoplastic drugs and cancer metastatic to bone (osteoblastic lesions). AFP (oncofetal antigen) is produced by fetal liver, yolk sac, and intestinal epithelium and disappears from blood soon after birth; it is not present in healthy individuals. It is increased in primary hepatocellular cancer, embryonal cell (nonseminomatous germ cell) cancer, testicular tumors, and others. PSA (protein marker), which is more sensitive than PAP, increases in prostate cancer and in BPH. hCG (hormone marker), produced by placental syncytiotrophoblasts, is not usually found in sera of healthy, nonpregnant women but increases in seminomatous and nonseminomatous testicular cancer.

7. **(1)** PSA can be elevated in clients with BPH and those with prostatitis, as well as after prostate gland massage and it does increase with the increasing burden of the tumor, as in the reoccurrence of prostate cancer.

8. **(2)** Recommended screening for prostate cancer should begin at age 40 with DRE, with PSA testing to begin at age 50 if there are no risk factors or symptoms. Urinalysis and CBC are used in an annual physical as screening procedures, but are not indicated in screening for prostate cancer. *PSA test and DRE are indicated for men over 50 years.*

9. **(3)** The scrotal sac is asymmetrical, darker than body skin, and often appears reddened in red-haired men (abnormal finding if found in clients without red hair), and has a surface that may be coarse with small lumps on the skin that are sebaceous or epidermoid cysts that may have an oily discharge.

Disorders

10. **(2)** Sudden onset of pain with a firm, tender mass in the scrotum; pain is not relieved when the involved testicle is elevated to relieve pressure. Prehn's sign, passive elevation of the testes, is associated with epididymitis. The cremasteric reflex is absent. Testicular torsion is most common among neonates and adolescents, with highest incidence at time of puberty.

11. **(1)** The lack of pain, increase in size of scrotal contents and transillumination are characteristic of hydrocele. Orchitis and epididymitis are usually characterized by pain; orchitis most often is associated with parotitis or mumps. There is no history of injury and the scrotum would be tender to palpation.

12. **(1)** Circumcision is helpful in preventing phimosis and paraphimosis, as both are retraction dysfunctions of the prepuce. In phimosis, the foreskin is too tight to be retracted backward over the glans penis. In paraphimosis, once the foreskin has been retracted behind the glans penis, it is too constricted to return to a position of covering the glans penis.

13. **(3)** Acute epididymitis is characterized by an acute scrotal pain, dysuria, and enlarged unilateral scrotum with abdominal pain.

Scrotal pain is relieved when the involved testicle is elevated.

14. **(1)** A male will present with impotence and decreased libido. These same men will often have gynecomastia due to the low or absent production of gonadotropin. Males with Klinefelter's syndrome (a chromosomal abnormality with a karyotype of 47,XXY– 47,XXXXY) is the most common cause of male hypogonadism, with failure of both spermatic function and virilization.

15. **(1)** Impotence can be caused by antihypertensives such as propranolol (Inderal, Inderal LA). The nonselective β-blockers are believed to decrease vascular resistance and central effect. Erectile dysfunction is reported to begin at doses of 120 mg/day. Other causes include infections or vascular, psychological, and traumatic causes.

16. **(1)** Paraphimosis is a retraction disorder related to a constricted prepuce that can be relieved through circumcision.

17. **(2)** The prostate secretes fluid that is alkaline and helps sperm survive in the acid environment of the female reproductive tract. Androgens are produced by the Leydig cells of the testes. Sperm are produced in the seminiferous tubules of the testes.

18. **(4)** The DRE and levels of PSA are the primary indicators of prostatic cancer. This should be thoroughly evaluated. The other options listed are directed toward treatment of BPH. Only after prostatic cancer has been ruled out should these be utilized.

19. **(4)** This involves the differential diagnosis between epididymitis and testicular torsion. Irreversible damage will be done to the testicles if torsion is not released within 3–4 hours. Time should not be wasted with other treatments if torsion is strongly suspected.

20. **(1)** Testicular torsion and testicular cancer are considerations that are potentially curable but must be treated early. Hydrocele, epididymitis, and inguinal hernias also require referrals but do not require immediate attention.

21. **(2)** In suspected acute prostatitis, only a rectal exam should be performed, if at all. Vigorous massage must be avoided because of the risk of inducing bacteremia. A urine culture, urethral cultures for gonorrhea and chlamydia, and blood collection for BUN and creatinine are indicated to help make the diagnosis.

22. **(3)** BPH is commonly seen in men over 50 years old. Bladder cancer should be ruled out as a diagnosis.

23. **(1)** All of the symptoms listed can be found in the client with prostate cancer, but only the symptoms listed in Option #1 are localized. Many times the client will be asymptomatic.

24. **(1)** Varicocele presents as described, whereas a hernia may transilluminate, and sometimes bowel sounds can be auscultated in the scrotum. Hernias vary in size with Valsalva maneuvers. Tumors do not transilluminate.

25. **(2)** Phimosis is a retraction disorder of the penile foreskin or prepuce and can occur at any age and is usually the result of poor hygiene and chronic infection (the foreskin cannot be retracted back over the glans penis). Paraphimosis is the inability to retract the foreskin from behind the glans penis.

26. **(4)** Peyronie's disease is a fibrotic condition that causes lateral curvature of the penis during erection.

27. **(2)** Inflammation of the glans penis and prepuce usually is associated with poor hygiene and is usually found in men with poorly controlled diabetes and candidiasis.

28. **(1)** Candidiasis is the usual cause for balanitis, which is inflammation of the glans penis and prepuce, usually associated with poor hygiene and is also found in men with poorly controlled diabetes.

29. **(4)** In sexual dysfunction, erection, emission, or ejaculation may not be functioning due to multifactorial causes, such as vascular, neuropathy, or trauma. Peyronie's disease and priapism are examples of erection dysfunction.

30. **(3)** Epididymitis presents as described and, on palpation, the epididymis will often feel like a bag of worms in the scrotal sac rather than a fairly smooth cord.

31. **(3)** This is the correct definition of erectile dysfunction which statistics reveal that 40% of 40-year-old males and 70% of 70+ year-old males may experience. It involves a hemodynamic mechanism of smooth muscle relaxation which increases the amount of blood flow in the penis and ultimately causes venous trapping (compression of the subtunical venules) causing rigidity.

32. **(1)** Priapism is a condition of prolonged penile erection related to venous obstruction and unrelated to sexual arousal.

33. **(3)** Males with undescended testicles are more prone to developing prostate cancer. The other conditions listed are not causes of prostate cancer.

34. **(1)** Antihypertensive drugs, such as propranolol (Inderal, Inderal LA), can cause impotence.

35. **(1)** This is the age group (15–35) that is affected by testicular cancer, and self-examination can be valuable in securing early diagnosis and treatment. PSA testing is recommended at age 50 and a DRE at age 40.

36. **(1)** Cirrhosis and diseases of the hepatic system are often a cause of gynecomastia. It is thought that cirrhosis and other hepatic disease alter the estrogen-androgen ratio. None of the other diseases has been implicated in gynecomastia.

37. **(2)** Gynecomastia is the result of an increased estrogen-to-androgen ratio in men, and as a result their breast cancers are receptor positive.

38. **(4)** Prostate cancer in men is usually found in those over the age of 50 years, and causes rapid onset of urinary obstructive symptoms. On palpation, asymmetrical, discrete, hard nodule(s) are located. An increase in size of the prostate of >4 mm.

39. **(4)** Rapid onset of obstructive symptoms of urinary output would indicate a fast-growing tumor or obstruction of the urinary

tract. All the other symptoms are indicative of BPH, tumor, or stricture of the urinary tract.

40. **(4)** Testicular cancer is primarily found in young men and presents as nonpainful nodules of the involved testicle. Trauma is not a causal factor.

41. **(2)** Acute bacterial prostatitis is caused by an infection in the urinary tract moving up the urethra into the prostate. The most common organisms are *Escherichia coli*, *Pseudomonas*, and *Streptococcus faecalis*. The condition tends to occur in men between 30 and 50 years old but can be associated with BPH in older men. Chronic bacterial prostatitis is characterized by recurrent urinary tract infections, with the usual course of antibiotic treatment lasting for 12 weeks (due to blockage of the antibiotics by fibrosis in the prostatic tissue).

42. **(1)** Usually orchitis presents with a tender unilateral swollen testicle within 7–10 days of mumps (parotitis). An elevated serum amylase is associated with inflammation of the salivary glands, i.e., mumps.

43. **(2)** NGU is often asymptomatic and as such is difficult to diagnose. NGU commonly has a clear discharge and usually is caused by chlamydia. Gonococcal urethritis produces a yellow, purulent discharge. If there is a discharge, NGU is hard to differentiate from gonorrhea without a culture. Reiter's syndrome is also associated with untreated chlamydia infections of the urogenital tract.

44. **(1)** *Chlamydia trachomatis* is the most common organism in males with NGU.

45. **(3)** Cryptorchidism is the result of undescended testes, either bilateral or, more often, affecting the right testis. Normally, descent is in the seventh to eighth month of gestation.

46. **(1)** AFP (onocefetal antigen) is produced by fetal liver, yolk sac, and intestinal epithelium and disappears from blood soon after birth and is not present in healthy individuals but increases in primary hepatocellular cancer, embryonal cell (nonseminomatous germ cell) cancer, testicular tumors, and others. PAP is an enzyme marker. An increased value is the result of increased metabolism and catabolism of cancer cells of the prostate; in three fourths of clients the cancer aries in the posterior lobe of the prostate. This marker is also used to monitor therapy with antineoplastic drugs and cancer metastatic to bone (osteoblastic lesions). PSA (protein marker), which is more sensitive than PAP, increases in prostate cancer and in benign prostatic hypertrophy. ALP increases in osteosarcoma, hepatocellular, metastatic to liver, and primary or secondary bone tumors.

47. **(3)** The mumps virus is responsible for causing orchitis. Arbovirus and echovirus are implicated in meningitis/encephalitis. Rubeola is associated with complications of otitis media, pneumonia, croup, and encephalitis.

48. **(3)** Obstructive symptoms are common in BPH. Dribbling, hesitancy, loss of normal urine stream, and recurrent urinary tract infections are present in chronic bacterial prostatitis. Dysuria, urgency, frequency, nocturia, and suprapubic heaviness are common symptoms of cystitis. Fever, chills, flank pain, headache, malaise, and costovertebral angle tenderness of acute onset with or without hematuria are indications of pyelonephritis.

49. **(3)** The symptoms described are consistent with testicular torsion. This is an emergent and surgical problem and the client should be referred immediately.

50. **(2)** This is considered a urologic emergency because the circulation to the penis may be compromised, as well as because of the inability to void. The client should be referred immediately to a physician.

51. **(4)** Dysuria is one of the most common complaints of young men with gonorrhea. There are no lesions, rash, or urinary dribbling along with the yellow discharge.

Pharmacology

52. **(1)** Doxazosin (Cardura) is also used as an antihypertensive agent; the client may be experiencing orthostatic hypotension. The other answers are directed toward evaluating his BPH, which has already been diagnosed.

53. **(3)** Antifungals (e.g., topical nystatin [Mycostatin] or Ciclopirox [Loprox]) are the treatment of choice. If the infection is recalcitrant, give oral fluconazole (Diflucan) 150 mg/day or itraconazole (Sporanox) 100 mg/day. All the other treatments are inappropriate.

54. **(1)** The client is presenting with classic symptoms of acute bacterial prostatitis. The treatment of choice is TMP-SMX. It is important to treat the client for at least 30 days to prevent relapse. Treatment is started pending the results of the culture and sensitivity.

55. **(2)** The client is presenting with classic symptoms of epididymitis. The treatment of choice is TMP-SMX. Nitrofurantoin is a urinary antiseptic, doxazosin is given for BPH, and oxbutynin is indicated for incontinence or enuresis. On differential diagnosis, the gradual onset of pain, voiding problems, urethral discharge, and swelling are more indicative of epididymitis than testicular torsion.

56. **(3)** It is important that women of child-bearing age are not exposed to the sperm of a client on finasteride. Pregnant women and those of child-bearing age should avoid handling crushed tablets.

57. **(4)** The recommended treatment is for at least 30 days to prevent recurrence. Clients may require continued suppression therapy for an extended period of time.

Women's Health

Physical Examination & Diagnostic Tests

1. When obtaining a cervical specimen for a Pap smear, the nurse practitioner:

   1. Lubricates the speculum with a water-soluble lubricant to assist in the insertion of the instrument.

   2. Utilizes the cervical brush when obtaining the cervical cells on a prenatal client due to the presence of the cervical mucous plug.

   3. Uses warm water to lubricate the speculum to assist in the insertion of the instrument.

   4. Completes the bimanual portion of the examination first in order to determine the relative position of the cervix to assist in a comfortable insertion of the speculum.

2. To promote client comfort prior to performing a pelvic exam, the nurse practitioner:

   1. Asks the client to bear down slightly as the speculum is inserted.

   2. Has the client empty her bladder.

   3. Explains each step of the procedure in a calm manner.

   4. Carefully reassures the client that the exam will only take a few minutes.

3. What finding is considered a normal surface characteristic of the cervix?

   1. Small, yellow, raised round area on cervix.

   2. Red patch areas with occasional white spots.

   3. Friable, bleeding tissue at opening of cervical os.

   4. Irregular, granular surface with red patches.

4. The primary role of a breast ultrasound is:

   1. Used as a screening test for breast cancer.

   2. Used for definitive diagnosis of breast cancer.

   3. Used to determine if a breast lesion is cystic or solid.

   4. Used to locate small lesions prior to surgery.

5. The optimal time to perform a hysterosalpingogram (HSG) is:

   1. During menses.

   2. Immediately after ovulation.

   3. After menses, but before ovulation.

   4. 3–4 days prior to menses.

6. Which statement about mammography is **false**?

   1. Mammography detects all breast cancers.

   2. Mammography should be accompanied by breast exam.

   3. Negative mammography should not delay biopsy of a clinically suspicious mass.

   4. Mammography is a cost-effective method to screen for breast cancer.

7. The use of potassium hydroxide (KOH) when doing a wet mount assists in the diagnosis of:

   1. Bacterial vaginosis and candida vaginitis.

   2. Trichomonas and chlamydia.

   3. Syphilis and gonorrhea.

   4. Herpes and condyloma.

8. The nurse practitioner is reviewing the lab results of an 18-year-old client seen recently for a Pap smear. The results are as follows: Classification—high-grade squamous intraepithelial lesion; endocervical cells seen; adequate smear.

The nurse practitioner phones the client and tells her which of the following?

   1. "Your Pap smear was normal. Follow up in one year, sooner if problems arise."

   2. "Your Pap smear shows invasive cancer. I would like you to see a gynecologic oncologist for treatment."

   3. "Your Pap smear shows abnormal tissue that needs to be evaluated. Please schedule an appointment for a colposcopy."

   4. "Your Pap smear shows a minor abnormality. Sometimes this can signify a disease process just beginning. Please schedule another Pap smear in 4 months for follow-up."

9. A 27-year-old client reports the desire to become pregnant. She and her husband have had regular, unprotected intercourse for more than 1 year. The nurse practitioner completes a thorough history and gynecologic exam, which appear normal. What diagnostic test might you order early in your work-up?

   1. Hysterosalpingogram.

   2. Tests for antisperm antibodies.

   3. Semen analysis.

   4. Endometrial biopsy.

10. When describing the findings from a normal breast examination, the nurse practitioner documents on the client record:

   1. Left nipple everted, several coarse black hairs arising from the areola, enlarged axillary lymph nodes palpated bilaterally, and tender nodes in supraclavicular area.

   2. No dimpling or retraction; 1-cm hard, fixed, stellate mass noted next to nipple with scant nipple discharge; no pain or tenderness on palpation.

   3. Right breast slightly larger and denser than left with no nipple discharge, right areola dark pink in color and inverted, left areola dark brown in color and everted, breasts tender to palpation with no axillary nodes noted.

4. Pendulous breasts with no dimpling, retraction, nipple discharge, or areas of discoloration; numerous small nevi near areola with Montgomery's tubercles noted, no supraclavicular or axillary lymph nodes palpated.

11. In an infertility work-up, what is the best way to evaluate ovulation?

    1. Hysterosalpingogram.

    2. Postcoital test.

    3. Endometrial biopsy.

    4. Basal body temperature (BBT) chart.

12. The nurse practitioner is reviewing the lab work of a 61-year-old adult client seen recently for a Pap smear. She has been treated for breast cancer with mastectomy and tamoxifen (Nolvadex). She is not and never has been on hormone replacement therapy (HRT). The results of her Pap smear are as follows: atrophic changes; scant endocervical cells; adequate smear. What is appropriate for the nurse practitioner to tell the client when she phones her with her results?

    1. "Your Pap smear is slightly abnormal. I would recommend the use of some estrogen vaginal cream nightly for 3 weeks, then return to the office to have the Pap smear repeated."

    2. "Your Pap smear is normal but shows a mild thinning of the tissue. This is to be expected in someone who is not on hormones and does not pose a threat to your health. Please return to the office in 1 year for your annual exam, sooner if needed."

    3. "Your Pap smear shows that you don't have enough endocervical cells. Please make an appointment for endocervical curettage."

    4. "Your Pap smear is abnormal. This could signify a disease state of the cervix. Please schedule a colposcopy at your earliest convenience."

13. Which test is the "gold standard" for the diagnosis of chlamydia?

    1. Use of KOH wet mount "whiff" test.

    2. Presence of inflammatory cells in Pap smear.

    3. Direct fluorescent antibody (DFA).

    4. Culture with special media and collection technique.

14. The nurse practitioner is discussing mammography with a group of women. It is important for the nurse practitioner to advise the women that:

    1. A mammography should be done annually for all women of child-bearing age.

    2. All women over 40 years old should have a mammogram on an annual basis.

    3. A mammogram should be done annually after pregnancy, if the woman does not breast-feed.

    4. A mammogram should be done if there is any breast pain or nipple retraction.

15. Which is the most accurate statement regarding a reactive serologic test for syphilis?

    1. All reactive serologic tests require confirmation with a treponemal test.

    2. Reactive serologic tests are highly suspicious for active syphilis.

    3. A false-positive serologic test, although rare, can be unnecessarily traumatizing to a client.

    4. A reactive serologic test most likely implies the need for retreatment.

16. While working-up a client with secondary amenorrhea, the prolactin serum assay results show a level of 24 ng/ml. Appropriate management includes:

    1. Administering medroxyprogesterone acetate 10 mg bid × 5 days.

    2. Referring to a physician.

    3. Recording the results as within normal limits.

    4. Assessment for nipple discharge.

17. When evaluating a young adult with amenorrhea and normal secondary sex characteristics, the purpose of the progesterone challenge is to determine the presence of:

    1. Endogenous estrogen.

    2. Thyroxine.

    3. Prolactin.

    4. Adequate body fat.

18. A client comes in complaining of fatigue, breast tenderness, abdominal bloating, fluid retention, and irritability about a week prior to the onset of her menses. This has been occurring for the past 4 months. What is the most important information for the nurse practitioner to obtain to assist in determining the diagnosis of premenstrual syndrome (PMS)?

    1. Occurrence of symptoms in the menstrual cycle.

    2. Severity of the symptoms.

    3. Number and frequency of symptoms over past 4 months.

    4. Presence or absence of anxiety or depression.

Normal Gynecology

19. The endometrial cycle is often described in three phases. Select the correct phases:

    1. Follicular, menstrual, and luteal.

    2. Proliferative, luteal, and menstrual.

    3. Follicular, secretory, and menstrual.

    4. Proliferative, secretory, and menstrual.

20. The nurse practitioner understands that PMS occurs with greatest frequency and severity in the:

    1. Late luteal phase.

    2. Follicular phase.

    3. Proliferative phase.

    4. Ovulatory phase.

21. Which hormone is **not** released from the anterior pituitary gland?

    1. Follicle-stimulating hormone (FSH).

    2. Luteinizing hormone (LH).

    3. Oxytocin.

    4. Prolactin.

22. The primary function of FSH is:

    1. Stimulation of maturation of ovarian follicles.

    2. Milk secretion.

    3. Triggering ovulation.

    4. Inhibiting release of LH from the pituitary gland.

23. In the ovarian cycle, what phase begins with ovulation and ends with the onset of menses?

    1. Follicular phase.

    2. Ovulation.

    3. Proliferative phase.

    4. Luteal phase.

24. Which is **not** a risk factor for heart disease in the postmenopausal female?

    1. Hyperlipidemia.

    2. Cigarette smoking.

    3. Hormone replacement therapy.

    4. Diabetes mellitus.

25. An adult client's last menstrual period (LMP) was 2 months ago. She has a Paragard T 380 intrauterine device (IUD) in place for the last 4 months. She is complaining of nausea, fatigue, breast tenderness, and abdominal bloating. Her physical exam reveals the following:

    • Abdomen: within normal limits (WNL)

    • Pelvic: cervix—positive Chadwick's sign, IUD strings seen protruding from the cervical os

    • Uterus: enlarged, approximately 7 weeks' size, nontender

    • Adnexae: nontender, without mass, no cervical motion tenderness (CMT)

The most likely diagnosis is:

1. Uterine fibroid.

2. Ovarian cancer.

3. Dislodged IUD.

4. Pregnancy.

26. What function do the Bartholin's glands have in reproduction?

    1. Prevent vaginitis by maintaining adequate pH.

    2. Prepare the mucous plug that occurs during early pregnancy.

    3. Produce an alkaline secretion that enhances sperm viability.

    4. Produce small amounts of hormones necessary for ovulation.

27. Which is **not** a risk factor for osteoporosis?

    1. Cigarette smoker.

    2. Caucasian.

    3. Alcohol consumption.

    4. Obesity.

28. A young woman complains to the nurse practitioner that she is experiencing headaches, irritability, decreased appetite, and fatigue about 1 week prior to her menses. Appropriate management includes:

    1. Treating the PMS with increased protein and salt in the diet.

    2. Incorporating daily regular aerobic exercise into her lifestyle.

    3. Ordering a complete blood count (CBC), SMAC-12, and urinalysis.

    4. Supplementing the diet with an additional 1–2 gm of vitamin C.

29. A middle-aged female presents with dysfunctional uterine bleeding. A hormonal profile reveals increased FSH and LH levels. The most likely cause for these findings is?

    1. Hypothalmic disorder.

    2. Onset of climacteric.

    3. Premature ovarian failure.

    4. Anterior pituitary disorder.

30. While assessing a 16-year-old girl, the nurse practitioner was asked about douching. What information would be used in the nurse practitioner's teaching plan?

    1. Douching during menstruation is safe.

    2. Due to vaginal discharge, daily douching is important.

    3. Hypoallergenic douches include flavored or perfumed types.

    4. Douching removes natural mucus and upsets normal vaginal flora.

31. A 29-year-old female client presents to the family planning clinic for her annual exam. She had a tubal ligation postpartum 6 months ago. She has been feeling tired, nauseated, and is slowly gaining weight. She had one menses postpartum, 4 months ago. The nurse practitioner notes the following on physical exam:

    - Abdomen: bowel sounds × 4, soft, no hepatosplenomegaly, palpable mass in lower abdomen, measures 14 cm, no tenderness

    - Pelvic: Bartholin's, urethral, and Skene's glands (BUS) normal; Cervix— os closed, smooth, pink mucosa

    - Bimanual: uterus enlarged, nontender, smooth contours, no CMT

    - Adnexae: not palpable

    What is the likely diagnosis?

    1. Pregnancy.

    2. Uterine fibroid.

    3. Premature menopause.

    4. Colon cancer.

Gynecologic Disorders

32. During a yearly physical examination, a nurse practitioner asks a woman if she has any problems or questions about sexual function or activity. Initially, the client hesitates but, with further questioning and discussion, she states that she is unsure if she has ever experienced an orgasm before. The nurse practitioner suspects:

   1. Vaginismus.
   2. Primary orgasmic dysfunction.
   3. Secondary orgasmic dysfunction.
   4. Dyspareunia.

33. The nurse practitioner is talking with a young women who has been diagnosed with herpes simplex type 2 (genital). In discussing her care, it would be important for the nurse practitioner to include what information?

   1. The initial lesions are usually worse than lesions that occur with outbreaks at a later time.
   2. Her sexual partner will not contract it if she does not have sex when the lesions are present.
   3. This condition can be treated and cured if she takes all of the antibiotics for 2 weeks.
   4. If in the future she becomes pregnant, she will have to have a cesarean delivery.

34. The definition of bacterial vaginosis is:

   1. A syndrome resulting from homeostatic disruption in the vagina.
   2. Vaginitis caused by a flagellated protozoan.
   3. A bacterial sexually transmitted disease (STD) that can be symptomatic or asymptomatic.
   4. A virus characterized by recurrent outbreaks and remissions.

35. A 22-year-old married client complains of severe dysmenorrhea. Her gynecologic exam is normal. Which management protocol is preferred?

   1. Assess for contraceptive interest and, if interested, suggest use of oral contraceptives (OC).
   2. Suggest use of prostaglandin synthetase inhibitor.
   3. Suggest over-the-counter use of ibuprofen.
   4. Assess exercise patterns and use of relaxation techniques.

36. Which is **not** a criterion for the diagnosis of bacterial vaginosis?

   1. Positive amine test (whiff test).
   2. Presence of clue cells.
   3. Vaginal pH >4.5.
   4. The presence of pseudohyphae.

37. A client with a history of dilatation and curettage (D&C) after a first-trimester spontaneous abortion and subsequent amenorrhea would lead the nurse practitioner to suspect which problem?

   1. Polycystic ovarian syndrome.
   2. Asherman's syndrome.
   3. Hypogonadism.
   4. Premature ovarian failure.

38. The LH/FSH ratio in polycystic ovarian syndrome (Stein-Leventhal syndrome) is:

   1. 1.5:1.
   2. 3:1.
   3. 6:1.
   4. 1:3.

39. What is a criterion for diagnosing polycystic ovarian syndrome?

   1. Weight loss.
   2. Hyperprolactinemia.
   3. Laboratory evidence of increased estradiol.
   4. Chronic anovulation.

40. The most common cause of dysfunctional uterine bleeding is?

    1. Thyroid disorder.

    2. Blood dyscrasia.

    3. Anovulation.

    4. Uterine tumor.

41. A 30-year-old female individual presents with scant pubic hair, minimal breast development, absent cervix, and uterus with a 46,XY karyotype. Your diagnosis is:

    1. Turner's syndrome.

    2. Müllerian agenesis.

    3. Testicular feminization.

    4. Gonadal dysgenesis.

42. The most common cause of a breast mass in clients ages 15–25 is:

    1. Fibroadenoma.

    2. Intraductal papilloma.

    3. Infiltrating lobular carcinoma.

    4. Fibrocystic breast syndrome.

43. An effective treatment for primary dysmenorrhea is:

    1. Nonsteroidal anti-inflammatory analgesics.

    2. Tranquilizers.

    3. Progestins.

    4. Steroids.

44. What is a cause of secondary amenorrhea?

    1. Testicular feminization.

    2. Hypogonadotropic hypogonadism.

    3. Congenital absence of uterus.

    4. Extreme exercise.

45. A young woman comes into the clinic for a well-woman checkup. She states that, about 3 weeks ago, she had a sore on her labia that went away. It was not particularly painful, did not itch, and there did not seem to be any residual problems from it. The nurse practitioner treats this woman by:

    1. Ordering the treponemal-specific test (FTA-ABS).

    2. Swabbing the area of the lesion for a viral culture.

    3. Advising her to notify her sexual contacts to determine if they have had any symptoms.

    4. Ordering nystatin (Mycostatin) cream to be applied to the area three to four times a day.

46. A high-school athlete presents to the clinic with concerns regarding her menstrual periods. She states she has not had a period in the past 2 months. She has been in training and running about 3 miles a day for the past 3 months. She has lost approximately 15 lbs. Her height is about 63 inches and she currently weights 100 lbs. The best response by the nurse practitioner is to:

    1. Determine the client's percentage of body fat and body mass.

    2. Obtain FSH serum levels.

    3. Determine serum levels of hCG.

    4. Order thyroid function tests.

47. Which is **not** a risk factor for the development of cervical cancer?

    1. Human papillomavirus (HPV).

    2. Virginal status.

    3. Multiple sexual partners.

    4. Previous high-grade squamous intraepithelial lesion (HSIL).

48. A young woman is complaining of tenderness and burning of her vulva. On examination the vulva is edematous and excoriated. The nurse practitioner performs a wet mount prep of the vaginal secretions. It reveals pseudohyphae and spores. The diagnosis for this client is:

    1. Vulvovaginal candidiasis.

    2. *Chlamydia trachomatis*.

    3. Bacterial vaginitis.

    4. Gonorrhea.

49. The leading cause of death in female genital cancers, excluding breast, is:

    1. Ovarian cancer.

    2. Endometrial cancer.

    3. Cervical cancer.

    4. Vulvar and/or vaginal cancer.

50. A young woman presents with complaints of an irritation in the vaginal area. This is the first time it has occurred. On vaginal examination, the cervix is inflamed and friable. Flagellated protozoa are seen on the wet prep. The most likely diagnosis is:

    1. Trichomoniasis.

    2. Mucopurulent cervicitis.

    3. Chlamydia.

    4. Bacterial vaginosis.

51. A 26-year-old female client presents to the emergency room and is seen by the nurse practitioner. The client had a gradual onset of abdominal pain, starting in the periumbilical region and now in the right lower quadrant. It is accompanied by nausea, anorexia, constipation, and low-grade fever. The physical exam confirms the diagnosis of acute appendicitis. What diagnostic studies are **least** useful in confirming this diagnosis?

    1. CBC, with differential.

    2. Flat plate of abdomen, kidney-ureters-bladder (KUB).

    3. Pelvic ultrasound.

    4. Pregnancy test.

52. Which is **not** a risk factor for endometrial cancer?

    1. Obesity.

    2. Birth control pill use.

    3. Unopposed estrogen use.

    4. Advancing age, >50 years.

53. Which statement is true regarding the diaphragm?

    1. May be inserted up to 24 hours prior to intercourse.

2. May be inserted any time up to 6 hours prior to intercourse.

3. Should be removed within 1 hour after intercourse.

4. May only be left in place up to 12 hours.

54. A contraceptive method that is associated with an increase in urinary tract infection is the:

    1. Intrauterine device.

    2. Diaphragm.

    3. Norplant.

    4. Oral contraceptive pills.

55. Which is **not** a risk factor for ovarian cancer?

    1. Family history of ovarian cancer.

    2. Advancing age, >50 years.

    3. Birth control pill use.

    4. Positive BRCA 2 gene.

56. What is the most common female genital malignancy, excluding the breast?

    1. Ovary.

    2. Endometrium.

    3. Cervix.

    4. Vulva/vagina.

57. A 20-year-old female college student presents to urgent care with new onset of painful sores in the vulva. These erupted yesterday and are associated with exquisite pain, fever, and flu-like symptoms of headache, general body aches, and mild dysuria. She has a new sexual partner and thinks she saw a sore on his external genitalia after coitus. The examination reveals vesicular lesions covering the labium; extreme tenderness to palpation of the external genitalia; normal BUS; normal vaginal inspection with a mild leukorrhea; normal cervical mucosa; and slightly tender minimally enlarged inguinal lymph nodes bilaterally. What is the likely diagnosis?

    1. Gonorrhea.

    2. Chlamydia.

3. Herpes simplex virus.

4. Lymphogranuloma venereum.

58. A 21-year-old female client is seen for her annual gynecologic exam. She is sexually active, rarely uses condoms for STD prevention, and has multiple sexual partners. She smokes one pack per day, admits to a sedentary lifestyle, and eats two meals per day, most often at fast food restaurants. Her exam is negative for any abnormality. Her family history and personal medical history are negative for major disease. There are no menstrual abnormalities; her LMP was 1 week ago. The nurse practitioner has done her Pap smear. Which would **not** be appropriate for this client?

1. Cultures for gonorrhea and chlamydia.

2. Lab testing: glucose, cardiac risk profile, and TSH.

3. Human immunodeficiency (HIV) titer and rapid plasma reagin (RPR).

4. Counseling on safe sex practice and contraceptive information.

59. Which is **not** considered to be a risk factor in the development of breast cancer?

1. Early menopause.

2. High-fat diet.

3. Advancing age.

4. Early menarche.

60. A 32-year-old female client, G2 T1 P1 A0 L2, is seen in the clinic by the nurse practitioner for her annual exam and is requesting information on preconception counseling. She has been on oral contraceptives for 3 years without complications. During the past year, she has started an exercise program at a health club 5 days a week and is eating three nutritionally sound meals daily. She has lost 33 lbs and is now at her ideal body weight. She quit her job as a postal worker and now stays home with her children. As part of her preconception care, what should the nurse practitioner recommend?

1. Start prenatal vitamins with folic acid.

2. Discontinue exercise.

3. Update measles-mumps-rubella (MMR) vaccine.

4. Genetic counseling due to advanced maternal age.

61. The initial work-up for dysfunctional uterine bleeding should include:

1. Referral for diagnostic dilatation and curettage.

2. Referral for endometrial biopsy to rule out cancer.

3. CBC, pregnancy test, endocrine studies.

4. Coagulation studies, STD cultures.

62. Which is **not** a risk factor for breast cancer?

1. History of maternal breast cancer— premenopausal onset.

2. First pregnancy after age 35.

3. Late menopause, after age 54.

4. Fibrocystic breast disease.

63. A 20-year-old female client presents for her first well-woman exam; she is not sexually active and never has been. Her family history and past medical history are negative for any gynecologic diseases. Her menses occur every 28 days, lasting 5 days, with a relatively moderate flow and no significant abdominal cramps. Her physical exam/visit today should include which tests?

1. Pap smear.

2. Cultures for gonorrhea and chlamydia.

3. Stool hemoccult.

4. Baseline mammogram.

64. What is the leading cause of death for females in the United States?

1. Breast cancer.

2. Colon cancer.

3. Heart disease.

4. Stroke.

65. During a gynecologic exam at the family planning clinic, an underweight 17-year-old presents with bruising around her upper torso and genitalia. She is minimally interactive and avoids eye contact as much as possible. Priority intervention should focus on:

    1. Lab work to rule out bleeding disorder.

    2. Nutritional assessment to determine possible anemia.

    3. Determination of possible physical abuse.

    4. Finding out if she has a support system.

66. Reactive cellular changes noted on a Pap smear are most often associated with:

    1. Inflammation.

    2. Use of estrogen vaginal cream.

    3. Drying artifact.

    4. Use of OCs.

67. Risk factors for cervical disease include:

    1. Pregnancy after 35 years of age.

    2. Viral exposure.

    3. Low parity.

    4. Prolonged contraceptive use.

68. What is the most common cancer in females in the United States?

    1. Breast cancer.

    2. Colon cancer.

    3. Malignant melanoma.

    4. Lung cancer.

69. A 48-year-old female client presents to the clinic with the following list of complaints: hot flashes, no menses for 14 months, insomnia, crying spells, irritability, decreased libido, and fatigue. At the end of her history and physical exam, she begins to cry and tells the nurse practitioner that she thinks she's going crazy; she then begs the nurse practitioner to tell her what is wrong. Which is **inappropriate** for the nurse practitioner to do at this point?

    1. Obtain lab tests, including FSH and LH.

    2. Discuss HRT, including risks and benefits and short-term and long-term treatment strategies.

    3. Provide antidepressant therapy and a referral for counseling sessions for depression.

    4. Provide the client with written information regarding menopause and the options for treatment of symptoms.

70. Follow-up care for a client with chancroid should include:

    1. Screening for HIV as well as syphilis.

    2. Mandatory notification and treatment of all sexual partners.

    3. Screening for lymphogranuloma venereum.

    4. Culture for gonorrhea.

71. During her annual exam, a 39-year-old female complains of recent breast changes. She states that her breasts are painful and frequently feel "lumpy." Because of this, she has stopped doing monthly breast self-examination (BSE), feeling that it is a waste of time. What would be the most appropriate advice to offer her?

    1. Stress the importance of continuing monthly BSE to detect unusual lumps because she knows the feel of her breasts.

    2. Suggest she at least do BSE every 2 months.

    3. Suggest she start getting mammograms to establish some baseline data about her breasts.

    4. Determine when her breasts are nontender and least "lumpy" and change her schedule for BSE.

72. During a breast exam on a young adult female, a 2-cm painless lobular mass in the right breast that is firm and freely mobile is noted on palpation. Appropriate management includes:

    1. Continued observation and rechecking in 3 months.

    2. Referral for a mammogram.

    3. Referral for probable surgical excision.

    4. Detailed family history to determine breast cancer risk.

73. A woman with bilateral breast implants asks if it is really necessary to do monthly BSE because she does not know what to feel for. The most appropriate response would be:

    1. Suggest she involve her sexual partner in assessing her breasts on a regular basis.

    2. Review the steps in BSE until she feels comfortable with the process.

    3. Acknowledge the difficulty of doing BSE after implant surgery.

    4. Explain the usefulness of regular mammograms for implant clients.

74. An adult client comes to the clinic complaining of abnormal vaginal discharge (dark watery brown) along with postcoital bleeding. The nurse practitioner suspects the possibility of cancer of the cervix. During the vaginal exam, suspicious physical results would be:

    1. Soft, sill-shaped cervix.

    2. Very firm cervix with an ulcer.

    3. Vague lower abdominal discomfort.

    4. Tender, enlarged lymph nodes.

75. A postmenopausal female is worried about pain in the upper outer quadrant of her left breast. The nurse practitioner should:

    1. Do a breast exam and order a mammogram.

    2. Explain that pain is related to hormone fluctuations and order laboratory studies.

3. Reassure the client that pain is not a presenting symptom of breast cancer and check for proper fit of the brassiere.

4. Teach the client BSE.

76. A 22-year-old female client comes to the nurse practitioner's office with a complaint of 1 day of fever of 102°F, a diffuse macular rash, vomiting, headache, and decreased urinary output. The history obtained by the nurse practitioner must include:

    1. Whether the client's immunizations are up to date.

    2. If the client is currently menstruating.

    3. If the client has a history of tuberculosis.

    4. What type of contraception the client uses.

77. A young female client presents to the nurse practitioner's office with a complaint of abdominal pain. In the United States, this diagnosis results in about 1 death per 1000 and therefore must be considered early in the decision process:

    1. Irritable bowel syndrome.

    2. Appendicitis.

    3. Pyelonephritis.

    4. Ectopic pregnancy.

78. A young adult female client presents with a history of vaginal itching and heavy white discharge. The client gives a history of no sexual activity. On exam, the nurse practitioner finds a red, edematous vulva and white patches on the vaginal walls. There is no odor to the discharge. The nurse practitioner expects what factors in the client's history?

    1. A vegetarian diet.

    2. Recent diarrhea.

    3. Early menopause.

    4. Recent antibiotic use.

79. A young female client comes to the office complaining of vaginal bleeding. The client states that she has used five tampons in the past 3 hours. She admits to sexual activity and takes oral contraceptives. On further questioning, the client states that she started her last pack of contraceptives "about 2 weeks late." The nurse practitioner should:

    1. Perform a STAT urine pregnancy test.

    2. Perform a STAT CBC.

    3. Discuss proper use of OCs.

    4. Send the client for a pelvic sonogram.

80. The nurse practitioner knows that the majority of breast cancers occur in which area of the breast?

    1. Upper inner quadrant.

    2. Upper outer quadrant.

    3. Beneath the nipple and areola.

    4. Lower outer quadrant.

81. The client presents with dysfunctional uterine bleeding and has been found to have endometrial cancer. She returned to the nurse practitioner because she does not understand how this is possible when the Pap smear 6 months ago was negative. The best response is:

    1. Uterine cancer develops quickly.

    2. Pap smears are difficult to read and mistakes can happen.

    3. Pap smears are not useful in detecting uterine cancers in most cases.

    4. The previous pap smear did not have an adequate sample.

Pharmacology

82. A 42-year-old female client presents to the office with complaints of dysuria, urinary frequency, and urgency. These symptoms began early this morning. She leaves a clean-catch midstream urine which shows the following: white blood cells (WBCs) too numerous to count (TNTC)/high power field (HPF), 4–5 red blood cells (RBCs)/HPF, positive nitrites. A urine culture is set up and will be ready in 3 days. Which is NOT a correct treatment for an uncomplicated lower urinary tract infection?

    1. Phenazopyridine (Pyridium) 200 mg 1 tab PO tid × 2 days.

    2. Trimethoprim-sulfamethoxazole (Bactrim DS) 1 tab PO bid × 5 days.

    3. Ceftriaxone (Rocephin) 1 gm IM.

    4. Nitrofurantoin (Macrobid) 1 tab PO bid × 5 days.

83. A 46-year-old female client is being seen in the clinic by the nurse practitioner. She was last seen 2 weeks ago for an upper respiratory tract infection and was treated with amoxicillin (Amoxil) 250 mg PO tid × 10 days. She completed her medication last week but now is aware of vaginal itching and a cottage cheese–like vaginal discharge. She states that she has never experienced such intense itching before. She is in a mutually monogamous relationship. Her LMP was 2 weeks ago. Her partner had a vasectomy 2 years ago. Wet mount with KOH shows negative whiff test, rare clue cells, positive lactobacilli, positive hyphae and spores, few WBCs, and no trichomonads. She is leaving tomorrow for a week-long cruise. She is not on any medications, and has no known drug allergies. Your treatment for this problem is:

    1. Metronidazole (Flagyl) 500 mg PO bid × 7 days.

    2. Clindamycin (Cleocin) vaginal cream one applicator full vaginally qhs × 7 days.

    3. Fluconazole (Diflucan) tablet 150 mg 1 tab PO one time.

    4. Hydrocortisone (Cortaid) 1% cream apply sparingly bid × 7 days.

84. A 25-year-old female client presents with complaints of a malodorous vaginal discharge described as white and watery. She douches with vinegar and water every 2 weeks. She uses a diaphragm for contraception. She and her boyfriend have

been sexually active for 2 years, using condoms for STD prevention with every act of coitus. She denies any dyspareunia. Her LMP was 1 week ago, and there are no noted changes in her normal menstrual pattern. Her wet mount with KOH results show a positive whiff test, TNTC clue cells/HPF, no lactobacilli, no hyphae or spores, no trichomonads, and few WBCs. Treatment for this client is:

1. Doxycycline (Vibratabs) 100 mg PO bid × 10 days.

2. Terconazole (Terazol 7 cream) 1 applicator full per vagina qhs × 7 days.

3. Acyclovir (Zovirax) 200 mg 1 PO q4h × 5 days.

4. Metronidazole (Metrogel) vaginal cream 1 applicator full per vagina qhs × 5 days.

85. A 55-year-old female client is being seen in the clinic for her annual exam. She went through a natural menopause 5 years ago and has never been interested in hormonal therapy. She smokes one pack per day, does no formal exercise. She is a G2 T2 P0 A0 L2. Her family history is positive for osteoporosis in her mother and myocardial infarction in her father, and negative for any cancers. She has a normal physical exam today and had a negative mammogram yesterday. She is now interested in hormonal therapy but wants to know what her alternatives are. Which choice **has not** been clinically proven for prevention of osteoporosis or cardiovascular disease?

1. Conjugated equine estrogen (Premarin) 0.625 mg 1 tab PO qd and medroxyprogesterone acetate (Provera) 2.5 mg 1 tablet PO qd.

2. Weight-bearing exercise three times weekly, calcium 1500 mg PO qd.

3. Discontinue cigarette smoking.

4. Wild Mexican yam cream apply to skin three times daily.

86. A young female is seen in the STD clinic. She noticed some itchy bumps in the vulvar area and is concerned that they could be cancer. On careful inspection the

nurse practitioner notes the following: five cauliflower-like warty, pinkish colored lesions in the lower introitus; two smaller lesions nestled anterior to the hymeneal ring of the vagina and cervix fail to reveal any abnormalities. A wet mount with KOH is negative. A culture for gonorrhea and chlamydia was obtained, a Pap smear done, and an HIV titer and RPR drawn. Which is **not** an appropriate treatment for this client?

1. Podophyllin (Podoben) application; wash off in 6 hours with soap and water.

2. Trichloroacetic acid application; do not wash off.

3. Cryotherapy with liquid nitrogen to lesions.

4. Benzathine penicillin 2.4 million units IM weekly × 3 weeks.

87. A young adult female client is being seen in the urgent care unit by the nurse practitioner. She is complaining of vaginal itching, thick yellow mucous discharge, and urinary discomfort. She is sexually active and uses condoms with one of her partners, but not both. On physical exam, the abdomen is negative; the pelvic exam reveals the BUS WNL, cervix has a mucopurulent discharge exuding from the os, the mucosa is friable to palpation; the bimanual exam is negative. Cultures were taken but are not yet available. Wet mount with KOH reveals a negative whiff, few clue cells, TNTC WBCs/HPF, no yeast, and no trichomonads. What is the likely diagnosis and appropriate treatment?

1. Chlamydia; give azithromycin (Zithromax) 1 gm PO single dose.

2. Chlamydia; give ceftriaxone (Rocephin) 125 mg IM.

3. Herpes simplex virus; give acyclovir (Zovirax) 200 mg 1 cap PO q4h × 5 days.

4. Trichomoniasis; give metronidazole (Flagyl) 2 gm PO single dose.

88. An adult female client is seen in the family planning clinic for a consultation on contraception. She is using birth control pills but forgets to take them because her work schedule changes very week. She is looking for an effective method that will be easy to remember. She has been married for 14 years, is G2 T2 P0 A0 L2, and is a nonsmoker. She has a negative past history for any major diseases and has a negative gynecologic history for abnormalities. She has never been treated for an STD and is in a mutually monogamous relationship. She is needle phobic and faints when she has to have blood drawn. What contraceptive method would be a good choice for the client?

   1. Depo-Provera injection every 3 months.

   2. Norplant implantation system for 5 years.

   3. Intrauterine device.

   4. Diaphragm.

89. A young adult female client is being seen at the family planning clinic by the nurse practitioner. The client wants birth control pills but has heard that they are dangerous to one's health. When asked for clarification, she lists the following: weight gain, ovarian cancer, heavy or irregular periods, and infertility. The nurse practitioner tells her: "I can see that you are concerned about your health . . ."

   1. "There are a lot of fallacies about birth control pills. They actually are felt to reduce the risk of ovarian cancers, help to regulate the bleeding, and are not associated with causing infertility. There can be a minor increase in body weight of 3–5 lbs."

   2. "Perhaps you would be better off trying the Norplant system or Depo-Provera."

   3. "What you have heard is true. They can be dangerous to your health and many people experience these problems."

   4. "There are a lot of fallacies about birth control pills. While ovarian cancer and infertility are risks that are taken with the use of the birth control pill, they do not cause weight gain or bleeding changes on periods. Pap smears done every year will detect such things as ovarian cancer."

90. A 41-year-old female client is seen in the family planning clinic. She is seeking information about contraceptive methods because her Norplant system is due for removal next month. She is in a new sexual relationship and plans to use condoms for STD prevention. She is in excellent health, is a nonsmoker, and is nulliparous. Her menses are every 28 days, with light flow. Which is **inappropriate** for the nurse practitioner to recommend?

   1. Oral contraceptives.

   2. IUD.

   3. Norplant system.

   4. Depo-Provera injections.

91. An adult female client is on oral contraceptive agents. She calls into the clinic with complaints of bleeding through the first $2\frac{1}{2}$ weeks of every package of pills. She has been on this pill for 4 months and takes them at the same time every day. Her present pill is a low-dosage monophasic pill. She is not on any other medications and denies any adverse effects to the birth control pills. She would like to remain on oral contraceptives if possible. The nurse practitioner's advice should include:

   1. Discontinue the pills and do not restart them. An alternative contraceptive method should be used.

   2. Change to a higher dosage, higher progestational agent.

   3. Try taking the pills first thing in the morning on an empty stomach to improve metabolism of the agents.

   4. There is no cause for concern; breakthrough bleeding is a normal side effect of oral contraceptives.

92. An adult female client is seen by the nurse practitioner at the family planning clinic. The client notes heavy, irregular menses. There has been an increase in facial acne and facial/abdominal hair growth over the past few years. She is G1 T1 P0 A0 L1, and is not planning future pregnancies. After a normal pelvic exam, the client

decides she wants oral contraceptives. A good choice in pill would be:

1. Loestrin 1/20.

2. Triphasil.

3. Demulen 1/35.

4. Birth control pills are inappropriate for this client.

93. A 41-year-old female client is seen for her 6-week-postpartum exam by the nurse practitioner. She is breast-feeding without difficulty and plans to continue for a year. She wants to begin using a contraceptive and plans no further pregnancies. Which is an inappropriate choice for this client?

1. Depo-Provera 150 mg IM injection every 3 months.

2. Intrauterine device.

3. Progestin-only oral contraceptive.

4. Combined oral contraceptive.

94. A 38-year-old female client is seen for her 6-week-postpartum exam by the nurse practitioner. The client was breast-feeding for a short time but discontinued 4 weeks ago. Her menses have resumed. She is contemplating another pregnancy in a year or so, but if she became pregnant before that she wouldn't mind. She is seeking contraception. She smokes one pack per day. Her exam is normal, with the uterus being well involuted. Which is **contraindicated** in this client?

1. Progestacert IUD.

2. Oral contraceptive agents.

3. Depo-Provera injection.

4. Condoms and spermicide.

95. A 25-year-old female client is seen by the nurse practitioner for her annual exam. The client is interested in contraceptive choices. She just quit smoking and is well motivated to remain a nonsmoker. She is on phenobarbital and phenytoin (Dilantin) for seizure control. She is G3 T2 P0 A1 L1. She may be planning future pregnancies but is unsure at this time. She is in good health other than the seizure disorder, and

has a normal exam. What contraceptive method is contraindicated in this client?

1. Diaphragm.

2. Depo-Provera injection.

3. Intrauterine device.

4. Norplant implantation system.

96. A 22-year-old female client presents to the urgent care department and is seen by the nurse practitioner. She is complaining of abdominal pain, low-grade fever, and mucopurulent vaginal discharge. Her symptoms began 3 days ago and are getting worse. She has a new sexual partner and has not used condoms with him yet. Her menses just ended; she is on OC agents. She denies nausea, vomiting, or anorexia. Her exam reveals findings consistent with pelvic inflammatory disease (PID). Cultures were taken for gonorrhea and chlamydia. Which represents an **inappropriate** treatment plan for the nurse practitioner to follow?

1. Ceftriaxone (Rocephin) 250 mg IM.

2. Doxycycline (Vibratabs) 100 mg PO bid × 10 days.

3. CBC, erythrocyte sedimentation rate.

4. Hospitalization.

97. An older female client is seen by the nurse practitioner for her annual exam. She has been on HRT for 6 months, having started herself on the pills left over by her deceased mother. She brings the pills with her, as she wants to remain on these and requests a prescription for Estrace 1 mg daily. She has an intact uterus, is in excellent health, and denies any complaints. She does not have any contraindications to the use of HRT. Her exam is normal. Which represents an **incorrect** and potentially dangerous plan for the nurse practitioner to follow?

1. Endometrial biopsy.

2. Prescription for Estrace 1 mg daily plus medroxyprogesterone acetate (Provera) 2.5 mg daily.

3. Prescription for Estrace 1 mg daily.

4. Instruct the client on the risks and benefits of HRT.

98. An older adult female client is seen for follow-up to discuss her HRT with the nurse practitioner. She needs a refill on her HRT but is not sure it is working right. She continues to feel hot flashes, moodiness, and decreased libido, and has many sleep disturbances. She is on Premarin 0.625 mg daily and Provera 2.5 mg daily. She denies any vaginal bleeding. Which is **not** an acceptable choice for the client?

    1. Premarin 0.9 mg 1 tab PO qd and Provera 5 mg 1 tab PO qd days 1–12.

    2. Premarin 0.9 mg 1 tab PO qd and Provera 5 mg 1 tab PO qd days 16–25.

    3. Premarin 0.3 mg 1 tab PO qd and Provera 2.5 mg 1 tab PO qd.

    4. Premarin 1.25 mg 1 tab PO qd and Provera 10 mg 1 tab PO qd days 1–12.

99. Which is **not** a contraindication to the use of HRT in the postmenopausal female?

    1. Recent deep vein thrombosis.

    2. Chronic active hepatitis.

    3. Controlled hypertension.

    4. Undiagnosed abnormal genital bleeding.

100. A young adult female client presents to the clinic with complaints of a malodorous, yellowish vaginal discharge and vulvovaginal itching. She has never had a gynecologic exam and is extremely apprehensive. She is sexually active and has had a new sexual partner for 2 months. She states that they use condoms most of the time and are not interested in alternate forms of contraception at this time. Her LMP was 1 week ago. Her wet mount with KOH shows few clue cells, moderate lactobacilli, few WBCs, no yeast, and TNTC mobile trichomonads. Appropriate treatment for this client would include:

    1. Metronidazole (Flagyl) 2 gm PO single dose.

    2. Metronidazole (Metrogel) vaginal cream 1 applicator full per vagina qhs × 5 days.

    3. Fluconazole (Diflucan) 150 mg PO single dose.

    4. Terconazole (Terazol) vaginal cream 1 applicator full per vagina qhs × 7 days.

101. Which dose of conjugated equine estrogen (Premarin) is the minimal effective dose to prevent osteoporosis?

    1. 0.3 mg.

    2. 0.625 mg.

    3. 0.9 mg.

    4. 1.25 mg.

102. A single woman presents for contraceptive counseling expressing preference for a diaphragm. Which factor in her history would make a diaphragm a poor choice?

    1. Three urinary tract infections in the past year.

    2. Strong desire to avoid pregnancy.

    3. Last two Pap smears showed atypical cells.

    4. Nulliparous cervix.

103. Combination oral contraceptive pills prevent pregnancy primarily by:

    1. Decreasing fallopian tube motility.

    2. Thinning of cervical mucus.

    3. Suppressing ovulation.

    4. Causing inflammation of the endometrium.

104. A young adult client is hesitant to be fitted for an IUD because of strong antiabortion views and asks your opinion. Which explanation most accurately describes the probable action of an IUD?

    1. Slows transport of ovum through the fallopian tube, causing it to age and die in transit.

    2. Prevents effective implantation of a fertilized ovum.

    3. Action is no different than that of spermicide.

    4. Mechanically blocks sperm from entering uterus.

105. What is a unique advantage of a Progesterone T IUD?

    1. Lowest failure rate of IUDs.

    2. May be left in place for up to 10 years.

    3. Decreases menstrual blood loss and dysmenorrhea.

    4. Must be replaced annually.

106. An older female client is seen by the nurse practitioner for her annual exam and needs a refill on her HRT. She is feeling well and has not voiced concerns. The client had a total abdominal hysterectomy and bilateral salpingo-oophorectomy 2 years ago for benign fibroids. Her exam is normal. She takes conjugated estrogen (Premarin) 0.625 mg days 1–25 and medroxyprogesterone acetate (Provera) 10 mg from days 16–25. What changes would be appropriate for the nurse practitioner to make in the HRT regimen?

    1. No changes needed; the client is doing well on the present regimen.

    2. Premarin 0.625 mg daily and discontinue the Provera.

    3. Premarin 0.625 mg daily and Provera 2.5 mg daily.

    4. Premarin 0.625 mg days 1–25 and Provera 5 mg days 16–25.

107. Which statement about progestin-only pills is true?

    1. Women who are breast-feeding should not use progestin-only pills.

    2. Ovulation suppression is as effective with progestin-only pills as with combined oral contraception pills.

    3. There is an increased incidence of functional ovarian cysts.

    4. The risk of ectopic pregnancy is lower for women using progestin-only pills.

108. Before prescribing HRT, which clinical approach should have the highest priority?

    1. The decision about use should rest primarily with the client after providing appropriate education and counseling.

    2. For most women the benefits of HRT far outweigh any possible side effects, so HRT should be actively encouraged.

    3. Involving the sexual partner in the counseling session is likely to lead to a higher compliance rate for HRT.

    4. Education regarding HRT should include a thorough review of risk factors and possible side effects in order to avoid liability issues.

109. The most common side effect associated with depomedroxyprogesterone (DMPA; Depo-Provera) is:

    1. Nausea.

    2. Acne.

    3. Menstrual cycle changes.

    4. Increased menstrual cramps.

110. The beneficial effects of estrogen on high-density (HDL) and low-density (LDL) lipoprotein fractions include:

    1. An increase in HDL and an increase in LDL.

    2. A decrease in HDL and a decrease in LDL.

    3. An increase in HDL and a decrease in LDL.

    4. A decrease in HDL and an increase in LDL.

111. The nurse practitioner is teaching a client about taking alendronate (Fosamax); her information includes:

    1. Take it midmorning.

    2. Take with food.

    3. Take with a full glass of orange juice.

    4. Remain upright after taking medication.

112. The addition of a progesterone to an estrogen regimen in a postmenopausal woman with a uterus reduces the risk of:

    1. Endometrial cancer.

    2. Cervical cancer.

    3. Gallbladder disease.

    4. Breast cancer.

113. The treatment of choice for trichomoniasis is:

    1. Azithromycin (Zithromax) 1 gm PO single dose.

    2. Ofloxacin (Floxin) 500 mg PO single dose.

    3. Metronidazole (Flagyl) 2 gm PO single dose.

    4. Clindamycin (Cleocin) 300 mg PO single dose.

114. A 25-year-old woman comes into the office with complaints of profuse malodorous discharge. The nurse practitioner's diagnosis is bacterial vaginosis. The nurse practitioner would:

    1. Advice the client to notify her sexual contacts regarding the diagnosis.

    2. Treat the problem with metronidazole (Flagyl) 2 gm for one dose.

    3. Initiate a treatment with doxycycline (Vibramycin) 100 mg PO bid × 7 days.

    4. Determine the presence of pregnancy prior to initiating a course of treatment.

115. A young woman who is taking a low-dose OC calls the clinic in a panic stating that she forgot her pill 2 days ago. She is taking phenytoin (Dilantin) for seizure activity and has been seizure-free for over a year. "What should I do about my pills?" The most appropriate response should be:

    1. Advise her to take the forgotten dose today along with the regular dose.

    2. Refer her to her physician for advice about the Dilantin.

    3. Advise her to continue pills, but to use another contraceptive through the rest of this cycle.

    4. Advise her to come to the clinic for a "morning-after" pill.

116. A vaginal culture has confirmed the presence of chancroid in a homeless woman who presented with a painful genital ulcer. The treatment regimen of choice should be:

    1. Ceftrixone (Rocephin) 250 mg IM in a single dose.

    2. Erythromycin (E-Mycin) 500 mg PO qid × 7 days.

    3. Metronidazole (Flagyl) 2 mg PO in a single dose.

    4. Clindamycin (Cleocin) cream 2% 1 full applicator (intravaginally) × 5 days.

117. A young adult female presents to the office for evaluation of abdominal pain. The client admits to recent sexual activity and states that she does not have her partner use condoms. On exam, the nurse practitioner finds vaginal discharge and CMT. Other than sending cultures to the lab, the nurse practitioner would treat this client with:

    1. Penicillin G, 2.4 million units IM.

    2. Metronidazole (Flagyl), 500 mg PO bid × 7 days.

    3. Ceftriaxone (Rocephin), 125 mg IM and azithromycin (Zithromax) 1 gm PO.

    4. Acyclovir (Zovirax) 400 mg PO bid × 7 days.

118. When assisting a woman to decide whether to initiate HRT, which state is true?

    1. Estrogen replacement delays the onset of menopause.

    2. Estrogen and progesterone cause vasomotor symptoms.

    3. Estrogen increases HDL cholesterol levels.

    4. Estrogen replacement with progesterone increases the risk of ovarian cancer.

16 ▷ Answers & Rationales

Physical Examination & Diagnostic Tests

1. **(3)** Lubricants, such as Vaseline or K-Y gel, should not be used if a cervical specimen is being obtained for analysis. The cervical brush should not be used on pregnant clients. The bimanual exam is performed after the internal vaginal exam.

2. **(2)** To aid in the examination, an empty bladder will provide for client comfort and will assist the nurse practitioner in making a more accurate assessment during the bimanual portion of the exam. Options #1 and #3 help reduce the client's anxiety, which ultimately may assist in the achievement of comfort.

3. **(1)** A nobothian cyst is a small, white or yellow, raised round area on the cervix. The surface of the cervix should be smooth and may have a symmetrical, reddened circle around the os (squamocolumnar epithelium). The other options are all unexpected, abnormal findings.

4. **(3)** A breast ultrasound is used to determine if a lesion is solid or cystic. Ultrasound misses 50% of lesions <2 cm. The test is not sensitive enough to be used for routine screening and cannot replace mammography. The definitive diagnosis of breast cancer is the breast biopsy.

5. **(3)** The HSG is used to document the presence of a normal uterine cavity and the patency of the fallopian tubes. A contrast dye is injected into the uterus and x-rays are taken to assess anatomy. The best time to do this test is 2–5 days after menses but before ovulation.

6. **(1)** Approximately 10% of breast cancers are not seen mammographically.

7. **(1)** KOH lyses epithelial and white blood cells making it easier to visualize *Candida* (yeast). *Candida* cells are resistant and remain intact. KOH also assists with diagnosing bacterial vaginosis by alkalinizing vaginal discharge, causing a distinct fishy odor. This is a positive amine or whiff test.

8. **(3)** The Pap smear is a screening test for cervical cancer and precancerous states. The diagnostic test needed to confirm the diagnosis of a high-grade lesion is the colposcopy with guided biopsies. The results of this test are clearly abnormal and must be acted upon. Waiting a year could be deleterious to the client's health. This is not a Pap smear report that one would choose to redo in 4 months; the client needs a diagnostic test, not another screening test. This is not a diagnosis of cervical cancer on this Pap smear; therefore, a referral to a gynecologic oncologist is premature at this time.

9. **(3)** All of the above tests may be included in the work-up for infertility. Because male factors account for 35–40% of infertility, a semen analysis should be done early in the work-up. HSG and endometrial biopsy are tests that require scheduling at specific times of the menstrual cycle. Tests for antisperm antibodies would be done if the postcoital test revealed abnormalities.

10. **(4)** In Option #1, the abnormal finding is the enlarged lymph nodes. In Option #2, the abnormal finding is the fixed, stellate mass with nipple discharge. In Option #3, the asymmetrical size is normal but not the different colors of the areola and unilateral nipple inversion. Longstanding nevi and Montgomery's tubercles are normal in Option #4.

11. **(4)** The BBT chart is one of the most important ways to evaluate ovulation. Clients should be instructed on the first visit how to use the special BBT thermometer and record the findings on the BBT chart. The remaining answers, which are possibly part of an infertility work-up, are not methods to evaluate ovulation.

12. **(2)** Atrophic changes on the cervix of a postmenopausal female are to be expected, as is the paucity of endocervical cells. Due to her past medical history of breast cancer, she is not a candidate for the use of estrogen vaginal cream, nor is the Pap smear interpretation abnormal. Endocervical curettage is used as a biopsy technique for sampling tissue from the endocervical canal; however, it is not appropriate to recommend this invasive procedure for someone with scant endocervical cells, but rather for one with abnormal endocervical cells. Since this Pap smear report really is not classified as abnormal, there is no need to recommend a diagnostic procedure for the client.

13. **(4)** Culture is the only certain or definitive method of diagnosis. It is a collected cervical specimen, and the results take about 2–6 days to obtain. The DFA is fast and has good sensitivity and specificity.

14. **(2)** Mammography should be done on a regular basis, with baseline screening around age 35, then a mammogram every 2 years. After age 40, it should be done on an annual basis. It should be done regardless of breast-feeding, and the client should not wait until a mass or other symptoms are present.

15. **(1)** Serologic tests are good screening tests, but positive results require following-up with a treponemal test to detect specific antibodies.

16. **(2)** Serum prolactin assay levels >20 ng/ml indicate the need for medical referral, usually to an endocrinologist. The most common cause of hyperprolactinemia and galactorrhea (milky breast discharge) is a pituitary tumor or lesion of the hypothalamus. Other causes may be hypothyroidism, medications (narcotics, tranquilizers, antihypertensives), and OCs.

17. **(1)** The initial work-up for this client includes determining the prolactin level by evaluating serum concentrations and determining the presence of endogenous estrogen. If the woman experiences withdrawal bleeding after the administration of PO or IM progesterone and the prolactin level is normal, this woman is producing estrogen and can be considered anovulatory. Absence of withdrawal bleeding with normal prolactin level requires further work-up.

18. **(1)** The occurrence of the symptoms in the menstrual cycle will assist the nurse practitioner to make a diagnosis of PMS. The client should keep track on a calendar as to when each symptom occurs, and disappears, and the onset and completion of menstrual flow.

Normal Gynecology

19. **(4)** Inside the uterus, the lining first proliferates and begins preparation for implantation. During the secretory phase, glandular epithelium develops, further enhancing the lining. If no fertilized egg arrives for implantation, the lining sloughs off; this is the menstrual phase.

20. **(1)** Premenstrual syndrome occurs approximately 5–11 days prior to the onset

of menses (late luteal phase) and is gone within 1–2 days of the onset of menses. This phase is progesterone dominant. The follicular phase is estrogen dominant.

21. **(3)** Oxytocin is released from the posterior pituitary. FSH, LH, and prolactin are all released from the anterior pituitary gland. The other hormones released from the anterior pituitary are thyroid-stimulating hormone (TSH), adrenocorticotropic hormone (ACTH), and growth hormone.

22. **(1)** FSH stimulates the maturation of ovarian follicles, resulting in a dominant follicle. Milk secretion is dependent on prolactin. The production and release of luteinizing hormone is regulated by estrogen. Luteinizing hormone is responsible for ovulation.

23. **(4)** The ovarian cycle is divided into three phases. The follicular phase begins on the first day of menses and continues until day 14, when ovulation usually occurs. Immediately after ovulation, the empty follicle begins to enlarge and develops into a corpus luteum, which releases increasing amounts of progesterone. If implantation does not occur, the corpus luteum regresses, causing the onset of menses. This phase, from ovulation to menses, is the luteal phase.

24. **(3)** HRT reduces the risk of heart disease in the postmenopausal female.

25. **(4)** Pregnancy is the most likely diagnosis in this client, given the list of symptoms and physical findings. She certainly could have a uterine fibroid; however, it is not contributing to the symptoms listed. Ovarian cancer could present with nausea, fatigue, and abdominal bloating; however, it would cause neither the enlarged uterus nor the positive Chadwick's sign. A dislodged IUD will usually change the position of the IUD, thereby causing the strings to be less visible or causing the IUD itself to be expelled into the vagina or endocervical canal.

26. **(3)** Maintaining an alkaline pH is important to promote viability of sperm that are deposited into the vaginal vault.

27. **(4)** Obesity is not a risk factor for osteoporosis. Cigarette use, Caucasian race, and alcohol consumption, in addition to others not listed here, are considered to be risk factors for osteoporosis.

28. **(2)** Conservative management for PMS includes daily exercise, support and reassurance that her problems are not uncommon, and education about symptoms to assist the client to obtain some type of control to help her to adapt to the situation. A low-salt diet is encouraged and a diuretic (hydrochlorothiazide [HCTZ]) may be ordered to deal with water retention along with vitamin B_6 (50–100 mg/day) and vitamins A and E for breast symptoms.

29. **(2)** As the function of the ovaries declines and the amount of circulating estrogen begins to fall, the middle-aged female may begin to experience the symptoms commonly associated with menopause. The body's feedback system will attempt to stimulate the ovaries and increase estrogen level. FSH and LH levels rise in response to these efforts.

30. **(4)** The vagina naturally cleanses itself and therefore douching is not necessary unless prescribed by a health care provider to treat a medical condition. Douching should be avoided during menses to prevent infection.

31. **(1)** Pregnancy is the most likely diagnosis, requiring a pregnancy test and pelvic ultrasound to confirm it. Even though she has had a tubal ligation, failure rates of 1 in 300 have been reported. This client could have uterine fibroids; however, they do not generally present with this symptom complex and are not associated with amenorrhea, although they do cause uterine enlargement. Premature menopause could cause all these symptoms, including amenorrhea, but not the enlarged uterus. Colon cancer can present with these symptoms, and could certainly be responsible for an abdominal mass, but not uterine enlargement or amenorrhea.

Gynecologic Disorders

32. **(2)** Dyspareunia is painful intercourse and vaginismus is painful vaginal spasms upon penetration. Primary orgasmic disorder is when an individual has never achieved orgasm, usually a lifelong problem. Secondary orgasmic dysfunction refers to an acquired problem of loss of orgasmic function after an individual has experienced orgasm.

33. **(1)** The initial outbreak is usually the worst. It can be transmitted even when there is no lesion present, and it cannot be cured. Vaginal delivery is allowed, if there are no genital lesions at the time of labor.

34. **(1)** Bacterial vaginosis results when the normal environment in the vagina is disrupted. The normal vaginal lactobacilli are decreased or absent, and there is an overgrowth of many different types of anaerobic bacteria. Trichomoniasis is caused by a flagellated protozoan, and gonorrhea is caused by a bacteria and may be asymptomatic. The virus that causes recurrent outbreaks of genital lesions is herpes genitalis type 2 (HSV-II).

35. **(1)** OCs will reduce prostaglandin production, which is thought to be the primary cause of dysmenorrhea.

36. **(4)** The criteria for the diagnosis of bacterial vaginosis are characteristic milky homogeneous discharge, pH >4.5, amine odor (positive whiff test) with addition of KOH, and the presence of epithelial cells studded with coccibacilli that obscure the borders (clue cells). Pseudohyphae are present in candidiasis.

37. **(2)** In Asherman's syndrome, a normally functioning uterus has been damaged and scarred secondary to instrumentation, usually a D&C. Ovulation may be occurring normally, but there is no healthy endometrial lining to shed, so clients do not menstruate. Asherman's syndrome is a problem with the uterus. The others, polycystic ovarian syndrome, hypogonadism, and premature ovarian failure, are problems with the ovaries.

38. **(2)** The LH/FSH ratio in polycystic ovarian syndrome is 3:1. The normal LH/FSH ratio is 1.5:1.

39. **(4)** The criteria for the diagnosis of polycystic ovarian syndrome are onset of menstrual irregularity, increased body weight, physical and laboratory evidence of androgen excess, chronic anovulation, and normal prolactin levels. Estradiol is not increased but may be decreased.

40. **(3)** Ninety per cent of dysfunctional uterine bleeding is caused by anovulation. The lack of progesterone allows asynchronous, excessive proliferation of the endometrium. This tissue is fragile and the normal hemostatic mechanism is altered. Thyroid disease, blood dyscrasias, and uterine tumors can mimic dysfunctional uterine bleeding and must be excluded.

41. **(3)** A female-appearing person with a 46,XY karyotype is referred to as having androgen insensitivity syndrome, or testicular feminization. This maternal X-linked recessive disorder accounts for approximately 10% of all cases of amenorrhea, and these appear normal until puberty. These clients present with amenorrhea, scant or absent pubic hair, and abnormal or no breast development. Persons with Müllerian abnormalities have a normal XX karyotype with abnormalities of fallopian tubes, uterus, and upper vagina occurring in fetal development. In Turner's syndrome, there is congenital absence of ovaries due to loss of one X chromosome.

42. **(1)** The most common breast mass in young women <30 years old is the fibroadenoma. This benign breast mass is the third most common breast mass after fibrocystic changes and carcinoma. Fibrocystic breast changes are seen most commonly in women 30–50 years old. Intraductal papilloma is a wart-like growth located in the mammary duct and occurs in women 40–50 years old. Malignant breast neoplasms occur most frequently in women over 40 and are rarely seen in women 15–25 years old.

43. **(1)** Nonsteroidal anti-inflammatory analgesics inhibit prostaglandin synthesis and are effective agents in primary

dysmenorrhea. The other agents listed have not demonstrated effectiveness in primary dysmenorrhea. Other measures to decrease discomfort are exercise, relaxation techniques, heat application, and low-dose oral contraceptives.

44. **(4)** Secondary amenorrhea is defined as no menses for three cycle lengths or 6 months in a woman with previously established menses. Exercise can cause an increase in estrogen and endorphin levels, which influences the release of gonadotropin releasing hormone (GnRH). Without appropriate GnRH release FSH and LH are not released appropriately, resulting in anovulation, which may lead to amenorrhea. The other conditions listed are causes of primary amenorrhea.

45. **(1)** This has the characteristics of a syphilitic lesion and needs to be evaluated. Only after determining the presence or type of STD can it be treated effectively. The herpes viral culture should be done while the lesion is present and the fluid from the vesicles can be obtained.

46. **(3)** Pregnancy is the most common cause of amenorrhea in young women. It is important to rule out pregnancy in a female client with a problem of amenorrhea, even if she is very athletic. Interviewing the client regarding her sexual practices is unreliable. The presence or absence of pregnancy should be determined prior to other diagnostic studies.

47. **(2)** A person who has never engaged in coital activity is not considered to be at risk for cervical cancer, due to the unlikelihood of exposure to HPV. In addition to others not listed here, the presence of HPV, multiple sexual partners, and/or previous HSIL are considered to be risk factors in the development of cervical cancer.

48. **(1)** The pseudohyphae and spores on the wet mount (KOH) are diagnostic for candida. *Chlamydia trachomatis* is diagnosed by direct immunofluorescence assay (DFA, or by chlamydia culture). Gonorrhea is diagnosed by a cervical culture, and bacterial vaginitis shows clue cells on the wet mount prep.

49. **(1)** Cancer of the ovary is the leading cause of death from female genital cancer, excluding the breast, in the United States.

50. **(1)** Flagellated protozoan confirms the diagnosis of trichomoniasis. The DFA test confirms chlamydia. Mucopurulent cervicitis is characterized by vaginal discharge and dysuria. Bacterial vaginosis is confirmed by gram stain and malodorous discharge with a fishy odor.

51. **(3)** The pelvic ultrasound is not a useful test to obtain for appendicitis, as it will not allow for adequate examination of the appendix. The CBC with differential is useful due to the expected rise in WBC, seen in this inflammatory state. The flat plate of the abdomen and KUB are very helpful to determine the extent of the problem and to rule out other diagnoses. Since pregnancy can cause these symptoms if complicated by an ectopic, the practitioner should consider it as part of the differential diagnosis.

52. **(2)** Birth control pills have been shown to reduce the risk of endometrial cancer. Obesity, unopposed estrogen use, and advanced age, in addition to others not listed here, are considered to be risk factors for developing endometrial cancer.

53. **(2)** The diaphragm may be inserted any time up to 6 hours prior to intercourse and should be removed no sooner than 6 hours after intercourse. The diaphragm should be left in place for no longer than 24 hours.

54. **(2)** Urethral discomfort and recurrent urinary tract infections are associated with diaphragm use and are the most common reasons for discontinuing use and changing birth control methods.

55. **(3)** Birth control pill use has been shown to reduce the risk of ovarian cancer. Family history of ovarian cancer, advancing age, and positive BRCA 2 gene, in addition to others not listed here, are considered to be risk factors for developing ovarian cancer.

56. **(2)** Endometrial cancer is the most common female genital cancer.

57. **(3)** Herpes simplex virus type 2 commonly presents dramatically in the newly infected primary outbreak. Gonorrhea generally is associated with a mucopurulent vaginal discharge and is not accompanied by vesicular lesions. Chlamydia can be associated with dysuria and, unless accompanied by PID, is not generally accompanied by fever or body aches, nor is it associated with vesicular lesions. Lymphogranuloma venereum is a rare disease classically accompanied by pustular enlargement of the lymph nodes, particularly the inguinal nodes. It is associated not with vesicles, but bubos.

58. **(2)** Screening lab blood work for glucose, cardiac risk profile, and TSH in this age group without any stated risk factors is not cost effective and is of little value. The client can be better served with a discussion regarding diet and exercise. Since this client is at risk for STDs, counseling and testing for these is a reasonable approach. Contraceptive information educates the client and allows her to make wiser choices in her family planning.

59. **(1)** Early menopause has not been associated with the development of breast cancer. High-fat diet, advancing age, early menarche, and others not listed here have been identified as risk factors in the development of breast cancer.

60. **(1)** The use of prenatal vitamins with folic acid prior to conception has been found to reduce the risk of neural tube defects in the fetus. It is important for the client to continue her exercise program, although some discussion about the type of exercise and any limitations are important once pregnancy is achieved. Since the client has had two previous pregnancies, it is likely that her rubella immune status has been determined; if she is found to not be immune to rubella, then an MMR should be recommended. This client is not of advanced maternal age and therefore does not require genetic counseling for this reason.

61. **(3)** Baseline lab work should be obtained to determine the presence of anemia, possible pregnancy, and/or endocrine dysfunction.

62. **(4)** Fibrocystic breast disease is not a risk factor for breast cancer. In addition to others, those listed in Options #1, #2, and #3 are considered to be risk factors for breast cancer.

63. **(1)** The recommended age for a female to begin screening Pap smears is at the onset of sexual activity or at 18 years of age. Since this client is 20 years old and has not had her first Pap smear yet, this would be the most appropriate test to perform. It is not necessary to perform STD screening on clients who have not been sexually active. Stool hemoccult testing and mammography are not recommended as screening procedures in the young adult.

64. **(3)** Heart disease remains the leading cause of death for females in the United States.

65. **(3)** The presence of bruising, particularly on genitalia, should raise suspicion of abuse. Combined with her nonverbal behavior, the bruising should prompt the nurse practitioner to explore the possibility of abuse.

66. **(1)** Reactive cellular changes are most commonly associated with inflammation, including typical repair. Other causes include atrophy with inflammation (atrophic vaginitis), IUD use, radiation, and diethylstilbestrol exposure in utero. OCs do not cause reactive changes, and estrogen vaginal cream may be used to improve atrophy.

67. **(2)** The exact cause of cervical disease is unknown. Evidence is increasing that sexually transmitted agents act as carcinogens. Exposure to herpes genitalis, HPV, and HIV is, therefore, considered a risk factor. Other risk factors are related to sexual activity, such as sex prior to 18 years of age, first pregnancy prior to 18 years of age, multiple sexual partners, high parity, and partners with carcinoma in situ of the penis.

68. **(4)** Lung cancer is the most common cancer in females in the United States.

69. **(3)** These symptoms are classic for menopausal syndrome, although it is true that there are some depressive symptoms listed. Antidepressant therapy and counseling for depression at this stage of treatment is not appropriate. Testing, teaching, and treatment in this case should be aimed at the menopause. The depressive symptoms will undoubtedly improve with greater understanding and treatment of the menopausal symptoms.

70. **(1)** Chancroid is well established as a cofactor for HIV transmission.

71. **(4)** Monthly BSE is the most effective way to pick up early breast changes.

72. **(2)** Symptoms are most likely indicative of benign fibroadenoma. Mammography is indicated. Surgical excision is unlikely for a young woman.

73. **(2)** She needs to become more knowledgeable about the normal feel of implants as well as her own breast tissue. Mammography is not a substitute for BSE.

74. **(2)** A very firm cervix along with a cervical lesion/ulcer is suspicious for cancer of the cervix, which can be confirmed with a Pap smear.

75. **(1)** This complaint is an indication for breast exam and mammography. Although pain is not a common presenting symptom, it can be. Teaching BSE is important but not the most important action in this situation; hormone levels can explain breast pain but should not be the first place to look for an explanation.

76. **(2)** Toxic shock syndrome occurs primarily in menstruating women ages 12–24 who use tampons. The diagnosis is made with the presence of fever over >102°F, macular rash, hypotension, and involvement of three or more organ systems.

77. **(4)** Over 16% of ectopic pregnancies present as surgical emergencies. In the United States, 1 in 1000 deaths from ectopic pregnancies occur as the result of blood loss.

78. **(4)** Almost half of all vaginal infections are due to candidiasis. The majority of women who develop the disease have recently taken antibiotics. It is not an STD.

79. **(1)** It is important to evaluate the client for threatened abortion as soon as possible. It is most likely too soon for the CBC to reflect blood loss. A pelvic sonogram will take longer than a urine pregnancy test, and it is imperative that the client be immediately referred for a D&C, if her pregnancy test is positive.

80. **(2)** The most common site for breast cancer occurrence is the upper outer quadrant, followed by the area beneath the nipple.

81. **(3)** Pap smears are crucial for the detection of cervical cancer but do not diagnose uterine cancer. In the early stages uterine cancer can be asymptomatic and would not be detectable even on bimanual examination.

Pharmacology

82. **(3)** Rocephin is a very effective drug for complicated urinary tract infection but is unnecessary in the uncomplicated lower urinary tract infection. Bactrim DS and Macrobid are both very effective for urinary tract infection treatment. Pyridium will help to make the client more comfortable until the antibiotic reaches effective levels for treatment.

83. **(3)** Fluconazole is now approved for single-dose oral treatment of uncomplicated vulvovaginal candidiasis. It is most convenient for this client, who is unlikely to be extremely compliant with vaginal creams, given the upcoming travel. She does not have any contraindications to its use. Metronidazole and clindamycin are treatments for bacterial vaginosis and not for *Candida* infections. Hydrocortisone is a topical steroid used for inflammatory dermatologic conditions, and, although it may help the itching, it would not treat the candidiasis.

84. **(4)** Metronidazole vaginal cream is the treatment of choice for bacterial vaginosis. The newest recommendations allow for its use once daily for 5 days. The use of doxycycline listed here is for treatment of uncomplicated vaginal *Chlamydia trachomatis*. Terconazole vaginal cream is used for vaginal candidiasis; acyclovir is used for treatment of herpes simplex infections.

85. **(4)** Although some authors may recommend herbal treatments for menopausal symptoms, there have not been any controlled studies regarding prevention of disease with this substance. Traditional medicine supports the use of HRT for prevention of osteoporosis and cardiovascular disease. The use of weight-bearing exercise and increased calcium intake has been shown to help maintain bone health. Cigarette smoking increases the risk for both osteoporosis and cardiovascular disease. This client can significantly reduce her risk of these two diseases by quitting her tobacco habit.

86. **(4)** Benzathine penicillin 2.4 million units IM is the treatment of choice for syphilis, but this client has condyloma acuminatum, not lata. Topical use of podophyllin, trichloroacetic acid, and cryotherapy are all accepted treatment modalities for condyloma acuminatum.

87. **(1)** Chlamydia will often times present this way; take note of the dysuria, mucopurulent discharge, and cervical friability. The treatment of choice in ambulatory care settings is single-dose therapy with azithromycin 1 gm PO. The treatment listed in Option #2 is for gonorrhea, not chlamydia. Herpes simplex virus will present with painful vesicles in the vulvovaginal region and is treated with acyclovir 200 mg 1 capsule PO q4h × 5 days for recurrences. Trichomoniasis can present this way; however, the absence of trichomonads on the wet mount is the key; the suggested treatment for trichomoniasis is metronidazole 2 gm PO in a single dose.

88. **(3)** The IUD would be a good choice for this client because it is extremely effective (>99%). There is not much she has to do to maintain it, and there are no injections involved for the insertion or removal. The

Depo-Provera injections, although being extremely effective (>99%), require an injection every 3 months, which could lead to decreased compliance by the client. The Norplant system of implants is also very effective (>99%), but it too requires injections for insertion and removal, and she is trying to avoid that. The diaphragm is a noninvasive contraceptive that is effective (88%), but it requires her to be a more active a participant in its use. None of these methods are contraindicated for this client, but an attempt should be made to help her choose one with which she is likely to be comfortable.

89. **(1)** Try to find out what the client has heard and dispel the fallacies if possible. Recent research supports the protective benefit by oral contraceptives from ovarian cancer as well as endometrial cancer. There is generally a reduction in the amount of menstrual bleeding and a regulation of the cycle. Minimal weight fluctuations are reported. Infertility is not associated with oral contraceptive use. To suggest either Norplant or Depo-Provera injections to someone who voices concerns about irregular menses or weight gain is sure to lead to an unhappy client, for these are quite common side effects of both methods. Options #3 and #4 are incorrect and misleading; Pap smears do not screen for ovarian cancer.

90. **(2)** The IUD is not recommended for use by an individual who is nulliparous nor for one who is not in a stable, mutually monogamous relationship due to the increased risk of complications. The use of oral contraceptives in a 41-year-old nonsmoker in good health is acceptable without concern. The client is already familiar with Norplant and may not be aware that she could have a new set of implants inserted when she has the others removed. Depo-Provera would be equally appropriate for this client.

91. **(2)** Very often, changing to a pill with a stronger progestational agent, or a different progestational agent, will resolve the problem of bleeding irregularities on oral contraceptives. There are so many choices one can make in the dosage or strength of a birth control pill that it is likely that her problem can be resolved

with a different pill. Taking them at a different time of day or on an empty stomach will do nothing to resolve the stated problem. The problem stated is not breakthrough bleeding, but rather prolonged bleeding likely secondary to poor endometrial support. If a change is not made in the pills, the client will continue to bleed in this fashion and may eventually develop anemia as a consequence.

92. **(3)** A pill such as Demulen 1/35 is a good choice for one with more androgenic characteristics due to the ability of this pill to exhibit a strong estrogenic effect with a moderate progestational effect. The Loestrin 1/20 is a poor choice for several reasons: the weaker dose of estrogen and progestin may not be adequate to support her endometrium, nor will it have a positive effect on the androgenic characteristics displayed by this client. Triphasil is a triphasic pill and does have a positive progestational effect that should support the endometrium well; however, the progestin in this pill tends to be slightly more androgenic, which is undesirable in this client.

93. **(4)** The use of combined oral contraceptives is not recommended for use with breast-feeding mothers due to the potential effect it can have on decreasing milk quantity and quality. Progestin-only oral contraceptives are cleared for use in nursing mothers because there has not been any proven deleterious effect on either milk quantity or quality. Depo-Provera and the IUD are also accepted contraceptive methods for use in lactating females.

94. **(2)** Oral contraceptives are contraindicated for use in a cigarette smoker who is 35 years or over. There is no contraindication to the use of Depo-Provera injection in the cigarette smoker. The Progestacert IUD would probably be a good IUD choice for this client because it is only approved for 1 year's use, and is safe in a cigarette smoker as well. The only contraindication to the use of condoms and spermicide is allergy to either substance.

95. **(4)** The Norplant implantation system is contraindicated in the person with seizure disorder on phenobarbital or Dilantin because there is potential for either reduced anticonvulsant effect or reduced contraceptive effect. This does not occur with Depo-Provera, allowing the client to use this method freely without concern. The IUD is not contraindicated for use with anticonvulsant medications, and the client is a good candidate for its use. The diaphragm is not contraindicated with the use of anticonvulsant therapy.

96. **(4)** It is not necessary to hospitalize the client with acute PID who is not vomiting or pregnant. If she does not respond well to outpatient treatment, then hospitalization can be recommended. The medications listed are the accepted treatment of choice for outpatient management of PID, and should be started before the results of the lab tests are available, based on the clinical presentation of the client. The CBC and sedimentation rate are helpful to track the WBC and inflammatory response of the body.

97. **(3)** The use of unopposed estrogen in the client with an intact uterus could put her at risk for endometrial hyperplasia or cancer. The addition of a progestin protects the endometrium adequately. The client is an excellent candidate for endometrial biopsy to document the status of the endometrium. This client also needs to be educated on the risks and benefits of HRT.

98. **(3)** The regimen of Premarin 0.3 mg has not been proven to be effective for prevention of osteoporosis or heart disease. In addition, lowering the dosage of the estrogen would not help the client's symptoms. The other dosage regimens listed are all acceptable choices for this client, proving that there are many effective ways for one to utilize HRT, allowing for individualization of the regimen to the client.

99. **(3)** Well-controlled hypertension is not a contraindication to the use of HRT.

100. **(1)** Metronidazole 2 gm PO single dose is the treatment of choice for trichomoniasis. Metronidazole vaginal cream does not effectively treat vaginal trichomoniasis. Fluconazole and terconazole are treatments for vaginal candidiasis.

101. **(2)** A dose of 0.625 mg of conjugated equine estrogen (Premarin) is the minimal effective dose to prevent osteoporosis.

102. **(1)** The diaphragm predisposes many women to UTIs. Some women are sensitive to the contraceptive creme/jelly. The diaphragm has been associated with toxic shock syndrome, hence its use should be avoided during menses and not left in place longer than 24 hours.

103. **(3)** The primary mechanism of action of oral contraceptives is suppression of ovulation. Ovulation is suppressed in 95–98% of clients. Should ovulation occur, the other mechanisms of action likely to prevent conception are thickening of cervical mucus, causing the endometrium to become atrophic, making the uterine environment unfavorable for implantation.

104. **(2)** Though still unproved conclusively, it is believed that the IUD probably causes inflammation of the endometrium, effectively preventing implantation.

105. **(3)** A progesterone-releasing IUD acts to decrease blood loss and cramping.

106. **(2)** The client no longer requires the use of Provera to protect the endometrium from the potential effects of estrogen; therefore, the progestin can be discontinued and the client given continuous estrogen therapy without concern. The other dosage regimens listed are appropriate for a client with an intact uterus on HRT.

107. **(3)** The progestin-only pill does not consistently suppress ovulation. This suppression only occurs in 40–60% of cycles. This makes the progestin-only pill less effective than combined contraceptive pills. Mechanisms of action that contribute to the progestin-only pill's effectiveness is creating an atrophic endometrium and possibly altering tubal physiology by decreasing ovum transport. Progestin-only pills contain no estrogen and are a good choice for the breast-feeding woman.

108. **(1)** Informed consent is essential. The pros and cons of HRT should be explained, but the choice is up to the client.

109. **(3)** Depo-Provera is frequently associated with menstrual cycle changes. In fact, this irregular bleeding is the most commonly cited reason for discontinuation. These menstrual cycle changes range from heavy, irregular bleeding to spotting and even amenorrhea. Nausea and acne are usually effects of estrogen and not seen in Depo-Provera.

110. **(3)** Repeated studies have demonstrated an increase in HDL and a decrease in LDL levels associated with postmenopausal administration of oral estrogens. This alteration in lipoprotein fractions has a beneficial effect on coronary artery disease and stroke.

111. **(4)** Clients taking alendronate (Fosamax) are instructed to take the medication upon arising, 30 minutes prior to eating, with a full glass of water. Clients should be instructed to remain erect after taking the medication to prevent esophageal irritation. Taking medication with food (reduces bioavailability by 40%), coffee or orange juice (decreases bioavailability by 60%), or after eating significantly reduces absorption.

112. **(1)** Women with a uterus taking unopposed exogenous estrogen have an increased risk of endometrial cancer. The addition of progesterone decreases this risk. The addition of progesterone may prompt bleeding, which many women view unfavorably. Progesterone does not affect cervical cancer, breast cancer, or gallbladder disease.

113. **(3)** Metronidazole (Flagyl) in a single 2-gm dose is the treatment of choice for trichomoniasis. An alternative is giving the 2 gm in divided doses the same day. This regimen causes less nausea and may improve compliance.

114. **(4)** Metronidazole (Flagyl) is the treatment of choice for bacterial vaginosis. However, pregnancy should be ruled out prior to

beginning treatment because metronidazole should not be used if there is any possibility the woman is pregnant. The sexual partners do not have to be treated, and doxycycline is not the drug choice.

115. **(3)** She requires added protection through this cycle because of the low-dose OC. Dilantin may also decrease effectiveness of OCs, especially low-dose.

116. **(1)** Because of homeless status, the nurse practitioner needs to use a single-dose treatment. Erythromycin, although a correct medication, is a poor dosing choice for this client.

117. **(3)** The most common cause of PID in sexually active women is gonococcal infections. Gonococcal infections are often accompanied by chlamydia, and they are usually both treated.

118. **(3)** The American College of Physicians recommends that HRT be considered for all women, as it is believed that it reduces the levels of LDLs while increasing the levels of HDLs.

17

Prenatal

Physiology of Pregnancy

1. Normal cardiovascular physiologic responses to pregnancy include:

    1. Increased heart rate, increased cardiac output, decreased blood volume, and systolic murmur.

    2. Increased heart rate, decreased cardiac output, increased blood volume, and systolic murmur.

    3. Increased heart rate, increased cardiac output, increased blood volume, and systolic murmur.

    4. Decreased heart rate, increased cardiac output, increased blood volume, and diastolic murmur.

2. How does progesterone effect the gastrointestinal system during pregnancy?

    1. Causes nausea and vomiting early in pregnancy.

    2. Causes hypertrophy and bleeding of gums.

    3. Delays gastric emptying time and decreases intestinal peristalsis.

    4. Causes diarrhea due to increased intestinal peristalsis.

3. A pregnant client has a hemoglobin of 11.7 gm/dl. Which factor explains this finding?

    1. Presence of iron deficiency anemia.

    2. The trimester of pregnancy.

    3. Physiologic anemia of pregnancy.

    4. Anemia of chronic disease.

4. Several physiologic changes in pregnancy may mimic heart disease. Which of the following is an abnormal finding in pregnancy?

    1. Third heart sound.

    2. Leg edema.

    3. Systolic murmur.

    4. Diastolic murmur.

5. Which of the following is **not** a common urinary system finding during pregnancy?

    1. Physiologic hydronephrosis.

    2. Increased glomerular filtration rate.

    3. Increased urinary frequency.

    4. Proteinuria.

6. Which laboratory finding remains unchanged during pregnancy?

    1. White blood cell (WBC) count.

    2. Red blood cell (RBC) volume.

    3. Fibrinogen level.

    4. Prothrombin level.

7. During pregnancy, estrogen is responsible for:

    1. Hyperpigmentation.

    2. Facilitating implantation.

    3. Reducing smooth muscle tone.

    4. Decreased uterine contractility.

8. Which is **not** a placental hormone?

    1. Human chorionic gonadotropin (hCG).

    2. Estrogen.

    3. Relaxin.

    4. Cortisol.

9. What is the function of the placental hormone relaxin?

    1. Causes changes in endometrium and relaxes smooth muscle.

    2. Stimulates the development of the ductal system of the breasts and causes hypertrophy and hyperplasia of the uterus.

    3. Aids in softening smooth muscle and connective tissue.

    4. Involved with metabolizing certain nutrients and aids in the growth of breasts and other maternal tissues.

10. The nurse practitioner understands that at 12 weeks of fetal development:

    1. Quickening is felt.

    2. Fetal heart tones should be heard with Doppler.

    3. Fetal heart tones are heard with the stethoscope.

    4. Respiratory movements occur.

11. A positive sign of pregnancy is:

    1. Softening of the cervix.

    2. Fetal heart beat.

    3. Enlargement of uterus and abdomen.

    4. Mother's perception of fetal movement.

12. The bluish discoloration of the cervix and vagina is known as:

    1. Goodell's sign.

    2. Chadwick's sign.

    3. Hegar's sign.

    4. Braxton-Hicks sign.

Prenatal Care

13. Dietary changes to reduce nausea and vomiting in pregnancy include:

    1. Consuming small, frequent, low-fat meals, and avoiding spicy foods.

    2. Avoiding carbonated beverages.

    3. Avoiding eating first thing in the morning.

    4. Increasing iron and prenatal vitamins to twice daily.

14. The average extra calories per day required for pregnancy are:

    1. 100 calories.

    2. 300 calories.

    3. 500 calories.

    4. 800 calories.

15. A 22-week pregnant client is planning a prolonged car trip. The nurse practitioner's recommendations would **not** include:

    1. Support stockings.

    2. Frequent (every 1–2 hours) walking.

    3. Wearing a seat belt.

    4. Knee-high stockings.

16. The recommended visits for a low-risk client at 28 weeks of pregnancy is every:
    1. 4 weeks.
    2. Week.
    3. 2 weeks.
    4. 6 weeks.

17. At 20 weeks' gestation, the nurse practitioner would expect to palpate the fundus at:
    1. The symphysis pubis.
    2. The umbilicus.
    3. Halfway between the symphysis pubis and the umbilicus.
    4. The xiphoid.

18. Which is **not** an expected complication of the pregnant client 35 years or older?
    1. Spontaneous abortion (SAB).
    2. Pregnancy-induced hypertension (PIH).
    3. Gestational diabetes.
    4. Anemia.

19. At an initial prenatal visit occurring in the first trimester, which blood test is not recommended?
    1. Antibody screen.
    2. Rubella.
    3. Maternal serum α-fetoprotein (MSAFP).
    4. Hepatitis B surface antigen.

20. The most common indication for genetic counseling is:
    1. Maternal age.
    2. Drug exposure during the first trimester.
    3. Increased maternal α-fetoprotein.
    4. History of previous stillbirth.

21. Clients at highest risk for having a child with Tay-Sachs disease are:
    1. Black.
    2. Jewish.

3. Oriental.

4. 35 years or older at conception.

22. The nurse practitioner teaches a prenatal client that a significant source of toxoplasmosis is:
    1. Rare hamburger.
    2. Fresh fruits.
    3. Raw oysters.
    4. Raw vegetables.

23. A pregnant diabetic client is in the clinic for a prenatal visit; she is at 34 weeks' gestation. She was last seen in the clinic 1 month ago and her dose of insulin had not changed from the previous month. This month her blood sugar remains in control with the same amount of insulin. The nurse practitioner would interpret this information as:
    1. This is normal and indicates the woman has been on her diet and her insulin needs are stable.
    2. The infant is developing well and his pancreas is assisting to control the increased blood sugar from the mother.
    3. With the developing fetus, there should be an increase in the serum glucose for increased nourishment.
    4. The mother may be developing problems with placental insufficiency and should be thoroughly evaluated.

24. Which finding would the nurse practitioner assess in a client with a ruptured tubal pregnancy?
    1. Sharp, stabbing pain localizing to left lower quadrant with blood pressure (BP) of 90/58.
    2. Board-like rigidity of the uterus with abdominal distention.
    3. Dilation of the cervix and rapidly falling BP and pulse.
    4. Serosanguineous vaginal fluid with grape-like vesicles.

25. A pregnant client at 20 weeks gestation comes into the clinic with complaints of vaginal bleeding for the past 6 hours, she also states she has had abdominal cramping prior to the beginning of the bleeding. Vaginal examination reveals a decrease in the uterine size, loss of pregnancy symptoms, and a closed firm cervix. The most likely diagnosis for this client is:

    1. Threatened abortion.

    2. Braxton Hicks contractions.

    3. Placenta abruptio.

    4. Missed abortion.

26. The nurse practitioner schedules a 38-year-old primigravida for an amniocentesis at 16 weeks' gestation. The nurse practitioner would explain that the purpose of this procedure is to:

    1. Assess for the possibility of twins.

    2. Determine the bilirubin level.

    3. Perform genetic studies.

    4. Assess lecithin-sphingomyelin (L/S) ratio.

27. Management of a client after an amniocentesis includes assessing for:

    1. Increased fetal activity.

    2. Elevated temperature.

    3. Spontaneous rupture of the membranes.

    4. Abnormal lung sounds.

28. What would be appropriate management for a primigravida at term who experiences rupture of the membranes?

    1. Begin timing contractions.

    2. Begin pushing.

    3. Take a warm bath.

    4. Refrain from sexual intercourse.

29. The nurse practitioner would note which finding as a possible sign of PIH?

    1. Urgency to urinate at night.

    2. Edema in the extremities and puffy face.

    3. Stomach cramps.

    4. Clear fluid discharge from the nipple.

30. During the first trimester, the nurse practitioner is discussing the monitoring of the growth of twins during the pregnancy. She would explain which test to the client?

    1. Nonstress test (NST).

    2. Sonogram.

    3. L/S ratio.

    4. Amniocentesis.

31. A woman who has missed her period for 5 weeks states that she has been having nausea with some vomiting in the morning hours. The woman also states that she may have a urinary tract infection due to frequency and fatigue. The nurse practitioner would recognize these symptoms to be:

    1. A possible systemic infection.

    2. Positive signs of pregnancy.

    3. Presumptive signs of pregnancy.

    4. Probable signs of pregnancy.

32. The nurse practitioner managing a pregnant client with sickle cell trait would include in the plan which information?

    1. Complete blood count (CBC) each trimester.

    2. Weekly nonstress test.

    3. Urine cultures each trimester.

    4. Frequent ultrasounds for growth.

33. Screening for gestational diabetes mellitus (GDM) during pregnancy includes:

    1. 1-hour postprandial 100-gm glucose screen for all women between 24 and 28 weeks' gestation.

    2. 3-hour 100-gm glucose tolerance test (GTT) at initial visit for all women with history of GDM.

    3. 1-hour postprandial 50-gm glucose screen at initial visit for women at risk.

    4. Glycosylated hemoglobin A_{1c} (HgbA_{1c}) for all women between 24 and 28 weeks' gestation.

34. A 23-year-old G3 P0 has a 1-hour postprandial 50-gm glucose screen result of

210 mg/dl. What is the next appropriate step to take?

1. Order a 3-hour 100-gm GTT.

2. Order a fasting blood sugar (FBS).

3. Order a HgbA$_{1c}$.

4. Refer immediately for diabetic treatment.

35. A teenager returns to the clinic for contraceptive follow-up after being on a low-dose oral contraceptive (OC) for 3 months. She complains of amenorrhea for 2 months, urinary frequency, and leukorrhea. Vaginal exam reveals uterus about 6 cm and the presence of Chadwick's sign. The first diagnostic test indicated should be:

1. Pregnancy test.

2. Complete blood count.

3. Microscopic urinalysis.

4. Culture for gonorrhea and chlamydia.

36. An adult female presents with her spouse for a prenatal visit. During the exam, you notice bruising of the abdomen and back. You also note that the spouse does most of talking during the history. The best approach to this situation is:

1. Ask the spouse to leave the room so you can do a pelvic exam.

2. Ask the woman to accompany you to the lab for blood work; ask about bruises.

3. Ask the woman about the bruises during the exam.

4. Do nothing; domestic violence is beyond the scope of your practice.

37. A pregnant employee who works at a day care center is concerned about a recent outbreak of "fifth disease." The nurse practitioner understands that:

1. Most parvovirus B19 infections in utero are associated with an increased number of congenital anomalies.

2. There are no isoimmunization-associated problems for the mother exposed to a young child with fifth disease.

3. Parvovirus B19 has caused hydrops fetalis and death in some fetuses who have been infected in utero.

4. The mortality risk for a fetus is extremely high, especially if the mother has never had fifth disease.

38. Which is an **abnormal** complaint in the second trimester of pregnancy?

1. Frequent uterine contractions.

2. Frequent fetal movement.

3. Calf cramps.

4. Heartburn.

39. Which statement is true about smoking during pregnancy?

1. The rate of spontaneous abortion among smokers is the same as in nonsmokers.

2. Risks of complications increase with the number of cigarettes smoked.

3. Discontinuation of smoking during pregnancy has no effect on pregnancy outcome.

4. There is not a relationship between smoking and sudden infant death syndrome (SIDS).

40. Chlamydia infections during pregnancy may be associated with:

1. Transplacental transmission to fetus.

2. Congenital anomalies of the eyes.

3. Premature rupture of membranes.

4. Fetal hydrops.

41. Cocaine use during pregnancy is associated with:

1. Abruptio placentae.

3. Postdate pregnancy.

3. Macrosomatia infant.

4. Maternal hypotension.

42. Which is **not** a normal cervical finding in the second trimester?

1. Cervix film.

2. Cervical dilation.

3. Cervix 2 cm long.

4. Cervix posterior.

43. During pregnancy, sexual relations are contraindicated:

    1. During the first trimester when there is a history of spontaneous abortion.

    2. After 36 weeks' gestation.

    3. With the diagnosis of placenta previa.

    4. With excessive maternal weight gain.

44. Which is an **abnormal** complaint in the first trimester of pregnancy?

    1. Nausea and vomiting.

    2. Fatigue.

    3. Vaginal bleeding.

    4. Low backache.

45. The recommended screening test for gestational diabetes is:

    1. 3-hour glucose tolerance test.

    2. 1-hour blood sugar measurement after 50 gm of glucose.

    3. 2-hour postprandial blood sugar measurement.

    4. Random blood sugar measurement.

46. Which is an **abnormal** complaint of the third trimester of pregnancy?

    1. Leukorrhea.

    2. Headache with blurred vision.

    3. Urinary frequency.

    4. Uterine contractions.

47. Which would be **incorrect** for the treatment of mild PIH?

    1. Modified bed rest.

    2. Monitor BP, weight, and urinary protein.

    3. Methyldopa (Aldomet) 250 mg PO tid.

    4. Diet and nutritional counseling to increase water intake, increase protein, and decrease salt intake to <2 gm/day.

48. What would be **incorrect** advice to the nonlaboring pregnant client upon the second-trimester diagnosis of a placenta previa?

1. Pelvic rest.

2. Report any bright red bleeding.

3. Planned cesarean section.

4. Follow-up ultrasound at 32 weeks' gestation.

49. The pregnant client wishes to have further information regarding exercise guidelines. She runs on the treadmill 4 mph for 30 minutes daily, then does 30 additional minutes of free weights and lower leg machines at the gym. General guidelines should include all **except**:

    1. Keep the heart rate <140 bpm.

    2. Limit free weight for upper body to <10 lb each.

    3. Limit exercise time to 30 minutes total.

    4. Avoid breathlessness and excessive heat.

50. Testing for gestational diabetes should be done:

    1. When a client has a history of a previous macrosomatia infant.

    2. If the client is obese.

    3. On all pregnant women.

    4. When the client has glycosuria.

51. Which is **not** a predisposing factor of PIH?

    1. Primigravida.

    2. Age >35.

    3. Multiple gestation.

    4. Hyperthyroidism.

52. For a pregnant client at 32 weeks' gestation with a BP of 140/92, weight gain the past 2 weeks of 4 lb, trace protein on urine dip, 1+ pitting edema in the feet, and 2+ reflexes, the probable diagnosis would be:

    1. Mild pregnancy induced hypertension.

    2. Severe pregnancy induced hypertension.

    3. Eclampsia.

    4. Hemolysis, elevated liver enzymes, low platelets (HELLP) syndrome.

53. The nurse practitioner is assessing a client who has a positive pregnancy test. The laboratory data indicate the mother's blood group to be O-positive and the father's to be AB-negative. What risk is there for this pregnancy?

    1. The mother may build up antibodies to the infant's blood if the infant is type B-positive, which will be significant in future pregnancies.

    2. The mother is Rh-positive; therefore, if the infant is Rh-negative there is an increased incidence of the infant building up Rh antibodies.

    3. Since the mother is O and the father is AB, there is an increased risk for the development of an ABO incompatibility.

    4. Type O blood is the dominant characteristic, the infant's blood will be in the O group, and there will be no complications.

54. A young adult client, G2 P1 A0 L1, 10 weeks' gestation intrauterine pregnancy (IUP) is seen for her first obstetric intake history and physical. She knows when she conceived, and denies any vaginal bleeding or abdominal pain. The client has a soft, nontender fundus that measures 14 cm, the adnexal exam is negative for mass or tenderness; no fetal heart tones (FHTs) are audible with the doptone. The most likely diagnosis seen on ultrasound is:

    1. Multiple gestation.

    2. Fibroid uterus.

    3. Ectopic pregnancy.

    4. 14-week viable IUP.

Pharmacology

55. Which immunization is contraindicated in pregnancy?

    1. Polio vaccine.

    2. Hepatitis B vaccine.

    3. Measles-mumps-rubella (MMR).

    4. Tetanus.

56. If studies in animals or pregnant women demonstrated evidence of fetal abnormality or risk, or if the potential for fetal risk clearly outweighs the possible benefit of the drug, the Food and Drug Administration (FDA) category for this drug is:

    1. B.

    2. C.

    3. D.

    4. X.

57. The nurse practitioner is aware that fetal exposure to tetracycline causes:

    1. Blindness.

    2. Hearing loss.

    3. Tooth discoloration.

    4. Limb deformities.

58. Which of the following may reduce the risk of neural tube defect when taken prior to conception?

    1. Vitamin A.

    2. Pyroxidine.

    3. Folic acid.

    4. Vitamin C.

59. The current recommendation for antepartum treatment of Rh-negative pregnant women, when the Rh status of the partner is unknown, with Rh immune globulin (RhoGAM) includes:

    1. Administration of 300 μg at 28 weeks and 36 weeks of pregnancy.

    2. Administration of 300 μm at 28 weeks of pregnancy to all Rh-negative women.

    3. Administration of 300 μg in each trimester.

    4. No administration is needed until postpartum.

17   Answers & Rationales

Physiology of Pregnancy

1. **(3)** In pregnancy, a hyperdynamic state is caused by an increase in blood volume, which results in a slightly increased heart rate and increased cardiac output. Systolic ejection murmurs are common and caused by increased flow across the pulmonic and aortic valves. Diastolic murmurs are abnormal and require referral.

2. **(3)** Progesterone affects the gastrointestinal system by decreasing smooth muscle tone, delaying gastric emptying, and decreasing intestinal peristalsis. hCG is associated with nausea and vomiting early in pregnancy. Estrogen causes the gums to become hyperemic, soft, and swollen with a tendency to bleed.

3. **(3)** The increase in plasma volume combined with a slower rise in red blood cell production produces a dilutional anemia. Hemoglobin and hematocrit decrease in relation to plasma volume. True anemia occurs with a hemoglobin <11 gm/dl and hematocrit <35%.

4. **(4)** Leg edema is due to increased venous pressure in the legs. Both components of the first heart sound become louder and there is an exaggerated splitting and a third heart sound gallop is common after midpregnancy. Systolic ejection murmurs are common and are due to the increased flow across the aortic and pulmonic valves. Diastolic murmurs are an abnormal finding.

5. **(4)** Changes in renal structure are influenced by estrogen, progesterone, increased blood volume, and uterine pressure. Changes in the collection system, such as dilatation of the renal pelvis and ureters, cause a physiologic hydronephrosis. The glomerular filtration rate does increase during pregnancy. Increased urinary frequency is related to increasing size of uterus and its pressure on the bladder. Proteinuria is abnormal except in very concentrated urine or in the first voided specimen upon arising. Proteinuria is a warning of impaired kidney function or PIH.

6. **(4)** RBC volume increases approximately 30%, and WBCs increase 5000–12,000/mm³. Fibrin, fibrinogen, and plasma levels of factors VII, IX, and X are also increased. Prothrombin levels remain unchanged.

7. **(1)** During pregnancy, estrogen is responsible for stimulation of melanin-stimulating hormone, thus resulting in hyperpigmentation. Progesterone from the corpus luteum and later the placenta is responsible for facilitating implantation, decreasing uterine contractility, and reducing smooth muscle tone.

8. **(4)** There are five placental hormones: hCG, estrogen, progesterone, human placental lactogen, and relaxin. Cortisol is not a placental hormone.

9. **(3)** Relaxin aids in softening smooth muscle and connective tissue in preparation for labor and delivery. Progesterone relaxes smooth muscle and causes changes in the

endometrium. Estrogen stimulates the development of the ductal system of the breasts and causes hypertrophy and hyperplasia of the uterus. Human placental lactogen is involved with metabolism of glucose, fatty acids, and amino acids. It also aids in the growth of the breasts and other maternal tissues.

10. **(2)** Fetal heart tones should be heard by 12 weeks' gestation and may be heard as early as 10 weeks. Quickening is felt at 16–20 weeks. Fetal heart tones can be heard by stethoscope at 20 weeks. Respiratory movements occur later in fetal development at approximately 24 weeks.

11. **(2)** Positive evidence of pregnancy are fetal heart beat, palpation of fetal movement by examiner, and visualization of the fetus (by ultrasonography). Amenorrhea, nausea, emesis, urinary frequency, fatigue, skin changes, and the mother's perception of fetal movement are presumptive evidence of pregnancy. Probable evidence of pregnancy are softening of the cervix, softening of the lower uterine segment, cyanosis of cervix and vagina, Braxton-Hicks contractions, ballottement, palpation of fetal outline by the examiner, and pregnancy tests.

12. **(2)** Chadwick's sign occurs at 6–8 weeks' gestation and is the bluish discoloration of the cervix and vagina. Goodell's sign is the softening of the cervix that is seen as early as 4 weeks' gestation. Hegar's sign is the softening of the lower uterine segment. Braxton-Hicks sign consists of contractions of the uterus that can occur as early as 16 weeks' gestation.

Prenatal Care

13. **(1)** Clients should eat frequent small meals to keep some food in the stomach at all times and to avoid stomach distention. Sipping on carbonated beverages may be helpful. Having crackers at the bedside to take before rising in the morning may be a successful preventative measure.

14. **(2)** The pregnant woman requires approximately 15% more calories per day than nonpregnant women. This is

approximately 300 calories per day and depends on the client's weight and activity level.

15. **(4)** Venous stasis occurs with prolonged sitting and may be a risk factor for thrombophlebitis. Support stockings and frequent walking should be encouraged. Knee-high stockings have elastic around the calf that may act as a tourniquet. They should be avoided during pregnancy. Seat belts are recommended.

16. **(3)** The American College of Obstetricians and Gynecologists (ACOG) recommends visits every 2 weeks starting at 28 weeks until 36 weeks. At 36 weeks, visits are weekly until delivery.

17. **(2)** The expected fundal height at 20 weeks' gestation is at the umbilicus. At 12 weeks, the fundus can be palpated just above the symphysis, and at 16 weeks between the symphysis and umbilicus. The fundus is palpated at the xiphoid at approximately 36 weeks.

18. **(4)** The risk for anemia in pregnancy does not increase with age. The risks for SAB, PIH, and gestational diabetes do increase with maternal age.

19. **(3)** Routine prenatal labs include CBC, blood type and Rh, antibody screen, hepatitis B surface antigen, syphilis screen, and rubella immune status. The MSAFP is done between 15 and 20 weeks. Before this, very little α-fetoprotein is produced by the fetus and results would be inaccurate.

20. **(1)** The largest group of women who potentially benefit from genetic counseling are those 35 and older. The number of births to women between 35 and 40 years old has increased by approximately 35% in the 1990s. The primary cause of congenital abnormalities in women older than 35 years is chromosomal abnormalities. The other answers are all reasons for genetic counseling, but to a much lesser degree.

21. **(2)** The incidence of the Tay-Sachs gene in the Jewish population is 1 in 30 as compared to 1 in 300 for the non-Jewish population.

22. **(1)** Undercooked red meat is a major source of toxoplasmosis. Pregnant women should be cautioned against eating undercooked meats. Cats are also shown to be hosts. Toxoplasmosis is spread through cat feces. Pregnant women should be warned about cleaning the litter box and about contaminated soil.

23. **(4)** In the last two trimesters of pregnancy, the insulin needs should steadily increase due to the insulin antagonism from the placenta, as well as from the fetus. By not increasing her need for insulin, she could be showing signs of placental insufficiency.

24. **(1)** The ruptured fallopian tube causes a sharp, sudden, stabbing pain. Symptoms of shock (decreased BP, increased pulse, and increased respirations) occur, as the client quickly becomes a surgical emergency. Board-like abdominal rigidity is often noted with abruptio placentae. Grape-like vesicles are associated with hydatidiform mole.

25. **(4)** A missed abortion is characterized by vaginal bleeding and a closed cervix. A threatened abortion has vaginal bleeding and cramping, but the symptoms of pregnancy are still present. Placenta abruptio is bleeding without pain and symptoms of pregnancy are present.

26. **(3)** The woman's age places her at risk for a Down's syndrome baby. The L/S ratio is tested in the third trimester for fetal lung maturity.

27. **(3)** Damage to the membranes is a possibility and a high-priority situation. Fever would not be an immediate problem. Fetal heart rate is monitored, not activity.

28. **(4)** Without the protective barrier of the amniotic membrane, the mother and the baby are susceptible to infection. The client should refrain from sexual intercourse due to the possibility of introduction of pathogens. Bathing would also be a hazard due to the possibility of contracting and infection from the bath water.

29. **(2)** Classic signs of PIH are generalized edema of the extremities and around the face, proteinuria, and hypertension. Stomach cramps could be an indication of early labor or gastrointestinal upset. Clear

nipple fluid would be an early sign of colostrum.

30. **(2)** The ultrasound test (sonogram) is used to assess growth of the fetus, position of the placenta, and position of the fetus. The NST is used to observe the response of the fetal heart rate to the stress of activity. The L/S ratio determines if there is sufficient surfactant. An amniocentesis is performed to obtain amniotic fluid for analysis at a later date in the pregnancy, if indicated.

31. **(3)** Missed menstrual periods, nausea, vomiting, frequency, and fatigue are presumptive signs (subjective) of pregnancy. Probable signs of pregnancy are objective, such as Chadwick's sign, ballottement, and positive pregnancy test. Positive signs of pregnancy are fetal heart rate or sonogram.

32. **(3)** Sickle cell trait occurs in 8% of American blacks. These women are asymptomatic, not anemic, and usually have no problems except under conditions of hypoxia. There is no difference in perinatal outcome and these women do not require frequent ultrasounds or nonstress testing. They are at increased risk for asymptomatic bacteriuria and require a urine culture each trimester.

33. **(3)** This is a standard screen for women at risk. It should also be done for all other pregnant women between 24 and 28 weeks' gestation.

34. **(2)** This is a standard diagnostic decision tree for a screen >200 mg. If the FBS is >130 mg, refer and/or consult with physician for treatment plan.

35. **(1)** This clinical picture is highly indicative or pregnancy.

36. **(2)** While Option #1 may work, it may also serve to arouse the spouse's suspicion and create a situation where you must then insist he leave or drop the request. Option #2 is best, as it gives a legitimate reason to quickly move the woman from the room, provides a moment of privacy to inquire about the bruises, and provides an opportunity to move the woman to a safe place if needed without creating confrontation.

37. **(3)** Most fetuses are not affected; however, some undergo isoimmunization, which leads to hydrops fetalis and death. The mortality risk is actually low and there are usually no associated congenital anomalies.

38. **(1)** Contractions could represent early premature labor and should be monitored to rule out early cervical change. Not all contractions are "Braxton-Hicks contractions," and they need to be taken seriously. The other symptoms listed are important to discuss and to rule out other associated symptomatology.

39. **(2)** The risk of complications and perinatal loss increases with the number of cigarettes smoked. Discontinuation or decrease in the amount of cigarettes smoked during pregnancy can reduce the risk of complications, especially for high-risk women.

40. **(3)** Premature rupture of membranes may be associated with chlamydia infections. Intrauterine transmission of *Chlamydia trachomatis* to the fetus has not been demonstrated. There is no evidence of fetal eye anomalies; however, without prophylaxis, conjunctivitis will develop in 30–50% of infants 7–days after birth.

41. **(1)** Use of cocaine during pregnancy is associated with placental abruption, spontaneous abortion, and preterm labor. Maternal blood pressure and heart rate are increased. The fetus is at risk for intrauterine growth retardation, fetal distress, seizures, and death.

42. **(2)** It is not considered normal or expected for one to have a dilated cervix at any time in the second trimester of pregnancy. The cervix will typically be firm, 2 cm long and posterior, as well as closed.

43. **(3)** In placenta previa, the placenta is improperly positioned in the lower uterine segment, covering all or part of the cervical os. There is an increased risk of bleeding. Management includes bed rest, no intercourse, no vaginal exams, instruction on what to do if bleeding occurs, and close fetal surveillance.

44. **(3)** Vaginal bleeding could represent a potential problem in the pregnancy during the first trimester. The other symptoms listed are important as well and warrant further discussion to rule out a problem.

45. **(2)** The recommended screening test for gestational diabetes is a blood sugar measurement 1 hour after 50 gm of glucose at 24–28 weeks of pregnancy. If the result of this test is 140 or above, then a 3-hour GTT is done.

46. **(2)** Headache associated with blurred vision could represent early symptoms of mild pre-eclampsia or PIH and warrant further work-up to rule out a problem. The other symptoms are not of concern if they are not associated with other symptoms as well.

47. **(3)** The use of medication is no longer felt to be useful in the treatment of mild PIH and, in fact, could be hazardous. The client is best treated conservatively with modified bed rest on the left side and dietary counseling, along with close monitoring of the BP, weight, and urinary protein. Close follow-up with examination for edema or symptomatic change and monitoring of the fetus are also performed.

48. **(3)** There is no reason to plan a cesarean section upon diagnosis of the placenta previa at this stage of the pregnancy, because the lower segment of the uterus goes through its final maturation between 28 and 32 weeks' gestation. There is an excellent chance that the placenta will migrate by the third trimester, thus allowing for vaginal birth, barring any other unforeseen factors.

49. **(3)** There is no reason to limit the amount of time for exercise, provided the client is feeling well. By keeping the heart rate below 140 bpm, there is less chance for internal overheating and exhaustion. The ACOG suggests limiting the free weight use of <10 lb to avoid undue stress and strain on muscles and ligaments. Avoidance of breathlessness and excessive heat will allow for better circulation to the fetus.

50. **(3)** Over one half of pregnant women who exhibit gestational diabetes lack the classic risk factors of family history of diabetes, unexpected stillbirth, prior macrosomatia infant, obesity, advanced maternal age, or glycosuria. The best answer is that all women should be screened for gestational diabetes.

51. **(4)** Predisposing factors in PIH include primigravida, <20 years or >35 years, women with vascular diseases (hypertension, systemic lupus erythematosis, diabetes mellitus, renal disease), family history, previous history of pre-eclampsia, and multiple gestation. Hyperthyroidism does not predispose to PIH.

52. **(1)** Mild PIH (pre-eclampsia) is consistent with a systolic blood presure ≥140 mm Hg or systolic rise ≥30 mm Hg, and/or diastolic blood pressure ≥90 or diastolic rise ≥15 mm Hg, weight gain >2 lb/wk, nondependent edema ≥1+ with normal reflexes. Severe pre-eclampsia symptoms include blood pressure ≥160/100, weight gain >2 lb/wk, generalized edema, proteinuria ≥3+, decreased urine output, and hyperreflexia. Eclampsia includes the above plus seizures. The HELLP syndrome includes signs and symptoms of severe pre-eclampsia, an enlarged and firm liver, epigastric or right upper quadrant pain, and, frequently, jaundice.

53. **(3)** There is an increased incidence of ABO incompatibility if the mother is blood group O and the infant is either blood group A or B. Rh incompatibility occurs only when the mother is Rh-negative and is carrying an Rh-positive infant. In the most common cases of ABO incompatibility there is a production of maternal antibodies against the A cells or the B cells.

54. **(1)** Multiple gestation will cause the uterus to enlarge faster than normal. It is not uncommon to have inaudible FHT with the doptone at 10 weeks gestation. A fibroid could cause the uterus to enlarge, however it is generally accompanied by firmness to palpation of the uterus. Ectopic pregnancy could be the cause of inaudible FHT but is usually accompanied by adnexal tenderness, mass or vaginal bleeding. A 14 week viable IUP should have audible FHT with the doptone.

Pharmacology

55. **(3)** The MMR is a live virus and is contraindicated in pregnancy. Polio, tetanus, and hepatitis B vaccine are inactivated bacterial or DNA-based vaccines and are safe when indicated.

56. **(4)** The FDA has five pregnancy risk categories for drugs. Category X indicates fetal risk outweighs any benefit and use in pregnancy is contraindicated. Category B drugs show no evidence of fetal abnormalities and risk to the fetus is relatively unlikely. Category C drugs have potential for animal fetal abnormalities and/or no adequate well-controlled studies available in pregnant women, but benefits of drugs are thought to justify risks to the fetus. Drugs classified as Category D demonstrate positive evidence of human fetal risk and should be used only in serious disease or life-threatening situations where safer drugs are ineffective.

57. **(3)** Tetracycline binds with developing enamel and discolors the deciduous teeth between 26 weeks' gestation and 6 months of infancy.

58. **(3)** Recent studies have confirmed that folic acid taken prior to conception can reduce the risk of neural tube defect.

59. **(2)** Current recommendations for RhoGAM is administration of 300 μg to all Rh-negative women at 28 weeks of pregnancy. This is considered protective for the remainder of the pregnancy.

18

Obstetrics, Postpartum, & Newborn

Disorders

1. During a postpartum assessment, the nurse practitioner notes a cluster of external hemorrhoids. Which statement made by the client indicates a need for additional teaching?

   1. "I can give myself an enema every other day to reduce constipation."

   2. "I can take sitz baths for pain."

   3. "I can decrease the swelling by using a topical hydrocortisone cream."

   4. "I can take a stool softener to decrease the pain of a BM."

2. A 28-year-old female client is seen by the nurse practitioner for an office visit. Her last menstrual period (LMP) was 8 weeks ago; she is complaining of left lower quadrant (LLQ) abdominal pain, spotting, and fatigue. Her pelvic exam reveals cervical os closed, minimal blood in vaginal vault; uterus minimally enlarged, mild cervical motion tenderness (CMT), left adnexal fullness and tenderness; right adnexa within normal limits (WNL). Vital signs are stable. The serum pregnancy test is positive. What is the most cost-effective and useful test for the nurse practitioner to order?

   1. Computed tomography (CAT) scan of the abdomen/pelvis.

   2. Barium enema.

   3. Pelvic ultrasound.

   4. Flat plate of the abdomen.

3. Ten days after delivery, a client is diagnosed with mastitis. The nurse practitioner would expect to find on the physical exam:

   1. Tender, hard, reddened breast.

   2. Dimpled skin on breasts.

   3. Lack of milk production.

   4. Nipple burning during feeding.

4. In discussing the timing of contractions with a client, the nurse practitioner explains "frequency" as the interval from the:

   1. Beginning of one contraction to the beginning of the next.

   2. Beginning of one contraction to the end of that contraction.

   3. End of one contraction to the start of the next.

   4. End of one contraction to the end of the next contraction.

5. Which is **not** an expected complication of the pregnant teen who is age 17 or less?

   1. Premature labor and birth.

   2. Anemia.

   3. Gestational diabetes.

   4. Pregnancy-induced hypertension (PIH).

6. The biophysical profile includes which of the following parameters?

   1. Fetal breathing movements.

   2. Fetal tone.

   3. Fetal amniotic volume.

   4. All of the above.

7. The most common reason for a nonreactive nonstress test (NST) is:

   1. Fetal hypoxia.

   2. Maternal drug use.

   3. Fetal inactivity or sleep.

   4. Congenital heart defect.

8. Which is **least** likely to be found in a client presenting with an ectopic pregnancy?

   1. Pain.

   2. Missed menses.

   3. Vaginal bleeding.

   4. Abdominal mass.

9. Which is **not** true about an ectopic pregnancy?

   1. 90% occur in the fallopian tube.

   2. They account for approximately 10% of maternal deaths.

   3. Prior history of pelvic inflammatory disease (PID) is reported in 50% of clients with ectopics.

   4. Previous ectopic pregnancy does not increase risk of another ectopic pregnancy.

10. A client presents to the clinic with a diagnosis of threatened abortion. The nurse practitioner describes this as:

    1. Vaginal bleeding with or without cramping and no cervical change.

    2. Vaginal bleeding with cramping and cervical change.

    3. Loss of pregnancy symptoms, decrease in uterine size, cervix closed and firm.

    4. Cramping, bleeding, incomplete expulsion of products of conception.

11. A predisposing factor in preterm labor is:

    1. Obesity.

    2. Previous spontaneous abortions.

    3. Prior preterm delivery.

    4. White race.

12. The ability of amniotic fluid to produce a ferning pattern when dried may be altered by:

    1. Meconium.

    2. Changes in vaginal pH.

    3. Presence of cervical mucus.

    4. Heavy contamination with blood.

13. Ten weeks into a client's pregnancy, she begins to experience vaginal bleeding. The client's human chorionic gonadotropin (hCG) levels remain elevated. The nurse practitioner would instruct the client to call the clinic if she develops signs of:

1. Nausea and vomiting.

2. Abdominal pain or cramping.

3. Urinary frequency.

4. Fatigue and tiredness.

14. Which statement is true regarding the course of pruritic urticaria papules and plaques of pregnancy (PUPPP)?

1. Perinatal mortality is increased.

2. Pruritis is increased postpartum.

3. Lesions first appear on abdomen.

4. Onset is usually in the first trimester.

15. Two to 4 months after delivery, an increase in scalp hair loss results from:

1. Increased number of hairs in telogen.

2. Hyperthyroidism.

3. Fatigue.

4. Sudden postpartum cardiovascular changes.

16. In a breast-feeding client having difficulty with milk production, the nurse practitioner understands that an increase in milk production will be produced by:

1. More frequent suckling of infant.

2. Longer duration of suckling.

3. Cessation of suckling for 24 hours.

4. Cold compresses to the breast.

17. During a breast exam on a lactating woman, which finding is cause for concern?

1. Leaking of "watery" fluid from left breast.

2. Cracked nipples that are tender to touch.

3. Bilateral warm breasts that are distended.

4. Inverted left nipple, flat right nipple.

18. A new first-time mother is being evaluated for a complaint of breast pain. Her infant is 3 weeks old and she is breast-feeding. The infant is gaining weight and seems satisfied after feeding. On exam the nurse practitioner finds a red, irritated nipple on one breast but no masses or tenderness to the breast itself. An important part of the nurse practitioner's evaluation is:

1. A mammogram of the breast.

2. Examination of the infant's mouth.

3. A stat complete blood count (CBC).

4. An analysis of the milk.

19. A client delivers a healthy newborn with a cleft lip and cleft palate during a home delivery. The new mother and baby visit the rural outreach clinic the next morning. What actions would promote maternal–infant bonding?

1. Point out the newborn's normal characteristics.

2. Explain to the mother how the problem is not significant.

3. Have the mother begin taking care of the newborn immediately after delivery.

4. Explain to the mother that orofacial surgery will completely correct the defect.

20. The nurse practitioner is measuring a newborn's frontal-occipital circumference (FOC). Correct technique involves:

1. Placement of the tape measure at the maximal occipital prominence, just above the eyebrows.

2. Placement of the cloth tape measure at a level 2 inches above the ears.

3. Using a cloth tape to prevent inaccuracy due to stretchable materials.

4. Having another person hold the tape in the center of the forehead and repeating the measurement.

21. Which newborn screening tests are mandatory state requirements?

    1. CBC and urinalysis (UA).

    2. Thyroid and phenylketonuria (PKU).

    3. PKU and α-fetoprotein.

    4. Glucose and thyroid studies.

22. The nurse practitioner notes an undescended testicle on a newborn. She understands that testicular function and the ability to produce healthy sperm as an adult may be impaired if the repair is not made by:

    1. 6 years of age.

    2. 2 years of age.

    3. 1 year of age.

    4. 6 months of age.

23. The most important obstetric measurement is the:

    1. Obstetrical conjugate.

    2. Diagonal conjugate.

    3. Midpelvis conjugate.

    4. Biparietal conjugate.

24. The nurse practitioner is examining a full-term infant who developed physiologic jaundice and is being treated with phototherapy. What is the mechanism of action of phototherapy in the treatment of this infant?

    1. The light is absorbed by bilirubin and promotes the conversion of a toxic bilirubin to an unconjugated product that can be excreted in the bile.

    2. It increases the hemolysis of the excessive red cells that are received by the full-term infant during labor and delivery.

    3. The ultraviolet light decreases the sensitivity to the destruction of red cells secondary to the Rh incompatibility.

    4. It increases the enzyme activity in breaking down the unconjugated bilirubin to a nontoxic form to be eliminated by the kidney.

25. The nurse practitioner is examining a 7-day-old infant who is bottle-fed and is developing a significant problem with jaundice. What is a primary concern based on this observation?

    1. The development of neonatal sepsis.

    2. There is an increase in destruction of fetal hemoglobin.

    3. The infant is not tolerating the formula.

    4. An exaggerated development of physiologic jaundice.

26. A 4-day-old infant who is being breast-fed begins to develop jaundice. What is a common theory regarding the precipitating cause of this jaundice?

    1. Decreased intake in the first few days and the subsequent weight loss.

    2. Decreased tolerance and digestion of the breast milk.

    3. Increased destruction of red cells with release of bilirubin.

    4. Antigen–antibody reaction increasing the destruction of fetal red cells.

27. Which infant is at an increased risk for the development of the "bronze baby syndrome?"

    1. Premature infant with ABO incompatibility.

    2. Oriental infant who is bottle-fed.

    3. Caucasian infant who is breast-fed.

    4. Presence of obstructive liver disease.

28. A mother brings her 6-week-old infant to the office with concern over the child's "constant crying." She states she did not have this problem with her other two children. She is bottle-feeding the infant and there is no problem with feeding. The infant has a bowel movement every day and the stools are soft. The infant is afebrile and there is no evidence of problems with the ears, throat, lungs, or abdomen.

Considering this information, what is the best diagnosis for this infant?

1. Infantile colic.

2. Spastic colon.

3. Infant stress syndrome.

4. Lactose intolerance.

29. The nurse suspects infantile colic in a 2-month-old infant. A complete physical examination does not reveal any abnormalities. What further investigation by the nurse practitioner is necessary?

1. Chest x-ray.

2. CBC and differential.

3. Blood culture.

4. Urinalysis.

30. The nurse practitioner is discussing with the parents the care of their 1-month-old infant who has been diagnosed with infantile colic. What is important to explain to the parents?

1. The problem may be decreased by not feeding the infant more often than every 3 hours.

2. There is no specific medication that is indicated to treat the problem.

3. The problem is often related to increased stress in the home; family therapy may be indicated.

4. The formula should be changed from a milk-based to a soy-based formula.

Pharmacology

31. Which medication would be considered safe for use after the first trimester of pregnancy?

1. Metronidazole (Flagyl).

2. Tetracycline (Achromycin).

3. Isotretinoin (Accutane).

4. Angiotensin converting enzyme (ACE) inhibitors.

32. For the client who wishes to breast-feed and take oral contraception, the pill of choice is:

1. A 1/35 preparation.

2. A triphasic preparation.

3. A progestin-only preparation.

4. A 1/50 preparation.

33. A pregnant client in the last trimester complains of a constant backache, especially aggravated by walking, moving, and bending. There is no radiation to either leg. In addition to rest, massage, and physiotherapy what would be appropriate to prescribe?

1. Acetaminophen (Tylenol).

2. Codeine.

3. Napoxyn (Anaprox).

4. Aspirin.

18 Answers & Rationales

Disorders

1. **(1)** An enema every other day to reduce constipation would negatively affect the normal bowel movement pattern and deplete the client's natural intestinal flora. Sitz baths, anti-inflammatory and analgesic topical ointments or sprays, along with stool softeners and increased bulk in the diet would be indicated in the management of the external hemorrhoids.

2. **(3)** This easy, inexpensive, and relatively noninvasive test will assist the nurse practitioner with confirming the diagnosis of ectopic pregnancy. It can be obtained quickly and is often available rapidly. The CT scan of the abdomen/pelvis will also show an ectopic, but it is neither cost-effective nor noninvasive. Neither barium enema nor a flat plate of the abdomen are of assistance in this case.

3. **(1)** Swelling, erythema, and pain are found in the upper, outer quadrant of the breast. Dimpled skin (orange peel appearance) is a potential sign of breast cancer. Nipple burning is related to positioning and initiation of the let-down reflex during feeding. Milk production starts about 4 days postpartum.

4. **(1)** Frequency of contractions should be timed from the beginning of one contraction to the beginning of the next contraction.

5. **(3)** The pregnant teen is at increased risk for premature labor, anemia, and PIH. There is no documentation that the pregnant teen is at greater risk of gestational diabetes.

6. **(4)** The biophysical profile includes observation of fetal respiratory movement, fetal tone, gross fetal movements, measurements of amniotic fluid volume, and fetal heart reactivity. Each parameter is given a score of 2 if present and normal if 8–10.

7. **(3)** The most common reason for a nonreactive NST is fetal sleep or inactivity. The fetal sleep–wake cycle ranges from 20–40 minutes. If reactivity is not demonstrated in 20 minutes, continuing to 40 minutes usually accommodates the sleep–wake cycles. Fetal hypoxia and maternal smoking and drug use certainly affect fetal heart rate but are not the most common causes. Infants with a congenital heart defect do not exhibit a significant incidence of nonreactive NSTs.

8. **(4)** Greater than 90% of clients presenting with ectopic pregnancies will complain of pain and report a missed period. Approximately 80% will describe vaginal bleeding; however, only 50% will have a palpable abdominal mass.

9. **(4)** It is true that 90% of ectopic pregnancies are found in the fallopian tubes. Clients with PID have a sevenfold increase in the rate of ectopic pregnancy. A previous ectopic pregnancy is a risk factor and does increase the risk of a subsequent ectopic pregnancy.

10. **(1)** A threatened abortion progresses to complete spontaneous abortion 50% of the time. Clinical findings are vaginal bleeding with or without cramping and no cervical change. Vaginal bleeding with cramping and cervical change is an inevitable abortion. An incomplete abortion is demonstrated by vaginal bleeding, cramping, and incomplete expulsion of products of conception. A missed abortion is diagnosed when products of conception are retained after fetal death. There is a decrease in uterine size, loss of pregnancy symptoms, and the cervix is often closed and firm.

11. **(3)** The history of preterm birth is associated with a 20−40% recurrence risk. Low prepregnancy weight and inadequate weight gain, not obesity, are associated with preterm labor. Maternal smoking, drug use (especially cocaine), low socioeconomic status, maternal age <17 and >35, and nonwhite race are all predisposing factors for preterm labor. Previous spontaneous or elective abortions are not risk factors.

12. **(4)** When air-dried, amniotic fluid produces a fern pattern. This microscopic arborization is accurate in confirming rupture of membranes in 90−95% of cases. Samples heavily contaminated with blood may not fern.

13. **(2)** Contractions, cramping, or continued bleeding may indicate a spontaneous abortion. The other symptoms are common in the first trimester.

14. **(3)** Lesions typically start on the abdomen, and spread to the thighs and possibly the buttocks. Onset of lesions is usually in the third trimester and usually resolves postpartum. There is no associated adverse perinatal outcome.

15. **(1)** Normally, 15−20% of hairs are in telogen. In late pregnancy, this is reduced to <10%. After delivery, the percentage increases, and by 2 months postpartum, 20% of hairs are in telogen; therefore, there is a marked increase in hair loss at 2−4 months after delivery.

16. **(1)** More frequent suckling will increase production of milk more effectively than increasing the duration of suckling. Stopping or decreasing breast-feeding or applying cold compresses to the breasts will decrease milk production.

17. **(2)** Cracked nipples are a sign of irritation and may eventually cause skin breakdown with severe pain.

18. **(2)** Breast irritation in nursing mothers is often caused by *Candida albicans*. The source of infection is most likely the infant's mouth (thrush).

19. **(1)** Initially after delivery, the mother needs an opportunity to accept the fact that her newborn has a congenital defect. Pointing out normal characteristics of the newborn will allow her to put the problem in perspective. Often, the mother will focus on the defect. Orofacial surgery will provide closure of the defect, but will not completely correct it, as scarring will undoubtedly occur.

20. **(1)** Using a paper or a plastic tape, rather than cloth, prevents error due to the stretching of the fabric. Measurements should be repeated to confirm accuracy. The tape should not lie over the ears.

21. **(2)** Neonatal screening for PKU and congenital hypothyroidism is done in all states. Other tests are up to the primary care provider. α-Fetoprotein is usually a maternal blood test done during the prenatal period to screen for genetic defects, primarily neural tube anomalies.

22. **(2)** Normal morphology and testes tissue development will be impaired if the testes are not descended by age 2. These children are at higher risk for the development of testicular cancer in the young adult male (20−30 year old).

23. **(2)** The diagonal conjugate is the most important, as it is the distance from the sacral promontory to the lower margin of the symphysis pubis. It determines the size of the pelvic inlet (≥11.5 cm is adequate size). The obstetrical conjugate is determined by adding 1.5−2.0 cm to the diagonal conjugate.

24. **(1)** Phototherapy is effective secondary to the absorption of the light by bilirubin across the infant's skin. The light energy is absorbed by bilirubin and promotes the conversion of bilirubin to a nontoxic form that can be excreted in the bile without the need for conjugation. The increase in hemolysis will increase the bilirubin level and this is physiological jaundice that is *not associated* with an Rh incompatibility problem.

25. **(1)** Jaundice occurring after the fifth day should be of concern due to the increased incidence of neonatal sepsis as the precipitating cause. Physiologic jaundice most often occurs at 2–3 days after birth and disappears by 4–6 days after birth. Increased incidence of physiologic jaundice may be associated with breast-feeding. The treatment, if any, of physiologic jaundice is controversial.

26. **(1)** Neonatal jaundice is more common in breast-fed babies and is thought to be due to the decreased intake in the first few days. It usually begins between 4 and 7 days after birth, and the bilirubin levels range from 10 mg/dl to 30 mg/dl. Increasing the infants' intake of water does not improve the condition. Breast-feeding may be temporarily interrupted; however, phototherapy is usually not necessary.

27. **(4)** Bronze baby syndrome describes a grayish brown pigmentation that occurs in neonates. This sometimes occurs in infants who are undergoing phototherapy, but is commonly associated with infants who have obstructive liver problems. The pigmentation is not permanent; however, it may last for several months.

28. **(1)** Infantile colic is unexplained crying and restlessness that lasts longer than 3 hours per day, 3 days a week. Most often it stops spontaneously around 3 months. Other causes, particularly infections, should be ruled out. Spastic colon and lactose intolerance are unlikely and would include problems with diarrhea and constipation.

Infant stress syndrome is not a valid problem.

29. **(4)** The most common other problem in these circumstances is a urinary tract infection. There is no evidence of an infection in any other of the common areas (i.e., ears, throat, lungs, or nerves). There is also the absence of any acute abdominal findings. In the presence of a fever or other positive findings, the practitioner should order a complete laboratory work-up to further evaluate the problem.

30. **(2)** After the infant has been carefully evaluated and there is no evidence of other problems, it is important to explain to the parents that there is no medication to treat the condition. The condition is not resolved by changing the feeding schedule of the infant, it is not related to stress within the home, and a change to soy formula will not solve the problem. It is important to explain to the parents that the colic most often resolves with no residual problems by the age of 3 months.

Pharmacology

31. **(1)** Metronidazole is safe after the first trimester. The other listed medications, in addition to others, are all known teratogens and are therefore contraindicated in pregnancy.

32. **(3)** Estrogen inhibits milk production. Progestin-only preparations are ideal for the breast-feeding client because they do not contain estrogen and, therefore, do not inhibit milk production. The other oral contraceptives listed contain estrogen in varying amounts.

33. **(1)** Acetaminophen can be prescribed to the pregnant client; aspirin should be avoided along with narcotics, such as codeine. Naproxyn (Anaprox) is contraindicated in the third trimester of pregnancy.

19

Mental Health

Psychosocial Examination & Diagnostic Tests

1. The mental status examination enables the nurse practitioner to identify:

   1. Intelligence quotient and reasoning.

   2. Abstract thinking and memory functioning.

   3. Reasoning and psychomotor skills.

   4. Memory functioning and intelligence quotient.

2. A client with a history of psychiatric problems arrives at the clinic shouting that he is a messenger of God and knows the meaning of the prophecies in Revelations. This behavior is assessed as:

   1. A delusion.

   2. A hallucination.

   3. Magical thinking.

   4. An illusion.

3. An assessment of a client experiencing auditory hallucinations would most likely reveal:

   1. Client mumbling to self, tilted head, eyes darting back and forth.

   2. Performance of obsessive-compulsive rituals of turning off and on a radio, talking to self.

   3. Hyperactivity, expansive mood, easy distractibility.

   4. Cool, aloof, unapproachable, avoiding enclosed areas.

4. The MAST and the CAGE are screening instruments for which disease process?

   1. Glaucoma.

   2. Depression.

   3. Alcoholism.

   4. Diabetes.

5. When receiving the records from another agency, the nurse practitioner notes on the summary sheet that the client has a dual diagnosis. This means the client has:

   1. Both manic and depressive symptoms of bipolar affective disorder.

   2. Two closely related psychiatric disorders (e.g., panic disorder and bulimia nervosa).

   3. Coexistence of both a psychiatric disorder (e.g., depression) and a substance abuse disorder (e.g., alcohol dependence).

   4. Coexistence of a personality disorder (e.g., borderline personality) and a psychiatric disorder (e.g., panic disorder).

6. A child is being evaluated for attention deficit hyperactivity disorder (ADHD). Which test is helpful in evaluating the difference between ADHD and a learning disability?

   1. Standardized IQ achievement test.

   2. Denver developmental screening test.

   3. Audiologic and visual testing.

   4. Complete neurologic examination.

7. While completing the history on an older adult, the nurse practitioner understands that when a client "makes up stories or answers" to the questions, this is known as:

   1. Perseveration.

   2. Confabulation.

   3. Echolalia.

   4. Alcoholic encephalopathy.

8. In taking a history from a client with depression, which is the most important question for the nurse practitioner to ask?

   1. Have you ever experienced hallucinations, delusions, or illusions?

   2. Have you ever been hospitalized in a psychiatric facility?

   3. Do you regularly take antidepressants or other medications?

   4. Have you thought about or attempted suicide?

9. While taking a history, the nurse practitioner is aware that the following drug is the most commonly first used by an adolescent:

   1. Nicotine.

   2. Alcohol.

   3. Marijuana.

   4. Crystal methamphetamine.

10. A common laboratory finding associated with bulimia nervosa is:

    1. Hyperkalemia.

    2. Hypochloremia.

    3. Elevated liver enzymes.

    4. Platelet abnormalities.

11. The nurse practitioner knows tolerance is suggested when a client gives a history of:

    1. The same dose of the drug has reduced effects.

    2. Less of the medication produces the desired effects.

    3. No withdrawal symptoms when the drug is stopped.

    4. Increasing side effects with an increase in the dosage of drug.

12. Which statement is correct about mental health in the older adult and supports research findings in the literature?

    1. Self-esteem does not decline as a person ages.

    2. Older adults are consistently concerned about their physical appearance.

    3. Older adults have a negative self-image in comparison with younger adults.

    4. Learning ability is not maintained due to loss of short-term memory.

Psychiatric Disorders

13. An elderly client has been experiencing confusion. The nurse practitioner is trying to determine whether the confusion is

related to depression or dementia. In evaluating this client, what specific assessment finding would be helpful in making this distinction?

1. Determining whether confusion worsens in the evening.

2. Assessing early morning agitation, hyperactivity, and insomnia.

3. Noting signs of anger, hostility, and loss of control.

4. Assessing reality distortions and preoccupation with family matters.

14. A client calls the clinic and asks to speak to the nurse practitioner. When she answers the telephone, the client states that he is going to commit suicide. The priority goal is to:

1. Refer the client to an appropriate treatment facility.

2. Encourage ventilation of angry and depressed feelings.

3. Assess the lethality of the suicide plan.

4. Establish rapport with the client.

15. During an intake interview with a 26-year-old man diagnosed with generalized anxiety disorder, the nurse practitioner might observe what type of behaviors?

1. An inflated sense of self.

2. Constant relation to future events.

3. Inability to concentrate and irritability when questioned.

4. Nervousness and fear of the nurse practitioner during the interview.

16. An elderly woman answers the nurse practitioner's questions by mumbling in low tones with answers that seem inappropriate. What would be initial findings associated with a diagnosis of dementia?

1. Sees people floating across the ceiling of her room.

2. Has problems with cognition and confusion.

3. Hears voices at night telling her to change her clothes.

4. Shows fear when the nurse makes any movements toward her.

17. An older client comes to your office with the complaint of confusion. The daughter is concerned that her mother is developing Alzheimer's disease. Which of these assessments would indicate this client is experiencing delirium versus dementia?

1. The confusion has been slowly developing.

2. The confusion started after the client started taking cimetidine (Tagamet).

3. The client's attention span has not been affected.

4. The client's memory has been impaired.

18. While talking with a client about his chemical dependency, the client states, "I wish I would have never used cocaine. It has ruined my life!" What would be the most appropriate response by the nurse practitioner?

1. "You should think before you do something."

2. "Things will work out, don't worry."

3. "It sounds like you've thought a lot about your cocaine use."

4. "You shouldn't be so hard on yourself. You can change."

19. The nurse would expect which symptoms in a client with a diagnosis of schizophrenia?

1. High energy with varying sleep patterns and nonstop conversation.

2. Extreme and frequent mood swings with hyperactivity and difficulty concentrating.

3. Paranoia, delusions, hallucinations, and diminished self-care.

4. Antisocial behavior, manipulativeness, charisma, and ability to lie convincingly.

20. Dementia can be distinguished from delirium by:

    1. Dementia lasts days to weeks compared to delirium, which lasts months to years.

    2. Dementia is often associated with medications or systemic illness.

    3. Dementia exhibits a disturbance in attention that is not present in delirium.

    4. Dementia does not include altered perception, including hallucinations and illusions.

21. An elderly client is brought to the nurse practitioner by his family for evaluation of increasing confusion over the past few days. The client has a history of dementia; however, the family states that this is a definite change. What course of action would the nurse practitioner consider?

    1. Help the family look for a nursing home.

    2. Order an immediate magnetic resonance imaging (MRI) scan.

    3. Perform a comprehensive medication review.

    4. Refer the client to neurology.

22. A middle-aged, upper-middle class, married female presents to your clinic for the third time in 2 months with a complaint of headache, gastrointestinal upset with abdominal pain, and difficulty sleeping. Past exams have been essentially negative. You suspect the client suffers from depression, but she has been reluctant to complete even the briefest of screenings for this. Today, the client requests "something for sleep," again stating she "doesn't have time to take a bunch of tests." Which diagnosis seems most likely?

    1. Hypochondriasis.

    2. Domestic violence.

    3. Addiction.

    4. Irritable bowel syndrome.

23. An elderly client was taken to the clinic in a confused state that began suddenly 24 hours ago. She fails to be oriented to person, time, or place. She was incontinent of urine due to her confusion. She looks apathetic and is drowsy. The nurse practitioner would suspect:

    1. Delirium.

    2. Dementia.

    3. Depression.

    4. A psychotic disorder.

24. Which of the following groups of clients fall under mandatory reporting laws for abuse and neglect in a majority of states in the United States?

    1. Children, adult women, dependent elderly.

    2. Children, disabled individuals, adult women.

    3. Disabled individuals, adult women, dependent elderly.

    4. Children, disabled individuals, dependent elderly.

25. A mother brings her young child to the clinic, stating she fell off the porch swing. What assessment finding would cause the nurse practitioner to consider the possibility of child abuse?

    1. Mother is very upset and stroking her daughter's hair.

    2. Child is crying and says her head and arm hurt.

    3. Child has red, blue, and green colored bruised areas on her trunk.

    4. Child has a bruised, edematous area on forehead and shoulder.

26. In evaluating a 16-year-old female client, which symptom would indicate anorexia nervosa?

    1. Refuses to discuss questions pertaining to food.

    2. Reflects a positive body image.

    3. States she is eating very well but has episodes of vomiting.

    4. The family states she refuses to stop her severe dieting.

27. A mother is concerned about her child having nightmares. The nurse practitioner understands the difference between nightmares and night terrors is:

    1. Nightmares are vivid, frightening dreams recalled by the child.

    2. Nightmares rarely occur in children before age 4.

    3. Nightmares are accompanied by gross motor movements, labored breathing, and enuresis.

    4. Nightmares and night terrors are essentially the same and are unrelated to stressful events.

28. A 16-year-old adolescent is 54 inches in height. The nurse practitioner identifies the following as a positive effective coping behavior:

    1. Acts as the class clown.

    2. Has a rehearsed reply to teasing comments.

    3. Spends most of his free time watching television.

    4. Has predominantly friends that are short statured.

29. The nurse practitioner is examining an older adolescent who has been a long-term intravenous cocaine user. What other findings would alert the nurse practitioner to a frequent complication?

    1. Epistaxis and chronic rhinorrhea.

    2. Cardiac arrhythmias and hypertension.

    3. Chest congestion and wheezing.

    4. Hepatitis and cellulitis.

30. The nurse practitioner is comparing the typical signs of depression in the adolescent with the adult client. The depressed adolescent would present with:

    1. Lonely feelings.

    2. Sad, flat affect.

    3. Anger and acting-out behavior.

    4. Feelings of powerlessness and anxiety.

31. The effects of prenatal cocaine exposure on newborns includes:

    1. Increased incidence of prematurity.

    2. Large-for-gestational-age.

    3. Caput succedaneum.

    4. Hypotonia and lethargy.

32. While interviewing a teenager to determine her level of health, the nurse practitioner recognizes symptoms of anorexia nervosa. Which characteristics of anorexia nervosa would be noted in the admission assessment interview?

    1. Below to average intelligence.

    2. Increased libido.

    3. Vigorous daily exercise.

    4. Tachycardia.

33. The nurse practitioner expects a preschool child with ADHD to have:

    1. Delayed growth and development, especially language skills.

    2. Negativism, overactivity, and active curiosity.

    3. Diminished fine motor skills and frequent mood swings.

    4. Easy distractibility, impulsiveness, and fidgeting.

34. The nurse practitioner is completing a history and physical on a child who she suspects may be autistic. Findings associated with autism include:

    1. Delay in language development.

    2. Delay in physical growth.

    3. Overprotective parents who provide minimal social interaction for the child.

    4. Warm, cuddling child with excessive need for interaction.

35. The mother of a preschooler is concerned because her child has begun to stutter. The nurse practitioner should:

    1. Refer the child to a speech pathologist.

    2. Encourage the mother to correct the child when she stutters.

    3. Give the child verbal exercises to perform at home.

    4. Reassure the mother that stuttering is normal in a preschooler.

36. A teenaged female client is brought to the nurse practitioner for evaluation by her grandmother with whom she lives. The teenager has been vomiting and her grandmother believes that she is becoming confused. The grandmother relates that the client has been upset lately over a breakup with her boyfriend. What will the nurse practitioner investigate as a possible cause for this teenager's symptoms?

    1. Appendicitis.

    2. Ectopic pregnancy.

    3. Drug overdose.

    4. Sexually transmitted disease.

37. An adult client has a history of irritability, loss of appetite, inability to concentrate, and feelings of depression and "burn out" at work. Recently, he relates missing several days at work. He is doing and taking everything he can to relax. What would be an appropriate question to ask this client?

    1. "Do you drink alcohol or take drugs?"

    2. "Have you ever felt this way before?"

    3. "When you feel depressed, do you talk to your wife?"

    4. "Have you lost your job?"

38. A teenager comes to the office of the nurse practitioner and states that she was raped several hours ago by her boyfriend. The immediate action taken by the nurse practitioner is:

    1. Perform a pelvic examination to determine injuries to the client.

    2. Accompany her to the emergency department for an exam.

    3. Send her immediately for counseling to help her deal with this situation.

    4. Call the client's parents so they can be with her.

39. Physical findings of cocaine abuse include:

    1. Bradycardia, miosis, hypertension.

    2. Hypertension, tachycardia, tremor.

    3. Hypotension, bradycardia, abdominal cramps.

    4. Decreased level of consciousness, tachycardia, excessive salivation.

40. While interviewing an adolescent female presenting with her mother for birth control counseling and examination you detect signs of family tension. During the physical exam, while the mother is out of the room, the daughter admits to frequent marijuana use and occasional drinking. What assessment information would most confirm the presence of active or potential violence in the home?

    1. Signs of general neglect.

    2. Injuries at different stages of healing.

    3. Client's response to a direct question.

    4. Admitted fear of mother's boyfriend.

41. The parents of a 7-year-old boy ask advice regarding sugar intake stating the teacher has said not to allow the child to have any sugar products such as cookies at lunch due to behavior problems. Advice would include:

    1. The child needs further assessment for ADHD.

    2. Moderate sugar consumption rarely produces inappropriate behavior.

    3. Increase the protein and fat in his diet to decrease nerve overstimulation.

    4. Research has shown increased sugar intake directly affects cognitive performance.

42. Which neurotransmitters are associated with the etiology of acute mania in bipolar affective disorder?

    1. Epinephrine and norepinephrine.

2. Serotonin and dopamine.

3. Dopamine and norepinephrine.

4. γ-Aminobutyric acid (GABA) and renin-angiotensin.

43. All of the following behaviors meet the criteria for substance abuse in the *Diagnostic and Statistical Manual of Mental Disorders, Fourth Edition* (DSM-IV) **except**:

    1. Repeated arrests for drunk driving.

    2. Multiple absences from work due to substance use.

    3. Chronic anxiety attacks.

    4. Recurrent arguments with spouse about his/her drinking behavior.

Pharmacology

44. A client has been receiving fluphenazine (Prolixin) for the past 3 weeks. The nurse practitioner's assessment notes the following: temperature elevated (41°C), marked muscle rigidity, agitation, and confusion. The nurse practitioner understands these findings are often associated with the diagnosis of:

    1. Acute dystonia.

    2. Tardive dyskinesia.

    3. Neuroleptic malignant syndrome.

    4. Extrapyramidal disorder.

45. The preferred antidepressant for an elderly client is:

    1. Amitriptyline (Elavil).

    2. Sertraline (Zoloft).

    3. Trazodone (Desyrel).

    4. Haloperidol (Haldol).

46. A client has been referred to the nurse practitioner. The client's medical history reveals a long-term usage of antianxiety agents that the client considers harmless. The nurse practitioner understands that antianxiety agents can:

    1. Cause drug dependency.

2. Produce hepatotoxicity and nephrotoxicity.

3. Lead to functional damage of the cardiopulmonary system.

4. Cause profound dissociative personality problems.

47. An older female has a diagnosis of dementia and is taking haloperidol (Haldol) 2 mg HS. The nurse practitioner observes her engaging in a restless, repetitive movement with her legs. She states that, not only does she have ongoing movement, but she also feels jittery. The nurse practitioner would interpret this activity to be:

    1. Ataxia.

    2. Akathisia.

    3. Agitation.

    4. Dyskinesia.

48. What is the best initial treatment plan for a sleep disorder in the elderly client?

    1. Medicate with amitriptyline (Elavil).

    2. Medicate with trazodone (Desyrel).

    3. Discuss the importance of naps daily.

    4. Decrease noise and light in the environment.

49. An elderly client presents with a new symptom of acute confusion over the last 24 hours. Which assessment would be the priority for the nurse practitioner to evaluate during the examination?

    1. Drug history.

    2. Electrocardiogram.

    3. Mini mental status exam.

    4. Thyroid profile.

50. The nurse practitioner is aware that the following class of drugs is most likely to precipitate a hypertensive crisis in the elderly.

    1. Narcotic analgesics.

    2. Monoamine oxidase (MAO) inhibitors.

    3. Barbiturates.

    4. Phenothiazines.

51. The nurse practitioner knows that the following class of drugs would have the greatest effect on memory in the elderly client:

    1. Phenothiazines.

    2. Tricyclic antidepressants.

    3. Benzodiazepines.

    4. MAO inhibitors.

52. The nurse practitioner understands that adolescents who use lysergic acid diethylamide (LSD):

    1. Experience withdrawal symptoms within 24 hours.

    2. Develop tolerance quickly and need increased amounts.

    3. Experience flashbacks and depression.

    4. Experience disorientation and delusional feelings.

53. Of the following antidepressants, which one has the most sedating side effects making it a good sleeping agent?

    1. Fluoxetine (Prozac).

    2. Doxepin (Sinequan).

    3. Trazadone (Desyrel).

    4. Paroxetine (Paxil).

54. In the management of acute alcohol withdrawal delirium, a nurse practitioner may want to use all of the following drugs **except**:

    1. Chlordiazepoxide (Librium).

    2. Lorazepam (Ativan).

    3. Thiamine.

    4. Chlorpromazine (Thorazine).

55. The nurse practitioner's physical exam on an adolescent is as follows: disheveled appearance, 5-lb weight loss since last visit 2 months ago, pulse strong and regular at 128, +4 deep tendon reflexes (DTRs), nasal mucosa erythematous and ulcerated. His mother relates that he has been getting in trouble at school, avoids the family, has no appetite, and is not sleeping much at night. The nurse practitioner suspects drug use of:

    1. Heroin.

    2. Marijuana.

    3. LSD.

    4. Crack cocaine.

56. Which laboratory results would be **least** important to assess before placing a client on Lithium?

    1. Thyroid-stimulating hormone, triiodothyronine, thyroxine.

    2. Blood urea nitrogen, creatinine.

    3. Urinalysis, electrolytes.

    4. Alanine aminotransferase, aspartate aminotransferase, lactate dehydrogenase.

57. A client comes to the rural clinic having taken an undetermined amount of heroin. Prior to transferring the client to a psychiatric treatment facility, the nurse practitioner anticipates the drug of choice for an opioid overdose is:

    1. Clonidine (Catapres).

    2. Methadone (Dolophine).

    3. Naloxone (Narcan).

    4. Naltrexone HCl (Revia).

58. Benzodiazepines are useful in the treatment of all the disorders below, **except**:

    1. Alcohol withdrawal.

    2. Anxiety.

    3. Obsessive-compulsive disorder.

    4. Seizures.

59. When starting a psychotropic medication in the elderly, a good rule of thumb is:

    1. Start low, go slow.

    2. Higher doses are almost always needed.

    3. Side effects of psychotropic medications will usually not impact other medications.

    4. The same adult dosages can be used initially without any problems.

60. A client is a 20-year, 2-pack-a-day smoker with a history of chronic bronchitis. What is

the prescription to give to this client who wishes to stop smoking?

1. Nicotine polacrilex (Nicorette) gum 2-mg piece, chew for 30 minutes, q1–2h × 6 weeks, then q2–4h × 3 weeks, then q4–8h × 3 weeks, then discontinue.

2. Nicotine patch (Nicoderm) 21 mg/24 hr qd × 6 weeks, then 14 mg/24 hr qd × 2 weeks, then 7 mg/24 hr qd × 2 weeks, then discontinue.

3. Bupropion HCl (Zyban) 150 mg qd × 3 days, then 150 mg bid for 7–12 weeks and to stop smoking when medication is started.

4. Nicotine patch (Nicoderm) 14 mg/24 hr qd × 6 weeks, then 7 mg/24 hr qd × 6 weeks, then discontinue.

61. The nurse practitioner understands the following about the use of benzodiazepines in the older adult:

1. Withdrawal symptoms may occur within 24 hours of abruptly stopping the medication.

2. Adverse side effects are minimal and tend to minimize the incidence of falls and other injuries.

3. Long-acting medications (i.e., chlordiazepoxide [Librium]) are preferred over the shorter acting medications (i.e., lorazepam [Ativan]).

4. Larger doses are needed to maintain therapeutic levels for the anxious or agitated client.

19 Answers & Rationales

Psychosocial Examination & Diagnostic Tests

1. **(2)** The mental status examination provides a basic assessment of the client's intellectual functioning (reasoning, abstract thinking, memory). The intelligence quotient (IQ) is determined by psychological testing. Psychomotor skill assessment is part of a neurologic examination.

2. **(1)** Delusions are false, fixed beliefs that can be of a persecutory or grandiose nature. In this instance, the client is experiencing a delusion of grandeur. A hallucination is a false sensory experience. An illusion is a misinterpretation of reality. Magical thinking is when the client feels that his/her thoughts or wishes can control other people.

3. **(1)** The client experiencing the auditory hallucination will often look out into space and act as if he/she is listening to someone talking. This is associated with behaviors such as tilting the head, mumbling, and eye movement.

4. **(3)** The Michigan Alcoholism Screening Test (MAST) and the CAGE (Cut down, Annoyed, Guilty, Eye opener) are used to alert providers to possibility of alcoholism.

5. **(3)** Dual diagnosis involves both a psychiatric diagnosis and a substance abuse diagnosis.

6. **(1)** Children with learning disabilities and ADHD are often impulsive, inattentive, and overactive. Usually, children with ADHD do not have lower IQ achievement scores; however, children with a learning disability usually demonstrate a level of educational achievement substantially below that of the IQ.

7. **(2)** The fabrication of events or situations to fill in gaps in the memory, usually in a plausible way, is a classic definition of a client who is experiencing dementia due to chronic alcoholism. Clients with alcohol amnesic disorder, or Korsakoff's syndrome, may experience confabulation. Echolalia is the parroting or automatic, meaningless repeating of another's words. Perseveration is the involuntary persistent repetition of an idea or response (e.g., client keeps repeating the same phrase over and over).

8. **(4)** Although the other questions are important to ask during the initial history, it is most important to ascertain whether or not the client has contemplated suicide. In addition, determination of a specific plan and the means to do it are also involved in the questioning about suicidal ideation.

9. **(1)** Nicotine is known as the "gateway drug" and the first drug most commonly used by adolescents.

10. **(2)** The other abnormalities are not usually associated with bulimia. The hypochloremia is associated with the purging (self-induced vomiting).

11. **(1)** Tolerance exists when the same dose of the drug produces reduced effects, and is usually seen with the development of physical dependence.

12. **(1)** According to research, self-esteem, along with attitude and morals, are maintained as a client ages, and older adults tend to have a positive self-image when compared to younger adults. Learning ability is maintained, although more time is often needed for the early phases of the learning process. Retrieval of information in long-term memory is slower, and short-term memory is diminished.

Psychiatric Disorders

13. **(1)** Confusion can occur in both dementia and depression. However, with dementia, symptoms worsen at night.

14. **(4)** The nurse practitioner must first establish trust and rapport with the caller before an assessment can be made. If rapport is not established, the client will hang up the phone. The nurse practitioner understands that, by keeping the client talking, he is prevented from acting out the suicidal threat.

15. **(3)** Impaired concentration and irritability are major characteristics of generalized anxiety disorder. Clients are more focused on the here and now and have low self-esteem.

16. **(2)** Confusion and cognitive function problems (i.e., short-term memory loss) are initial signs of dementia. The severity of the symptoms is dependent upon what stage of cognitive degeneration the client is manifesting. The other options are characteristic of hallucinatory experiences and usually occur later.

17. **(2)** A history of a new medication with an abrupt onset of confusion must be reviewed closely. An adverse reaction of cimetidine (Tagamet) is confusion in the elderly. Dementia results in confusion, which develops slowly. The attention span and memory may be affected in each diagnosis.

18. **(3)** The nurse's statement acknowledges the client's feelings and is open ended, which promotes open discussion and helps the client clarify his feelings and thoughts. Option #1 is condescending and punitive. Option #2 offers false reassurance. Option #4 tends to discount the client's feelings.

19. **(3)** The characteristics of schizophrenia are delusions, tangential thought, suspiciousness, disorganized behavior, and hallucinations.

20. **(4)** People with dementia do not usually have altered perceptions that include hallucinations and illusions. Dementia does last months to years. Delirium is often associated with medications or systemic illness and a disturbance in the ability to pay attention.

21. **(3)** Drug effects are one of the most common causes of sudden increase in dementia in the elderly. Dementia has a gradual increase, and a sudden increase is a cause for concern. The nurse practitioner should question the family about any new addition to the client's medications and who helps the client take his medication. It should also include a "brown bag review" of the client's medications, both prescription and over-the-counter.

22. **(2)** The indicators to domestic violence in this case are the multiple vague physical complaints without supporting objective data, the suspected depression, and the reluctance to wait around in the clinic for extended periods of time. This client is on the verge of disclosing, if a provider would only ask her about domestic violence.

23. **(1)** Based on the acute confusion state and the incontinence, she is experiencing delirium. This is most likely secondary to a urinary tract infection. Dementia is more insidious versus acute. Depression and psychosis are not consistent with the assessments. The major symptoms in depression would include loss of interest, sleep disorder, decreased appetite, loss of concentration, inactivity, guilt, lack of energy, and potential suicidal thoughts. Psychotic disorders include thoughts and behavior indicating the client is not in touch with reality.

24. **(4)** The laws in most states require the reporting of suspected or actual abuse and neglect of any person considered to be dependent or with a reduced ability to make life choices. Children, disabled individuals, and dependent elderly fall into these categories. Very few states require reporting for adult women unless a weapon is involved; this is a different situation requiring a report.

25. **(3)** The nurse practitioner must determine whether the bruised areas match the type of trauma the parent describes. Bruises in various stages of healing turn different colors. Having different-colored bruises indicates the injuries have not occurred at the same time, which could be indicative of child abuse.

26. **(4)** Adolescents with anorexia nervosa will severely reduce their nutritional intake by dieting constantly on high fiber and low calories. They usually have an inappropriate body image.

27. **(1)** Nightmares peak in incidence around ages 3–4 years and are often associated with abandonment issues and posttraumatic stress disorder (following gun shootings, fires, abuse). Night terrors are typically accompanied by gross motor movements (sleep walking, enuresis), tachypnea, labored breathing, and tachycardia.

28. **(2)** Role playing and planning a rehearsed reply to teasing comments about short stature are helpful tools to deal with this issue. Although humor can be effective, constantly clowning around for attention is not positive coping behavior. Withdrawal (i.e., watching television or reading) is not effective coping and may indicate depression. Spending time and associating only with younger adolescents who are his height is not a positive coping behavior and may hinder normal maturation.

29. **(4)** More than 50% of intravenous cocaine users develop hepatitis, phlebitis, endocarditis, and acquired immunodeficiency syndrome (AIDS). Epistaxis, rhinorrhea, and nasal congestion are seen most often in intranasal users of cocaine. Chest congestion, wheezing, and eventual emphysema occur with chronic free-base (crack) smokers. Although cardiac arrhythmias, hypertension, and respiratory arrest can occur, they are not the common complications.

30. **(3)** Adults who are depressed typically display findings noted in Options #1, #2, and #4. Adolescents often act out in defense of trying to protect themselves from feelings of vulnerability and dependency. Noting signs of anger and frustration in the adolescent is important to evaluate, as the significance of the behavior may indicate symptoms of depression.

31. **(1)** The newborn exposed to cocaine is often premature, small-for-gestational-age, has low birth weight, and has a low Apgar score. Intrauterine growth retardation occurs along with symptoms of hypertonia, irritability, tremulousness, irregular sleeping patterns, and frequent gaze aversion.

32. **(3)** People with anorexia nervosa will exercise up to 4 hours a day. They are above average intelligence in most cases, suffer from bradycardia, and have decreased libido.

33. **(4)** In a preschool child, it may be difficult to distinguish ADHD, as problems of overactivity, inattention, and negativism are common. Language skill development along with fine motor skills are more likely found with learning disabilities. Active curiosity and negativism are normal behaviors for preschoolers.

34. **(1)** Autism is a developmental disorder that starts early in a child's life and is characterized by avoidance of eye contact, indifference to caregivers, language and communication delays, failure to develop a social smile, repetitive movements, and an excessive need for routine.

35. **(4)** Repetition of whole words and phrases is normal for preschoolers; therefore, it would be inappropriate to refer to a speech pathologist at this time. Parents should not correct or criticize the child. Verbal exercises are unnecessary and could be very stressful to the child.

36. **(3)** In teenage girls, the most common form of suicide attempt is by drug overdose. The combination of vomiting and confusion suggests a drug overdose.

37. **(1)** The nurse practitioner would suspect this client to have a diagnosis of substance-induced mood disorder. It would be appropriate to determine exactly how much, how long, and how often he consumes alcohol or any other drugs. The key points in the situation are the occupational burn out, depressive symptoms, and ineffective coping measures (taking and doing everything to relax, but with no relief).

38. **(2)** This client should be examined by emergency department personnel, many of whom are specially trained to collect the evidence needed to testify in court about the rape. The exam should not be done in the office unless the nurse practitioner has been trained in evidence collection and has a rape evidence collection kit. The exam must be done quickly, before evidence is destroyed. The client decides who should be called for support. While she is encouraged to call her parents, she is also offered the support of rape crisis and other resources.

39. **(2)** Bradycardia and excessive salivation are not found with cocaine abuse. There are no drug antagonists that can be used for cocaine overdose, although naloxone is given to reduce the concurrent toxic effects of other narcotic drugs that may be in the client's body system.

40. **(4)** While all of the answers may contribute to a clinician suspicion of family violence, the admission of genuine fear of a household member is considered an excellent indicator of actual or potential violence and the level of danger in a home.

41. **(2)** Woraich's 1994 study failed to demonstrate a link between sugar and behavior or cognitive performance. Further assessment is indicated before labeling as ADHD.

42. **(3)** Dopamine and norepinephine (drugs that stimulate the noradrenergic and dopaminergic receptors) can precipitate mania or hypomania in clients. GABA and acetylcholine may also be neurotransmitters involved in the process. In addition, stimulants such as amphetamines and cocaine can also cause manic-like symptoms.

43. **(3)** Chronic anxiety attacks are not part of the DSM-IV criteria for substance abuse.

Pharmacology

44. **(3)** The client is experiencing a rare problem called neuroleptic malignant syndrome. This client would require immediate referral and hospitalization. Acute dystonia, parkinsonism, and akathisia are associated with extrapyramidal disorder or acute movement disorder. Tardive dyskinesia occurs late in therapy and is often irreversible. Slow worm-like movements of the tongue are the earliest symptom, followed by grimacing, lip smacking, and involuntary limb movements.

45. **(2)** Zoloft's favorable side-effect profile makes it a useful alternative to the traditional tricyclic antidepressants. It has the shortest half-life of the currently marketed serotonin reuptake inhibitors. Elavil has the most anticholinergic and sedating side effects of the antidepressants. There may be pronounced effects on the cardiovascular system (hypotension). Geropsychiatrists agree it is best to avoid in the elderly. Desyrel is very sedating for the elderly client. Haldol is an antipsychotic medication.

46. **(1)** Physical dependence can occur, even with low doses of the medication. This is a particular problem in the elderly, who are sensitive to low dose ranges.

47. **(2)** Akathisia is a feeling of restlessness. Clients may complain of a feeling of muscular quivering. Ataxia is a disorder wherein muscular incoordination occurs with voluntary muscular movements. Agitation is a general assessment that may be part of the psychotic behavior. Dyskinesia is a defect in voluntary movement.

48. **(4)** Correction of environmental factors and treatment of underlying iatrogenic and medical problems should be addressed initially. Elavil can cause excessive somnolence. Desyrel may be of particular use when sleep disturbance is prominent; however, it does not address the best initial plan. The goal is to begin with good sleep hygiene prior to pharmacologic therapy. Eliminating naps during the day may be useful in facilitating sleep.

49. **(1)** Drug–drug interactions are a common cause of acute confusion in the elderly client. This assessment can minimize the need to do further costly interventions if the client only needs medication adjustment. The other options would be included in the plan after the drug history had been completed and had been ruled out as a potential problem.

50. **(2)** In combination with tyramine-rich foods that have undergone an aging process such as cheese, wine, beer, salami, and yogurt, catecholamines are released from the nerve endings causing a hypertensive crisis. The other drugs listed cause hypotension.

51. **(3)** The benzodiazepines cause sedation and decreased attention, which in turn affects the memory. Although phenothiazines and antidepressants may also cause sedation, they don't affect memory.

52. **(3)** Flashbacks, depression, and psychotic behavior can occur with LSD use. There are no withdrawal symptoms or physical dependence associated with use. Commonly, the adolescent remains oriented but experiences hallucinations and altered bodily sensations.

53. **(3)** Trazadone (Desyrel) has sedation as a side effect, which has made it less popular as an antidepressant; however, it is commonly prescribed for insomnia.

54. **(4)** All of the drugs listed above may be used in acute alcohol withdrawal delirium except chlorpromazine, which is an antipsychotic that has no use in the management plan.

55. **(4)** Often, some of the first indications of drug use in adolescents are related to a sudden change in behavior or school performance. Heroin use symptoms are constricted pupils, respiratory depression, needle tracks, and poor nutrition. Marijuana use symptoms are slow reflexes, tachycardia, conjunctival injection, nasal congestion, and increased appetite. LSD use symptoms are dilated pupils, reddened eyes, hypertension, increased appetite, and hallucinations. The use of central nervous system stimulants, like crack cocaine, leads to hypertension, weight loss, anorexia, insomnia, hyperreflexia, and a perforated or ulcerated nasal septum.

56. **(4)** It is **not** important to evaluate liver function before initiating treatment with lithium. The adverse side effects of lithium affect renal, cardiac, and thyroid function. Baseline electrolytes are also important to obtain.

57. **(3)** Naloxone is a narcotic antagonist and is used for the reversal of narcotic depression, including respiratory depression. Clonidine (Catapres) is a central α-agonist and is indicated for treatment of hypertension. Methadone is used in the treatment of opioid addiction. The Food and Drug Administration (FDA) has placed methadone in a special drug category that allows medically supervised administration of the drug to addicts with chronic, intractable addictions to heroin. Naltrexone's therapeutic classification is narcotic detoxification adjunct.

58. **(3)** Seizures, alcohol withdrawal, and anxiety are commonly treated with benzodiazepines. They are **not** the first drug of choice for obsessive-compulsive disorder; selective serotonin reuptake inhibitors are usually used.

59. **(1)** Dosages should be reduced by 30–50% to start therapy and gradually increased as necessary. Adverse effects are likely to occur because of slowed drug metabolism, which occurs with aging. These include hypotension, arrhythmias, and sedative and anticholinergic effects.

60. **(2)** A highly nicotine-dependent client benefits from intense counseling and prescription of alternative nicotine delivery during the smoking cessation process. The nicotine patch is usually the preferred form of replacement, as the gum is noncontinuous and withdrawal symptoms

may occur during nonchewing times. The nicotine patch delivers a fixed dose of nicotine on a continual basis, is applied once daily, and eliminates the gastrointestinal upset that often occurs with the gum. If this client insisted on using the gum, the dose should be 4 mg, not 2 mg. Option #4 is too low a dose to start on this client and is not the correct dosing schedule. Zyban (bupropion HCl) would be used in conjunction with the nicotine patch, and clients are to quit smoking 1–2 weeks after starting the Zyban, not immediately.

61. **(1)** Benzodiazepines should be tapered slowly in the older adult. Withdrawal symptoms occur within 24 hours in clients taking the shorter acting medications and may not occur for several days in clients taking long-acting medications. The adverse effects of oversedation, dizziness, confusion, and sometimes hypotension contribute to falls and other injuries in the elderly. In Option #3, short-acting medications are preferred. Typically, larger doses are not needed, but rather small initial doses with gradual increases.

20

Emergencies

1. While attending a rural public school, a 7-year-old child was bitten on the hand by a raccoon. At the rural clinic, the nurse practitioner cleansed the wound. The next action is:

   1. Administer tetanus antitoxin.

   2. Contact local animal control authorities.

   3. Administer rabies immune globulin (RIG) and human diploid cell vaccine (HDCV).

   4. Teach the family how to do hourly soaks to the hand using normal saline and peroxide.

2. A toddler is brought to the clinic with a history of an insect bite last evening. What presenting symptom would be associated with the bite of a brown recluse spider?

   1. Paresthesias in all extremities.

   2. Edematous, erythematous area with coalescing macules.

   3. Tissue sloughing in the bite area within 8–10 hours.

   4. Development of a central black eschar of "sinking infarct" within 6–12 hours.

3. The nurse practitioner understands that cat bites become infected more often than dog bites because:

   1. Dogs have a "cleaner mouth" than cats.

   2. Cat bites are often deep puncture wounds.

   3. Dog bites are usually on the face, which makes them less susceptible to infection.

   4. Cat bites are usually associated with clawing and spreading of microorganisms.

4. When do bites from insects, spiders, snakes, and bees most commonly occur?

   1. Fall.

   2. Spring to fall.

   3. Winter.

   4. Any time of the year.

5. An adolescent was bitten by a neighbor's dog 3 days ago. He has developed an infection in a large wound on his lower leg. What would be appropriate management of this client?

   1. Prescribe amoxicillin/clavulanate potassium (Augmentin) 250 mg PO tid × 14 days.

   2. Approximate the edges of the wound together with suture.

   3. Prescribe cephalexin (Keflex) 500 mg PO tid × 7 days.

   4. Have the adolescent return to the clinic for follow-up in 2 weeks.

6. Medical management for a brown recluse spider bite includes:

   1. Warm, moist soaks to the area.

   2. Ice pack and elevation of the area.

   3. Active and passive range of motion (ROM) to area.

   4. Avoidance of antihistamines.

7. A young adolescent has been bitten by a black widow spider while doing yard work. He is having a severe reaction; the nurse practitioner expects:

   1. Hypotension and shock.

   2. Localized pain, erythema, and edema in the area.

   3. Black eschar of sloughing tissue within 4 hours of the bite.

   4. Abdominal rigidity, nausea, and headache.

8. A scout leader is explaining about snakes and snake bites and relates the following to his group about the coral snake, "Red on yellow, kill a fellow; red on black, venom lack." Later on, one of the boys is bitten by a snake described a having broad rings of red and black separated by narrow rings of yellow. The nurse practitioner understands that this client will probably experience all **except**:

   1. Numbness and change in sensation.

   2. Local swelling at the fang mark site.

   3. Dizziness and diplopia.

   4. No symptoms, as the snake was not poisonous.

9. A father brings in his 4-year-old son to the emergency room after having ingested a small bottle of aspirin. The nurse practitioner's priority is:

   1. Insert a nasogastric tube and attach to low suction.

   2. Give 16 oz of orange juice.

   3. Give 8 oz of milk.

   4. Give 30 ml of syrup of ipecac followed by a glass of water.

10. The nurse practitioner is aware that the toxic symptoms of salicylate poisoning are:

    1. Tinnitus and nausea.

    2. Itching and blurred vision.

    3. Fruity odor to the breath.

    4. Fever and chills.

Answers & Rationales

1. **(3)** Any type of animal bite that might be associated with an animal that may potentially harbor rabies (skunks, bats, raccoons, foxes, coyotes, rats) should be treated with both active and passive rabies immunization. Tetanus antitoxin would be indicated if the client was not current on the immunization. Animal authorities would be called after the initial treatment to locate the animal and sacrifice it, so that the brain could be examined for rabies.

2. **(4)** Brown recluse spiders produce sharp pain at the instant of the bite, with subsequent minor swelling and erythema. Tissue necrosis may occur within 4 hours. A blue-gray to black macular halo may surround the bite, with eventual widening and sinking of the center of the lesion, leading to a "sinking infarct." This leaves a deep ulcer that takes weeks or months to heal.

3. **(2)** Deep puncture wounds are more likely to get infected with anaerobic organisms. Bites on the hand have the highest infection rate, whereas bites on the face have the lowest infection rate.

4. **(2)** Insects are more active, reproduce, and are present in greater numbers in the warm months (i.e., spring to early fall).

5. **(1)** Amoxicillin clavulanate potassium (Augmentin) is an excellent choice for the empiric treatment of animal bites. Keflex is not indicated due to resistant strains of *Pasteurella multocida*, an organism present in 25% of dog bites and 50% of cat bites. An infected bite should be followed-up on a daily basis until the infection clears. Open-wound management is indicated, not suturing.

6. **(2)** Heat application is contraindicated; ice packs are preferred, as is elevation, to decrease the edema. The area should be immobilized. Tetanus toxoid may be given along with antihistamines to reduce swelling and relieve itching.

7. **(4)** In addition to these symptoms, bronchospasm, hypertension, seizures, and altered mental status may occur. Black eschar is associated with a brown recluse spider bite.

8. **(4)** This was a poisonous coral snake bite. The typical symptoms are those listed plus the following: nausea, vomiting, and muscle fasciculations.

9. **(4)** An age-appropriate dose of syrup of ipecac followed by a glass of water would be indicated. The nurse practitioner would gavage the child, not insert a nasogastric tube and attach to suction.

10. **(1)** Tinnitus and nausea are toxic symptoms of salicylate poisoning. Fruity odor to the breath is usually associated with diabetic ketoacidosis.

21

Research & Theory

Research

1. When designing a research project that will involve clients, from the options presented, the most important point to be included in the written consent to participate is:

   1. The directions regarding the use of a black pen.

   2. The anticipated date for publication of the completed research report.

   3. The assurance of privacy and confidentiality.

   4. The number of previously published research studies about this topic.

2. When determining whether to incorporate a new procedure into your clinical practice based on the findings of a recent study, which of the following should you consider?

   1. The statistical significance of the findings.

   2. The statistical relevance of the findings.

   3. The statistical software program used.

   4. The statistical background of the researcher.

3. The research process is similar to the processes nurse practitioners use to provide client care in that both are decision-making processes that include the steps (in the order presented here) of:

   1. Assessing, teaching, evaluating, and discussing.

   2. Defining, planning, implementing, and charting.

   3. Questioning, evaluating, diagnosing, and teaching.

   4. Assessing, planning, implementing, and evaluating.

4. Both descriptive and inferential statistics are used in research. However, their purposes are different in that:

   1. Inferential statistics are used for assigning participant code numbers.

   2. Descriptive statistics are used for assigning participant code numbers.

   3. Inferential statistics are used for hypothesis testing.

   4. Descriptive statistics are used for hypothesis testing.

5. In an ambulatory care setting, the nurse practitioner might find it difficult to utilize nursing research because:

    1. The demands of providing primary care leave little time for research utilization.

    2. Procedures for research utilization have not been well defined in the literature.

    3. Research published in professional journals is too difficult to access by clinicians.

    4. Ambulatory care settings have little in common with the settings used for most research.

6. While nursing theories vary greatly in their perspectives of nursing care, all nursing theorists explicitly incorporate three key concepts. These three concepts, which are basic to nursing care, are:

    1. Individuals, families, and communities.

    2. Primary, secondary, and tertiary prevention.

    3. Past, present, and future well-being.

    4. Person, health, and environment.

7. The scientific method for conducting research uses the null hypothesis, which is statistically based. The correct format for the null hypothesis is:

    1. There are no significant difference between two groups.

    2. Group "A" is greater than group "B."

    3. Group "A" is less than group "B."

    4. There is a 95% probability that group "A" is different from group "B."

8. When evaluating claims made on advertisements, such as "Drug X has been used for 5 years with over 1 million doses administered in the United States, Canada, and Great Britain. Drug X stops heartburn, aids in digestion, and prevents esophageal reflux and is the 'treatment of choice' to relieve GERD," the nurse practitioner realizes that the claim is:

    1. Invalid, as there is no control or comparison group and no statistics are stated.

    2. Valid, as there are sufficient numbers of users who have had success.

    3. Invalid, because the level of significance is not mentioned to be at the 0.05 level.

    4. Valid, as the cohort and Hawthorne effects are operating.

9. In your practice, you have noticed that women clients who are pregnant and still in their teens generally seem to go into labor before their due date (as determined by ultrasound), while the women who are in their mid-20s usually go into labor at or after their due date. Which statistical analysis would answer the research question, "Among pregnant women in a nurse practitioner practice, is there a statistically significant difference between the length of gestation for women age 16 to 19 when compared to women age 23 to 26?"

    1. Multiple regression.

    2. Chronbach's alpha.

    3. The two-tailed t-test.

    4. Pearson's correlation.

10. The utilization of research in nursing practice can be equated with:

    1. The nursing process.

    2. The change process.

    3. Discharge planning.

    4. Family planning.

11. You are compiling monthly statistics for your practice, and one of the elements of your analysis is the cultural background of your clients. What level of data is "cultural background"?

    1. Nominal level data.

    2. Ordinal level data.

    3. Interval level data.

    4. Ratio level data.

12. A nurse practitioner practicing with a physician in general practice is compiling the practice statistics at the end of the month. The clients who received care range from infants to the elderly. Of the following

data from the monthly report, which are most likely to be normally distributed?

1. The lab tests scheduled for the clients.

2. The gender of the clients.

3. The primary diagnosis of the clients.

4. The age of the clients.

13. A nurse practitioner practicing with a physician in general practice is compiling the practice statistics at the end of the month. The clients who received care range from infants to the elderly. The nurse practitioner and the physician want to know the average monthly income of their clients. Which would be the most appropriate statistical measure of the "average income," assuming income was exact in dollars and cents?

1. The mean.

2. The median.

3. The mode.

4. The range.

14. A nurse practitioner is evaluating research articles for a utilization project. The majority of the articles report that either random selection or random assignment was used to select the sample for that study. Because certain procedures in research are used across disciplines, what can be assumed for studies where randomization has been used?

1. The ages of the research subjects in these studies will be negatively skewed.

2. The research subjects in these studies will automatically be half male and half female.

3. The ages of the research subjects in these studies will be positively skewed.

4. The researchers were attempting to obtain the most representative sample.

15. The ability to predict outcomes of care is desirable both in research and in practice. If a nurse practitioner wanted to create a theoretical model for a specific aspect of his/her practice to predict the client outcomes,

which statistical analysis methods would be used to analyze the clinical data?

1. Descriptive statistics.

2. Repeated measures t-test.

3. Multiple regression.

4. Chi-squared for independent samples.

16. Research articles are being evaluated for a utilization project. What can the nurse practitioner do if he/she does not understand the statistical procedures that were used for the analysis of data in an article?

1. Assume that the correct procedure was used, and read about the method or consult a statistician for an explanation of the statistics.

2. Assume that the article is beyond his/her ability to understand, so set that one aside and go on to the next article.

3. Assume that the correct procedure was used and, instead of reading the results section, read the discussion of the findings section.

4. Assume that the article is beyond his/her ability to understand and use someone else's critique of the reported study.

17. The nurse practitioner has determined that the office procedures for diagnosing and stabilizing new diabetics need to be evaluated and possibly changed. Which would be the best choice for the first phase of the evaluation?

1. Design and conduct a double-blind clinical trial.

2. Design and conduct a research utilization project.

3. Design and conduct a research project comparing men and women.

4. Design and conduct a study to test Callista Roy's theoretical model.

18. A nurse practitioner was reading a nursing research article in which there were no statistically significant findings. The most appropriate response would be:

    1. "Reading this article was a waste of my time."

    2. "Because of reading this article, there is no reason to conduct similar studies."

    3. "Reading this article raises new questions for my practice."

    4. "Because of reading this article, I will immediately change my practice."

19. The verification of the more abstract nursing theories (e.g., Martha Rogers) is often hampered by:

    1. The lack of adequate measures for the theoretical concepts.

    2. Prior studies that did not support the theory.

    3. The lack of adequate laboratory settings for conducting experiments.

    4. Prior studies that were conducted in other countries.

20. In a recently published study, the researcher reported "the statistical analysis used to identify the differences between the two variables was Pearson's correlation." Which most specifically tells what is wrong with this statement?

    1. Pearson's correlation can be used only with three or more variables.

    2. Pearson's correlation actually identifies the common factors between variables.

    3. Pearson's correlation can be used only when there is a single variable.

    4. Pearson's correlation actually identifies the relationship between variables.

21. Qualitative research studies are conducted by nurse researchers because:

    1. Qualitative studies help to identify and define nursing concepts.

    2. With qualitative methods, there are no concerns about the rights of research subjects.

    3. Qualitative approaches provide precise measures for statistical analysis.

    4. Nurse researchers find qualitative research designs easier to use.

22. The normal ranges of blood chemistry values are most like which statistical concept?

    1. The standard error.

    2. The mean.

    3. The standard deviation.

    4. The median.

23. The five major sequential steps of research utilization are:

    1. Establish a client relationship, perform a health assessment, make a diagnosis, devise a plan of care, evaluate the treatment.

    2. Identify the problem, assess published research, design the innovation, evaluate, decide whether to adopt the innovation.

    3. Review the popular literature, review the practice's clients, summarize of the findings, evaluate, do client teaching.

    4. Review the client's lab reports, complete a thorough health assessment, diagnose, implement the treatment, evaluate.

24. Both *qualitative* and *quantitative* research methods are used in nursing research because:

    1. Master's-prepared nurses conduct quantitative studies, while doctorally prepared nurses conduct qualitative studies.

    2. Master's-prepared nurses conduct qualitative studies, while doctorally prepared nurses conduct quantitative studies.

    3. They complement each other because they produce different types of findings about the same concepts.

    4. They complement each other because they produce the same types of findings about different concepts.

25. Nursing research subscribes to the scientific method for the design of research studies. The advantage of this is that:

    1. Nursing research is based on logically constructed arguments.

    2. Nursing research is designed to answer any research question.

    3. Nursing research findings are precise and need not be duplicated.

    4. Nursing research findings are generalizable to all client populations.

26. With the restructuring of health care delivery and a shift in the provision of nonacute care from the hospital to ambulatory care settings and the home, previous nursing research that was conducted in hospitals:

    1. Now becomes applicable to all in-hospital providers of care.

    2. Remains relevant in the new settings; client care is unchanged.

    3. Should be applied directly to client care provided in the new settings.

    4. May no longer be applicable to the delivery of client care.

27. Nurse researchers strive to substantiate causality so that client outcomes can be consistently predicted. For the nurse practitioner, the ability to predict the outcomes for every client could mean that:

    1. The appropriate treatment would be prescribed for clients.

    2. No further studies would need to be conducted about treatments.

    3. The client's individual qualities would not need to be considered.

    4. Treatments would not need to be individualized for each client.

28. The reason that quantitative research articles always have a section containing descriptive findings is that descriptive data analysis:

    1. Provides the basis for making inferences about the findings.

2. May yield statistically significant findings that were unexpected.

3. Is conducted for predicting client outcomes in nursing settings.

4. Organizes the data for clearer understanding of subjects and variables.

29. The difference between univariate and multivariate studies is:

    1. The number of subjects in the sample.

    2. The number of variables being studied.

    3. The number of sites for collecting data.

    4. The number of statistical hypotheses.

30. The theoretical basis for nursing practice is:

    1. A relatively new approach to nursing care.

    2. Borrowed from other professions such as medicine.

    3. As old as formal nursing and began with Florence Nightingale.

    4. Unrelated to the conduct of nursing research studies.

31. The independent variable and the dependent variable of a research study might be thought of as:

    1. The cause (the independent variable) and the effect (the dependent variable).

    2. The median (the independent variable) and the mode (the dependent variable).

    3. The outcome (the independent variable) and the treatment (the dependent variable).

    4. The sample (the independent variable) and the population (the dependent variable).

32. *Variance* is a key statistical concept. How would current research methods change if there were no variance?

    1. We would need to increase the sample size in all of our research studies to 100 research subjects or greater.

    2. Since our current research methods do not depend on the presence of variance, we would not need to change our current methods.

    3. We would need to decrease the sample size of all our research studies to 15 research subjects.

    4. Since our current research methods are based on the presence of variance, we would not be able to use our current methods.

Theory

33. Basing nursing practice on nursing theory contributes to the professionalization of nursing practice by:

    1. Adapting the medical model to nursing care.

    2. Limiting the choice of treatments for clients.

    3. Determining what type of clients will be seen by the nurse.

    4. Providing a consistent perspective for providing care to clients.

34. A nurse practitioner has decided to incorporate a nursing theoretical model into his/her practice. The practice includes clients of all ages. Which nursing model is most applicable to an ambulatory care setting?

    1. Orem's Model of Self-Care.

    2. Roy's Adaptation Model.

    3. Roger's Unitary Person Model.

    4. King's System Model.

35. Which nursing theorist is considered to have general systems theory as philosophical orientation to her model?

    1. Sister Callista Roy.

    2. Martha Rogers.

    3. Rosemarie Parse.

    4. Betty Neuman.

36. Which nursing theorist addresses nursing outcomes in terms of primary, secondary, and tertiary prevention?

    1. Sister Callista Roy.

    2. Betty Neuman.

    3. Imogene King.

    4. Jean Watson.

37. Which nursing theorist's model primarily addresses health promotion?

    1. Jean Watson.

    2. Betty Neuman.

    3. N. J. Pender.

    4. Sister Callista Roy.

21   Answers & Rationales

Research

1. **(3)** By federal law, clients must be assured of their privacy and confidentiality. The other information is interesting and may be included, but is not required by federal law.

2. **(1)** In published research reports, of the choices listed, only the first choice is consistently reported by researchers. The clinical relevance is considered, not the statistical relevance. The specific program used does not make a difference, since all are based on the same statistical formulas. Researchers frequently work with statistical consultants, so a researcher's background is not a limitation to a published study.

3. **(4)** Only the last choice contains those elements common to both processes: assessing, planning, implementing, and evaluating.

4. **(3)** Neither type of statistics is used to assign participant code numbers. Descriptive statistics are used to describe the sample.

5. **(1)** Inadequate time can be a barrier to research utilization in any setting. The process of research utilization is well delineated by researchers. With the ever-increasing availability of professional journals via the Internet, access is rarely a problem. There is a considerable body of research that has been conducted in ambulatory care settings.

6. **(4)** All current theories incorporate person, health, and environment. Other concepts may or may not be explicitly included in nursing theories.

7. **(1)** The correct format for the null hypothesis is, "There are no significant differences between two groups." The alternate or research hypothesis may take the other forms.

8. **(1)** Even though the claims detail extensive use of "Drug X," there must be statistical evidence as demonstrated through the use of control or comparison groups that will render a level of significance.

9. **(3)** Only the t-test compares two independent groups on a variable.

10. **(2)** Incorporating research findings into practice often results in a change in practice. The nursing process is most like conducting research.

11. **(1)** The variable of "cultural background" is categorical data or nominal level data.

12. **(4)** The gender and primary diagnosis are nominal level data, and the lab tests would be skewed, while the age would approximate the normal curve.

13. **(2)** The median income would be most representative of the average because the income of 50% of the clients is above and 50% is below the median. The mean could be influenced by one client with a very high or very low income, and the mode only identifies the income that is reported most often. The range only identifies the lowest and the highest income and does not present an average.

14. **(4)** Randomization is a research technique used to increase the amount of control in any research design. The other three options are false; they do not occur because of randomization.

15. **(3)** Of the choices, only multiple regression examines the relationship between two or more variables in a way that permits prediction.

16. **(1)** In reviewing research, it is necessary to understand the statistical methods that the researcher used in order to determine the value of the study findings for the practice setting. The researcher's discussion may not provide the full extent of the findings, and someone else's critique may reflect a specific point of view that does not apply in every situation.

17. **(2)** As a first step, a research utilization project would provide a thorough review of the published literature on which to base a change. A full study may not be needed, and testing a theoretical model is not appropriate for this situation.

18. **(3)** The lack of significant findings is an important piece of information about the topic of the research, and definitely is not a waste of time. Particularly when findings are nonsignificant, more studies need to be conducted about this topic. Ideally, changes in practice are based on the findings of more than one study.

19. **(1)** The lack of adequate measures for theoretical concepts is a major roadblock in many areas of research, and particularly so with the more abstract theories. Prior studies always provide information about the theory, even when conducted in other countries. More abstract concepts tend not to be studied in lab settings.

20. **(4)** Correlations identify the relationships between variables. Two or more variables may be used. Factor analysis is used to identify common factors.

21. **(1)** The purpose of qualitative designs is to identify and define nursing concepts. Qualitative designs do not yield precise measures, are usually not analyzed statistically, are more difficult to use, and carry the same concerns about the rights of subjects as all other research designs.

22. **(3)** The normal ranges of blood chemistry values are based on studies that identified the standard deviation for each blood chemical. The mean and the median are averages, and the standard error is not applicable to this situation.

23. **(2)** This option contains the published steps. All other options are nursing actions taken on behalf of the client (in no particular order).

24. **(3)** The two methods complement each other because they produce different types of findings about the same concepts. The educational preparation of the researcher does not dictate the research method used.

25. **(1)** The scientific method is highly organized and is based on logical reasoning. Findings are rarely precise, and studies do need to be duplicated. Some questions are not answerable by our current research methods. Because of small samples and other limitations, many findings from nursing research are **not** generalizable.

26. **(4)** Such a drastic change in health care delivery may make previous studies no longer applicable to nursing care. Health care restructuring has changed the way client care is provided.

27. **(1)** The ability to always predict client outcomes would mean that every client would receive the exact treatment for that individual. Treatments would still have to be individualized, and individual qualities would need to be considered. Because new treatments are always being devised, there would be a need for ongoing research.

28. **(4)** Descriptive data analysis organizes the data, and it facilitates understanding.

Descriptive statistics cannot be used for significance testing or for making inferences; inferential statistics are used. Predictions are made from studies that use inferential statistics.

29. **(2)** "Variate" refers to the number of variables in the study.

30. **(3)** The theoretical basis for nursing practice began with Florence Nightingale and has been used for practice and for research for over a century. Nursing theories are specifically developed for nursing.

31. **(1)** The independent variable may be considered the cause or the treatment, and the dependent variable may be considered the effect or the outcome. The median, mode, sample, and population are not designations for the independent or the dependent variables.

32. **(4)** All our current research and statistical analysis methods rely on the presence of variance or variation; if variance is no longer present, our current methods could no longer be used. If there is no variance, a sample of one would be adequate.

Theory

33. **(4)** Theory-based practice contributes the consistent perspective that permits the comparison of care across settings. Theory-based practice does not necessarily limit treatments or determine client types. Theory-based practice specifically eliminates reliance on the medical model.

34. **(1)** Orem's theory focuses on the client participating and being in control of his/her own health care. Roy's model is most appropriate for acute care settings, Roger's for holistic health settings, and King's for a mental health setting.

35. **(4)** Betty Neuman's Health Care Systems Model, Imogene King's Systems Interaction Model, and Dorothy Johnson's Behavioral Systems are based on general systems theory. Roy's Adaptation Model is based on stress and adaptation as the framework. Martha Roger's Science of Unitary Human Beings and Rosemarie Parse's Human Becoming Model are based on a humanistic developmental framework.

36. **(2)** Betty Neuman identified the need to implement nursing interventions through use of one of more of three prevention modalities (primary, secondary, and tertiary prevention).

37. **(3)** Pender's Health Promotion Model is an excellent nursing model that readily fits into a nurse practitioner's scope of practice. The other theorist's models are Betty Neuman's Health Care Systems Model, Jean Watson's Human Science and Human Model of Caring, and Roy's Adaptation Model.

Issues & Trends

1. Considering the four advanced practice roles of clinical nurse specialist, nurse practitioner, certified nurse midwife, and nurse anesthetist, which role became accepted by and included into the practice arena without significant controversy?

   1. Clinical nurse specialist.

   2. Nurse practitioner.

   3. Certified nurse midwife.

   4. Nurse anesthetist.

2. Historically, who was one of the most outspoken opponents of the nurse practitioner role?

   1. Loretta Ford.

   2. Hildegard Peplau.

   3. Martha Rogers.

   4. Dorothea Orem.

3. Who started the first nurse practitioner program?

   1. Hildegard Peplau.

   2. Mary Breckenridge.

   3. Agnes McGee.

   4. Loretta Ford.

4. Which is the most important action in developing health policy skills in the nurse practitioner?

   1. Develop political allies in Congress.

   2. Work on a campaign.

   3. Support causes such as teen pregnancy or acquired immunodeficiency syndrome.

   4. Write letters and editorials.

5. Which is the least important barrier to collaborative advanced nursing practice?

   1. Prescriptive authority.

   2. Reimbursement privileges.

   3. Legal scope of practice.

   4. Political activism.

6. For the nurse practitioner to obtain reimbursement, an understanding of which is important?

   1. Minimum Nursing Data Set (MNDS).

   2. ICD-9-CM, CPT, and HCPC codes.

   3. HCPC codes and NANDA diagnosis.

   4. Medicare and Medicaid number.

7. Steps of the change process according to Kurt Lewin are:

1. Unsolving, mobilizing, recruiting, finalizing.

2. Building relationships, acquiring resources, choosing solution, stabilizing.

3. Unfreezing, moving, refreezing.

4. Forming, storming, norming.

8. What was the major impetus for nurse practitioner development?

1. Need for an expert nurse clinician.

2. Shortage of primary care physicians.

3. Trend for specialized nurses to diagnose and manage unstable acute and chronic clients.

4. Movement of graduate nursing education to diagnosis and treatment of major illness.

9. The nurse practitioner understands that Medicare B provides:

1. Hospitalization costs for the insured.

2. Health insurance benefits for low-income families.

3. Benefits that cover physicians, nurse practitioners, medical equipment, and outpatient services.

4. Outpatient laboratory services, radiography services, and skilled nursing care in appropriate facilities.

10. What is the impact of the Balanced Budget Act of 1997 on nurse practitioner practice?

1. Authorizes all states to provide nurse practitioners prescriptive authority.

2. Provides for only well visits and primary care services.

3. Prevents a physician from billing 100% for a nurse practitioner's services.

4. Allows direct Medicare payments to nurse practitioners in both rural and urban settings.

11. In the clinic, you have observed the following: one medical assistant is usually pleasant and helpful; the other is often abrasive and angry. The most important basic guideline to be observed by the nurse practitioner nurse who must resolve a conflict between two medical assistants is:

1. Require the medical assistants to reach a compromise.

2. Weigh the consequences of each possible solution.

3. Encourage ventilation of anger and use humor to minimize the conflict.

4. Deal with issues, not personalities.

12. A male nurse practitioner approaches another nurse practitioner who is his friend and tells him that one of the female physicians at the clinic often follows him into the supplies room and tells him how good looking he is. Yesterday, she patted his hand and said, "I wish we would get to know each other better. I would make it worth your while—better benefits at the clinic, more money." The male staff nurse asks his friend, "What do I do? I don't want to date her, but I don't want to lose my job. I just want her to leave me alone!" The best reply for the friend would be:

1. "Tell her that her behavior makes you feel uncomfortable and that you want her to stop."

2. "Go for it!! Date her and see if you get what she promises."

3. "Go to the human relations office at the agency right away and relate to them the entire situation."

4. "Contact your lawyer and get advice as soon as possible, in case she decides to turn the tables and accuse you of advances."

22 Answers & Rationales

1. **(1)** According to the National Commission on Nursing (1983) and the Task Force on Nursing Practice in Hospitals (1983), the clinical nurse specialist (CNS) role was accepted quite rapidly. The psychiatric CNS role is considered the oldest and most highly developed of the CNS specialities and helped initiate the growth of other CNS specialties.

2. **(3)** Martha Rogers argued that the development of the nurse practitioner role was a ploy to lure nurses out of nursing and into medicine, hence weakening and undermining nursing's unique role in health care. This led to a major division within nursing, which led to barriers to the establishment of nurse practitioner educational programs within the mainstream of graduate nursing education.

3. **(4)** Loretta Ford, R.N., Ph.D. and Henry Silver, M.D. established the first pediatric nurse practitioner program at the University of Colorado. Mary Breckenridge established the Frontier Nursing Service in the depressed rural mountain area of Kentucky, which led to training nurse midwives. Agnes McGee is credited with offering the first postgraduate program for the nurse anesthetist role at St. Vincent's Hospital in Portland, Oregon. Hildegard Peplau started the first psychiatric CNS program at Rutger's University.

4. **(1)** Although all of these answers are important for the nurse practitioner to develop policy skills, the most important is developing political allies. Having political allies in decision-making places (legislature) will enable the nurse practitioner to be active and informed regarding issues surrounding regulation, limitations on admitting privileges and prescriptive authority, and managed care.

5. **(4)** There are three major issues that are central to the expansion of the nurse practitioner role—prescriptive authority, reimbursement privileges, and legal scope of practice. Although political activism is important, it is not specific to collaborative practice.

6. **(2)** The ICD-9-CM (*International Classification of Diseases, 9th Edition*) codes are diagnostic codes that identify the condition, illness, or injury to be treated and are used for billing insurance carriers. CPT codes (Physicians's Current Procedural Terminology) specify the procedure or medical service given (over 7000 terms). Medicare and state Medicaid carriers are required by law to use CPT codes. The Health Care Financing Administration Common Procedure Coding System (HCPC) is used for reporting supplies and medical equipment.

7. **(3)** Lewin described three processes of change: unfreezing—involves breaking the habit, disturbing the equilibrium; moving—development of new responses based on new information with a change in attitudes, feelings, behaviors, or values; and refreezing—reaching a new status quo, stabilizing and integrating new behaviors with appropriate support that is available to maintain the change. Forming, storming, and norming refer to the stages of group process development. Option #2 lists Havelock's change theory steps.

8. **(2)** According to most sources, the nurse practitioner role developed due to a shortage of primary care physicians in the 1960s and 1970s, when medical specialization was the trend.

9. **(3)** Medicare is regulated by the federal government and includes the services described, plus outpatient laboratory and radiography. Hospitalization costs are covered under Medicare A.

10. **(4)** The Balanced Budget Act is a crucial and significant piece of legislation that allows direct payments to nurse practitioners at "80% of the lesser of either the actual charge or 85% of the fee schedule amount of the same service if provided by a physician." This does not change the "incident to" rule, which allows a physician to bill for 100% for a nurse practitioner's services (i.e., provided the physician is in

the suite at the time of the service and readily available to provide assistance).

11. **(4)** Conflict must be addressed directly by the nurse practitioner. The personal characteristics of each of the medical assistants must not enter into the conflict resolution process. Determine what is the issue of conflict and then work on possible solutions to resolve the issue. Compromise is just one method of conflict resolution wherein both parties must be willing to give up something.

12. **(1)** There are two ways to deal with sexual harassment at work: informally and formally through a grievance procedure. Always start with the direct approach; ask the person to STOP! Tell the harasser in clear terms that the behavior makes you uncomfortable and that you want it to stop immediately.

23

Legal & Ethical Issues

1. An occurrence-form professional liability insurance policy is preferred because:

   1. The amount of insurance money available to pay a claim increases with each renewal of the policy.

   2. The policy proceeds are available to pay claims regardless of when the claim is reported to the carrier.

   3. The carrier will be notified of a potential claim during the policy period.

   4. The coverage is broader than that provided by a claims-made policy form.

2. Early reporting of a potential professional liability claim is advantageous because:

   1. Insurance carriers have a 10-day reporting window after which the coverage is canceled.

   2. Documents and witnesses needed to defend the claim are more likely to be available at the time of the event.

   3. Your insurance premiums will be reduced upon a good-faith showing of cooperation with the carrier.

   4. Risk management personnel require such reporting in order to comply with Joint Commission on the Accreditation of Healthcare Organizations (JCAHO) mandates.

3. Your nursing license may be in jeopardy if:

   1. You appropriately delegate medication administration to a trusted RN employee, who administers a fatal dose.

   2. You delegate client assessment tasks to an LPN who has been floated to your outpatient clinic for the day.

   3. You provide nursing care services consistent with established standards of practice in your jurisdiction.

   4. The medical assistant in your supervising physician's office exceeds the scope of her authority, but you take prompt action to correct the problem.

4. Your client is a 46-year-old mentally challenged man who has been diagnosed with colon cancer. Consent for his corrective surgery should be obtained from:

   1. The client himself.

   2. The client's 84-year-old mother, who is his closest relative.

   3. The client's court-appointed guardian.

   4. The administrator of the group home where the client lives.

327

5. Your client is a 75-year-old woman with metastatic cancer. Her affairs are in order; she has arranged all her finances and her own funeral rites. She has systematically secured enough barbiturates to successfully end her life; she asks you to mix the drugs for her in some pudding to make them palatable for ingestion. Your best course of action would be:

   1. Mix the medications as requested and stay with her while she consumes the preparation.

   2. Consult with family and attending physician to warn them about the client's proposed course of action.

   3. Seek an immediate order for an antidepressant.

   4. Sit down with the client and conduct a physical and psychological needs assessment.

6. The Patient Self-Determination Act (PSDA) passed by Congress in 1990, resulted in which of the following policy changes?

   1. Hospitals are mandated to assist every client to create a "living will."

   2. Federally funded managed care organizations (MCOs) are required to inform subscribers about their rights under state law to create advance directives.

   3. Home health agencies are required to have "do-not-resuscitate" orders on file for all terminally ill clients.

   4. Hospitalized clients are obligated to select a surrogate decision maker to make health care decisions for them if they become incapacitated.

7. Both the Food and Drug Administration (FDA) and the Department of Health and Human Services (DHHS) have regulations governing research activities on human subjects. The principal investigator is responsible for:

   1. Securing a signed special research consent form.

   2. Reporting back to the Institutional Review Board if a subject is injured during the course of the study.

   3. Appearing before the Institutional Review Board to present the study and secure approval to proceed with subject recruitment at the facility.

   4. All of the above.

8. If you are served with a summons and complaint (i.e., lawsuit documents), the first step you should take is:

   1. Call the client to determine the basis for the action and what you allegedly did wrong.

   2. Call the client's lawyer (listed on the first page of the lawsuit) to get more information about the case.

   3. Call your insurance company for instructions on how to proceed.

   4. Confer with your colleagues and review the chart to see if you need to clarify your notes.

9. As a nurse practitioner in an impoverished rural area, you frequently encounter a female client in a situation of domestic violence with few community options for referral. Participating in community education forums and fund-raising for a safe house is an example of applying the ethical principle of:

   1. Autonomy.

   2. Nonmaleficence.

   3. Justice.

   4. Veracity.

10. Nurses practicing in expanded roles should carry professional liability insurance for which of the following reasons?

   1. Premiums are often modest and are a tax-deductible business expense.

   2. Even if the employer insures the nurse practitioner, there may be situations of conflict between employer and nurse necessitating separate legal counsel, a covered benefit under the policy.

   3. As roles expand, so does the liability potential.

   4. All of the above.

11. The confidentiality of medical records is always a valid concern, especially in this age of computerization, "smart cards" and fax machines. Release of medical information to third parties is:

1. A creature of state law, meaning that state statutes control the processing of such requests.

2. Prohibited without the informed consent of the client.

3. Automatic when the requesting party is a third-party payor or insurer.

4. Disallowed if the records contain proof of a diagnosis of acquired immunodeficiency syndrome (AIDS).

12. Which categories of persons are **not** included in the definition of disability under the Americans with Disabilities Act (ADA)?

1. Profoundly deaf employees.

2. Persons who are wheelchair-bound.

3. Current users of illegal drugs.

4. Persons with mental retardation.

13. If your client is having a problem with a managed care plan, you can offer to assist in the following ways:

1. Suggest that the client contact the customer service department (may be called "member services") at the plan to resolve the issue; a formal grievance filing may be necessary.

2. Remind the client who is a member of the "senior" plan for Medicare recipients, that he/she may complain to the federal Office of Personnel Management (OPM).

3. Remind the client that the state's insurance department also investigates complaints against health plans.

4. All of the above.

14. Health policy theorist Daniel Callahan believes that our health care system could be improved by:

1. Making the care of the chronically ill our first priority, so that these individuals are not abandoned by the health care system.

2. Making preventive care the first priority.

3. Maintaining the current allocation of dollars to high-tech care.

4. Leaving the system "as is" and letting market forces determine the allocation of health care dollars.

15. If a piece of equipment malfunctions while being used on a hospitalized client, the risk manager would probably recommend the following course of action:

1. Return the item to the manufacturer with a description of the problem and a request for analysis.

2. Tag and sequester the item at the facility and defer analysis pending risk management review of the litigation potential.

3. Send the item to the biomedical engineering department with a request for immediate equipment breakdown and troubleshooting.

4. Repair the item, either in-house or by an outside contracted firm, and return it to service as soon as possible.

16. Nurse expert witnesses are essential in the adjudication of most professional negligence claims against nurses. The following criteria for nurse experts are sought by attorneys:

1. Appropriate professional education, preferably at the technical level.

2. Relevant and recent professional work experience.

3. Ability to understand and articulate the legal issues involved in the claim.

4. Published authors of medical texts in the clinical subject areas.

17. Which federal law mandates the tracking of implantable medical devices?

1. The Administrative Procedures Act (APA).

2. The Patient Self-Determination Act (PSDA).

3. The Safe Medical Devices Act (SMDA).

4. The Omnibus Budget Reconciliation Act (OBRA) of 1987.

18. Which of the following are elements of a broad-based risk management program?

    1. A hazardous materials compliance program as part of a comprehensive safety and security system.

    2. An early-warning/incident reporting program to identify elements of risk.

    3. A system of contract review to avoid assuming liabilities that should be borne by others.

    4. All of the above.

19. The type of insurance coverage that is purchased (or self-insured) by an organization to handle employee job-related injuries is:

    1. Professional liability insurance.

    2. Business interruption insurance.

    3. Directors and officers insurance.

    4. Workers' compensation insurance.

20. While driving your personal vehicle on a job-related errand, you are struck by a semitrailer on the interstate. The car is totaled and you are severely injured. Which insurance policies will respond to these losses?

    1. Your personal auto policy and your employer's workers' compensation policy.

    2. The employer's business auto policy and workers' compensation policy.

    3. Your homeowner's policy.

    4. The semitrailer driver's personal auto policy.

21. Nurse practitioners with hospital privileges may be impacted by the part of the Health Care Quality Improvement Act known as the National Practitioner Data Bank. Which of the following statements about the Data Bank is **not** true?

    1. Professional liability insurance claims payments made on behalf of nurse practitioners must be reported to the Data Bank.

    2. The facility granting medical staff privileges must query the Data Bank

before approving a practitioner's privileges.

    3. The purpose of the Data Bank is to have a national source of information about malpractice claims, licensure actions, and restrictions on privileges so that practitioners may not easily move from one jurisdiction to another to escape quality review.

    4. Insurance companies report all malpractice payments made on behalf of affected practitioners, regardless of the amount of the payment.

22. In 1985 Congress took action against a phenomenon known as "patient dumping" by enacting what was known at the time as the COBRA law, now referred to as EMTALA, the Emergency Medical Treatment and Active Labor Act (EMTALA). Which statement about EMTALA is **not true**?

    1. The original purpose of the statute was to prohibit the transfer of uninsured and untreated clients from the emergency department of one hospital to another (usually the county hospital).

    2. Subsequent rules and case law have expanded the statute so that almost any unauthorized transfer of a client from one facility to another is potentially problematic.

    3. In order to effect a proper transfer, the forwarding facility need not notify or secure the acquiescence of the receiving facility.

    4. The transferring facility must utilize appropriate transport methods and send copies of clients' medical records.

23. You are a nurse practitioner wishing to effect change in the state's laws regarding the dispensing of prescription medications by nurse practitioners. You would take your case to:

    1. The state legislature.

    2. The state board of nursing.

    3. The state board of pharmacy.

    4. The nursing specialty organization.

24. The common meaning of "gag clauses" or "gag orders" in the managed care arena is:

    1. The MCO declines to publish, in its subscriber contracts, the treatments that are excluded from coverage under the plan.

    2. The MCO refuses to allow its member services personnel to answer certain subscriber questions about covered benefits.

    3. MCO contracts with providers disallow providers' offering treatment alternatives that the providers know are not covered by clients' plans.

    4. Providers are prohibited from offering experimental treatment to clients.

25. Under the Safe Medical Devices Act of 1990, the following health care providers or organizations are required to report the death of a client to the FDA if the death is related to the use of a medical device:

    1. Physicians' office staff.

    2. Hospitals, home health agencies, and ambulance companies.

    3. Nurse family members treating clients without compensation.

    4. Physicians making home visits.

26. A client receives a medication that was intended for another person. An appropriate way to document this event in the medical record would be:

    1. "Client was given x mg of y drug in error."

    2. "x mg y drug administered to client. No adverse effects noted. Physician notified."

    3. "Client received wrong medication. Incident report filed. Practitioner disciplined."

    4. "Practitioner inadvertently administered y drug to wrong client. Supervisor notified. Family threatening litigation."

27. The one reason that clients offer, above all others, for suing practitioners for medical negligence is:

    1. The care they received was substandard.

2. The provider made an honest mistake.

3. The client wasn't "heard" when he/she attempted to communicate with the provider.

4. The client participated fully in all aspects of medical decision making, but the results were disappointing.

28. Informed consent is based upon the ethical principle of:

    1. Beneficence.

    2. Respect for persons.

    3. Nonmaleficence.

    4. Autonomy.

29. The four elements of a professional negligence claim are:

    1. Duty, fulfillment of duty, professional relationship, and wrongful act.

    2. Professional responsibility, fault, harm to the client, and wrongful act.

    3. Duty, breach of duty, causal connection between the act and the harm, and harm to the client.

    4. Professional relationship, intentional wrongful act, proximate cause, and damage to the client.

30. You are making an initial home health care visit to an elderly lady whose spouse tells you that she is often confused. He answers all your questions and dominates the discussion. You proceed to do your initial assessment; the wife does seem to be oriented to time, place, and person. Who is the proper party to sign the written form to request/consent for services?

    1. The husband.

    2. The wife/client.

    3. The attending physician.

    4. The home health aide who will be providing continuing care.

31. An expert witness is usually required in a nursing negligence case because:

    1. Knowledge of medical or nursing facts is not considered intuitive to a lay jury.

    2. Jurors are allowed to use their "sixth sense" regarding the facts presented to them.

    3. Fact witnesses are not able to present an unbiased account of the circumstances in dispute.

    4. Appropriately credentialed experts have more credibility in the eyes of lay jurors.

32. The standard of care for a nurse practitioner, in a trial, will be established by expert witness(es). The expert opinion will be based upon:

    1. National norms for the specialty.

    2. Facility policies and procedures.

    3. Professional literature.

    4. All of the above.

33. Alternative Dispute Resolution (ADR) is a process where the parties to a dispute resolve their differences outside of a court trial. Advantages to this system of problem solving include all **except**:

    1. The parties usually prefer the process because they have their opportunity to be heard in a less formal and less intimidating environment.

    2. The process is often less time-consuming and less costly than traditional litigation.

    3. Damage awards are less likely to include nonfinancial compensation.

    4. Insurers are amenable to working with mediators with a track record of fairness and successful case resolution.

34. The statute of limitations is:

    1. The state law which prescribes the time frames within which a nursing negligence action may be filed.

    2. The law which states that minors have no legal authority to sue nurses for malpractice.

    3. The law which limits the right of clients to sue nurse practitioners for negligent acts.

    4. The federal law which limits a nurse practitioner's right to countersue a client for malicious prosecution.

35. You are a family nurse practitioner driving along the interstate on your way to a nursing seminar. You observe a head-on collision and decide to stop to render aid. Which statement is **false** with respect to your potential liability for malpractice?

    1. You had no legal obligation to stop to render assistance; if you had driven by the accident, there would be no liability on your part.

    2. If you provide appropriate nursing care, gratuitously, you will be protected from liability under your state's Good Samaritan Law.

    3. Even if you act in a grossly negligent manner, the Good Samaritan Law will shield you from liability.

    4. The protections afforded by the Good Samaritan Law may differ from state to state; you should research your state's law on the subject.

36. If you are subpoenaed to appear for a deposition in a nursing negligence case, appropriate preparation is prudent. One of the following tips would probably not be suggested by your attorney. Which piece of advice is **not** appropriate?

    1. Discreetly chew gum to calm your nerves and dress for dinner because depositions usually take all day and you won't have time to change.

    2. Review the client's medical record and any other materials suggested by your attorney prior to your appearance for questioning.

    3. Take as much time as you need to think about your response before answering; don't let an attorney put words in your mouth.

4. Be straightforward and truthful; remember that "I don't know" and "I don't remember" are acceptable responses.

37. Which of the following documentation tips is **not** a good idea?

1. Carefully document your criticism of a fellow provider's clinical decision in the client's medical record. This will protect you if your treatment decisions need to be defended later.

2. Use standard abbreviations in the medical record so that subsequent readers will have no doubt as to your meaning and intent.

3. Document telephone conversations with the client and/or the family in the medical record. Be particularly vigilant about recording changes in the client's medications.

4. Document noncompliant client behaviors in the medical record; be thorough, yet factual.

38. If a client is under the age of majority in your state, what factors would you consider in order to determine if the client is "emancipated" and able to consent to medical treatment?

1. Whether the client is married.

2. Whether the client is in the military.

3. Whether the client is living outside the "care, custody, and control" of a parent or guardian.

4. All of the above.

39. In 1987, and again in 1994, Congress acted to update many of the regulations that govern the provision of long-term care services. If you are an employer or nurse manager in this environment, you need to know that:

1. Nursing assistants working in long-term care facilities must be formally trained and certified.

2. Clients or residents have specific rights, such as information about their physical condition, medical benefits, and associated costs.

3. New and swifter sanctions are available to reviewers to impose upon facilities with deficiencies.

4. All of the above.

40. You are employed as a nurse practitioner in a private medical office. You notice all the activity at the front desk where some clients are checking in for appointments; staff are scheduling tests; and telephone advice triage is in progress. To preserve client confidentiality, you could implement which of the following changes?

1. Orient the fax machine and computer monitor such that incoming reports or other data cannot be read by non–staff members.

2. Do all telephone scheduling from a more secure location, such as a conference room in the back office.

3. Create a more private space to confer with clients who need follow-up information or explanations of tests or treatments.

4. All of the above.

41. As a nurse-employer, you would be well advised to have procedures in place to appropriately terminate an employee. To avoid a charge of discrimination, or a claim for wrongful termination, you should be particularly sensitive to the protections afforded to select groups. Which of the following is **not** a protected class under the antidiscrimination statues?

1. Pregnant women.

2. Gay men.

3. Those age 40 and older.

4. The handicapped.

42. Which activity could be considered grounds for a sexual harassment claim?

    1. A male employee tells an off-color joke to another man. The joke is overheard by a female co-worker who seems to appreciate the humor in it. The joke-telling is an isolated incident.

    2. A nurse-supervisor conducts an employee performance review. The supervisor does not mention a prior social relationship with the employee; the ratings are appropriate for the level of performance; the employee receives a salary increase.

    3. A co-ed locker room is decorated with multiple centerfold photos from a popular men's magazine. The female employees find this offensive and have filed several complaints.

    4. A nurse is complimented on her appearance and asked on a date by her boss. She informs the boss that she is married and not seeking another relationship. The incident is forgotten.

43. Your client is a comatose lady who needs a feeding tube inserted for long-term nutritional needs. Her husband presents you with a document that he says is his wife's living will. It is signed by him, and sets out, so he says, the wishes of his wife with respect to the feeding tube. The living will is not a legally binding document because:

    1. The wife did not sign the document.

    2. The husband is not authorized to execute a living will on behalf of his wife.

    3. This type of advance directive must be signed by the individual while he/she is legally competent to execute documents.

    4. All of the above.

44. A nurse practitioner is helping out at a clinic for homeless women. A diabetic client, in her third trimester of pregnancy, has been reasonably compliant with respect to insulin therapy. Now, however, she has announced her intent to abandon her insulin regimen because she has heard on the streets that some drugs are harmful to fetuses. Which option is **not** legally appropriate for the nurse practitioner, as her health care provider, to consider?

    1. Seek the support of the clinic's attorney to file a petition for court-ordered treatment for the client.

    2. Attempt to engage the client in dialogue to provide her with accurate medical information.

    3. Detain the client in the homeless shelter and administer the insulin, with or without her consent.

    4. Confer with social services to find an appropriate interim placement for the client until her medical and legal issues can be sorted out.

45. The purpose of the Americans with Disabilities Act is:

    1. To level the playing field with respect to employment and other opportunities for disabled people.

    2. To create a federal entitlement program for people with AIDS.

    3. To guarantee wheelchair access to every residential and commercial building.

    4. To authorize interpreters for deaf employees at all private businesses.

46. As a result of the U.S. Supreme Court's ruling on assisted suicide, the current state of the law on this topic is:

    1. Assisted suicide is still a criminal offense in most jurisdictions.

    2. A physician may prescribe a fatal dose of medication with the concurrence of the ethics committee.

    3. A nurse practitioner may prescribe a fatal dose of medication with the concurrence of the supervising physician.

    4. A pharmacist may instruct a client how to mix and ingest a fatal dose of prescription medication.

47. A professional negligence or medical malpractice case is a civil action. The difference between a civil lawsuit and a criminal lawsuit is:

    1. The damages sought in a civil suit are monetary; one private party sues another for money.

2. If you are convicted in a criminal case, you are still covered by your professional liability insurer.

3. In a criminal case, your state sues you for money; other penalties do not apply.

4. In a civil suit, if you do not prevail you could be incarcerated.

48. Which of the following is **not** a form of alternative dispute resolution (ADR)?

1. Mediation.

2. Binding and nonbinding arbitration.

3. Settlement conference.

4. A jury trial.

49. It is particularly important for nurses who care for children to have adequate professional liability insurance coverage because:

1. Damages are always higher when a child is the injured party.

2. Juries tend to award fewer dollars to injured children because the children are eligible for a variety of social programs that cover their medical expenses.

3. The statute of limitations is often tolled (put on hold) until the minor reaches majority, so the time frame within which the child can file a lawsuit is extended.

4. Insurers are sensitive to the increased risk posed by minor claimants so the coverage is difficult to obtain.

50. A health care provider has a duty to disclose certain information to the client as part of the informed consent process. Exceptions to this duty would include all of the following **except**:

1. The client has waived the right to receive the data.

2. It is a bona fide emergency situation.

3. The provider believes that the information would be harmful to the client and invokes the therapeutic privilege.

4. The client is 80 years old and the elderly are unable to comprehend complex medical facts.

51. Before contemplating providing a detailed reference on a former employee, it would be important to consider the following:

1. Check the requirements of the Human Resources Department of your employer.

2. If the comments are perceived as negative, and the former employee becomes aware of them, you could subject yourself to suit for defamation.

3. If the employee exhibits unsafe client care practices, it may be wiser to risk legal action from the employee than to subject future clients to this unsafe practitioner.

4. All of the above.

52. The primary purpose of a pre-employment physical is:

1. Identify existing health problems that might adversely affect the company's insurance rates.

2. Determine the mental status of the applicant.

3. Determine if the applicant is physically capable of doing the job.

4. Document any existing disabilities and recommend accommodations.

53. A nurse practitioner involved in work-related surveillance knows that the records related to this activity must be held for how many years after employment?

1. 5 years.

2. 25 years.

3. 30 years.

4. Can be destroyed only after the employee's death.

54. The nurse practitioner knows that when treating a work-related injury it is required that he/she:

    1. Document thoroughly because of the high probability of legal action.

    2. Communicate directly with the client's employer.

    3. File a report with the industrial commission documenting the injury and treatment.

    4. Notify the Occupational Safety and Health Administration (OSHA).

55. Which situation would be considered reportable under the Occupational and Safety Health Act?

    1. A 3-cm abrasion of the forearm.

    2. A warehouse worker with back strain reassigned to office work for a week.

    3. A twisted ankle that responded to ice and Ace wrap.

    4. A minor closed head injury with no loss of consciousness.

56. The purpose of an Occupational and Safety Health Administration 200 log is to record:

    1. Occupational injuries and illnesses.

    2. Only work-related deaths.

    3. Dangerous workplace situations.

    4. Lost work days.

57. The American Disabilities Act (ADA) regulates how employers treat the disabled. Under the ADA, disability is defined as a physical or mental impairment that substantially limits one or more major life activities of an individual or a record of a situation in which an individual is regarded as having such an impairment. This would include:

    1. A history of addiction.

    2. Paralysis.

    3. Bipolar disorder.

    4. All of the above.

58. Bioethical practice dilemmas are best described as situations in which proposed treatment alternatives are:

    1. Ranked from most to least acceptable.

    2. Not appealing to involved parties.

    3. Lacking acceptance by anyone.

    4. Less than perfect approaches to the situation.

23 ▸ Answers & Rationales

1. **(2)** The most important advantage of an occurrence policy is that the coverage is available regardless of how long it takes to become aware of a claim (the long "tail" of a medical malpractice claim). The limits do not automatically increase. The carrier need not be notified during the policy period, as is required with claims-made coverage. The coverage under each policy may be as broad as the carrier allows.

2. **(2)** Fact witnesses and necessary paperwork are always easier to discover the closer in time you seek them after a medical misadventure. Memories are fresh and documents are less likely to be misplaced or destroyed. There is no rigid reporting window required by insurance carriers; they do want to be notified in a timely manner. Insurance premiums may be reduced if an insured's track record is clean (i.e., no claims), but not by mere compliance with policy requirements. Risk management employees prefer early notification so that damage control efforts may be implemented promptly, not for regulatory reasons.

3. **(2)** Assessment skills are presumed to be within the purview of the professional nurse, not those with fewer years of nursing education. Also, in this scenario, the LPN is an unknown entity to the delegator. Delegating to the LPN should be done cautiously after determining that person's skill level. Your license is not in jeopardy if you delegated appropriately, as in Option #1, but an error was made and is attributed to the delegatee. Activities in Options #3 and #4 are appropriate for the role.

4. **(3)** The client's capacity to consent is questionable; therefore, alternatives must be sought. If the client has a court-appointed guardian, as set out in Option #3, then that person is the decision maker. The court has already made a determination of the client's legal incapacity and appointed the person to whom you will look for consent. If there were no guardian, you would analyze whether the client himself may be able to consent or whether you would look to his mother as the most appropriate surrogate decision maker. The group home employee has no automatic legal authority to consent to treatment for any resident.

5. **(4)** Assisted suicide is still a criminal activity in most states (and in legal limbo in the others). Circumventing the client may seem to be an appealing option, but it substitutes paternalism for the autonomy we all claim as our due. A diagnosis of depression can hardly be made with inadequate data; the necessary information can only be determined by conferring with the client herself.

6. **(2)** MCOs are one group of health care organizations impacted by this law. All subscribers must be provided with the stated information at the time of enrollment. Advance directive documents, though extremely helpful in the health care setting, are never mandatory.

7. **(4)** These are the basic requirements for conducting research at health care facilities.

8. **(3)** Your insurance carrier is thoroughly familiar with the processes of handling a claim. They will assist you with every step of this fearsome activity; the first significant obligation they will meet is to put you in touch with your lawyer. Conferring with the client or the client's lawyer is never a wise move. Your colleagues can only offer moral support at this stage; your lawyer is the professional of choice at this time. Never, never even think about altering a record; it can turn a defensible case into a nondefensible one.

9. **(3)** Lobbying for underserved clients is an example of justice, which is the duty to treat all clients fairly, without regard to age, socioeconomic status, or other variables. Autonomy is the client's right to self-determination without outside control. Nonmaleficence is the duty to prevent or avoid doing harm, whether intentional or unintentional. Veracity is the duty to tell the truth.

10. **(4)** These are all valid reasons to protect your assets in the event of litigation. There is an opposing view regarding the need for professional liability insurance. Some professionals feel that, if there are few assets to protect, insurance is an unnecessary expense. Nurses with professional liability coverage ("deep pockets") could be retained as defendants in a case for a longer period of time.

11. **(1)** Look to state law to define the circumstances under which confidential medical information may be disclosed. There may be additional requirements imposed by federal regulations (e.g., the handling of certain psychiatric records), but the bulk of the rule-making on this issue is accomplished at the state level. There are exceptions to the requirement of client consent, such as communicable disease reporting to public health authorities and court-ordered record production. Third-party payors, although powerful with their fiscal controls, must produce some proof of client consent to acquire records. An AIDS diagnosis does not shield a record from production, although many states have enacted extra levels of protection for this information. Again, knowledge of state laws is helpful.

12. **(3)** The ADA does not protect this group of people. In fact, employers may test for illegal drug use; this is not considered a medical examination, which ordinarily is subject to specific requirements under the law.

13. **(4)** These are all ways to get satisfaction from a health plan. You could also offer to help explain clinical issues to plan personnel who may not be clinically oriented.

14. **(1)** Callahan believes that health care priorities need to be re-evaluated. He advocates spending first on chronic care (those who cannot be cured), then preventive care, and lastly on the high-cost, high-tech modalities that benefit few but consume enormous resources.

15. **(2)** The best immediate solution is to identify the item and remove it from service to avoid further client injury. Then the risk manager, in consultation with the facility's attorneys and/or insurers, will determine how to proceed with equipment analysis. Returning the item to the manufacturer removes it from your control and diminishes your opportunity to defend against a charge of user error. Immediate repair may fail to uncover the real cause of the client injury and impair a successful defense of a claim. If the litigation potential is high, the parties may wish to pool their efforts (and costs) to conduct a third-party review of the equipment. If litigation is likely, then it is also likely that the manufacturer and others in the distribution chain will be co-defendants with the facility and its staff.

16. **(2)** The level of education preferred is that of the Master's, not the Associate degree conferred on the technical nurse. The legal issues are the province of the attorneys and the judge; the nurse is expected to be the expert in the clinical issues. Published authorship, on nursing issues, do add an aura of credibility, but specific work experience coupled with the educational credentials are more appealing.

17. **(3)** The APA describes the workings of federal agencies. The PSDA deals with advance directives, and the OBRA '87 changed the rule dealing with long-term care.

18. **(4)** These and other elements combine to produce a program of systematic risk identification, analysis, treatment, and evaluation, with the overall goal of loss prevention.

19. **(4)** Liability insurance is acquired to protect the organization from suits by clients arising from negligent acts of employees. Business interruption coverage is usually purchased in tandem with fire insurance. It reimburses an organization for losses sustained while the business is partially or completely shut down after a catastrophic event. The organization's management team (CEO and senior staff) is insured against losses based upon business judgment errors through directors and officers (D&O) coverage. Workers' compensation is the line of coverage that protects employees after on-the-job injuries. It is a no-fault system (negligence is not a factor) that covers employee medical bills and pays a percentage of wages while an employee is unable to work.

20. **(1)** You were driving your personal vehicle, so your own auto insurer is "primary"; that is, it responds first to a loss. Since you were on company business, your injuries were sustained "within the course and scope of your employment" so there is coverage under the employer's workers' compensation policy for your medical bills and wage replacement. Depending on the circumstances and policy definitions, there could be some "excess" or additional coverage available under the employer's auto policy, but in no event would that carrier be primarily responsible for your losses. This is not the type of incident that homeowners' insurance is intended to cover. The semitrailer, presumably in use as a business vehicle, would not be insured under a driver's personal auto policy.

21. **(1)** At this point, the mandatory reporting affects only dentists and doctors. Other licensed practitioners are subject to permissive reporting.

22. **(3)** The forwarding facility needs to know whether the receiving facility has space for the new arrival and, more importantly, the ability to treat the particular illness for which the client needs therapy. A familiar example of a client transfer is that of the burn victim, for whom specialty care is mandatory and the locations of that specialty care are usually limited.

23. **(1)** Health care policy within the states is codified or enacted into law by the respective states' legislatures. The boards have significant input (hopefully) in the process, providing the research data and expert "testimony" that the legislatures need in order to make informed decisions. Nursing organizations should also be willing to provide background information and nurse experts to educate the lawmakers.

24. **(3)** The MCOs' cost-containment strategy is enhanced if providers practice within the treatment guidelines suggested by the plans. Providers who inform clients that a certain treatment regimen is the preferred alternative create difficulties if that alternative is excluded from coverage. MCOs usually clearly set out the exclusions in the plan documents, and member services personnel are expected to be able to explain the coverage to subscribers. Experimental treatment, if excluded, would be listed as such in the plan documents.

25. **(2)** These are three of the agencies required to report. Events occurring in the other settings are exempt from reporting requirements under this federal law.

26. **(2)** This is the most factual note; the writer does not apportionate blame or assume liability. The other notes would be "red flags" for a chart reviewer. The mention of an incident report makes it virtually impossible to protect these documents from disclosure, especially in those jurisdictions that still afford some protection to these internal early warning documents that seek to alert risk management personnel to a potential claim.

27. **(3)** Clients are often unable to evaluate the quality of the care they receive, but they do react to the way in which the care is delivered. Perceptions by clients of rudeness or "uncaring" on the part of the provider often spur clients to pursue legal action. Clients tend to be more forgiving of less-than-optimal outcomes if they have been involved in the process and are treated with respect.

28. **(4)** Making one's own decisions is the basis for informed consent and the ethical underpinning of the Patient Self-Determination Act. "Doing good" (Option #1), and its corollary "avoiding harm" (Option #3), are ethics principles usually cited as the basis for other health care activities, such as maintaining professional competency. Respect for persons is a more global ethical principle supporting much of a nurse's personal philosophy of caring.

29. **(3)** Usually phrased as duty, breach, proximate cause, and damages, these are the four elements of proof required to prevail in a medical negligence action. Intentional acts are not synonymous with negligent acts. Duty presumes a professional relationship and obligation to provide services. The breach is the error or mistake ascribed to the provider that results in the harm to the client.

30. **(2)** A competent adult client is the person to whom you look for consent to treat. It is only when the client is unable to consent that surrogate decision makers are sought. Individual states' laws need to be checked for the selection and priority of surrogate decision makers.

31. **(1)** Lay jurors are not expected to know the clinical facts and circumstances involved in a professional negligence claim. The expert witness is necessary to educate the jurors about those medical facts and to testify to the standard of care to be applied. Witnesses with direct involvement in the case are no less credible because of their involvement; their testimony, and personal bias, if any, will be evaluated by the jurors in the context of their roles.

32. **(4)** With respect to nursing specialties, the standard of care is usually a national one. Facility policies, books, and journals are important to review, and physician input may be sought. In some cases, physicians may even be allowed to testify about the standard of care.

33. **(3)** One particular advantage of ADR is the flexibility of the system. In mediation, for example, the mediator can assist with crafting a solution package that meets all the needs of a party, including such things as an apology from the health care provider.

Money isn't always the only answer. Insurers' goals, however, usually do focus on cash: avoiding huge damage awards to plaintiffs. If a mediator is successful in facilitating case settlements, the costs are usually significantly lower than the costs of a court trial. Insurers with an eye on the bottom line are not averse to these advantages.

34. **(1)** Statutes of limitations set out each state's rules for the timing of the filing of lawsuits, including malpractice actions. These statutes are procedural laws, in that they describe the "how-to" parameters within which legal rights may be exercised. Minority is considered a legal disability; other state laws usually define it and describe its effects. Rights to sue are not governed by statutes of limitations.

35. **(3)** Statutes may indeed differ from state to state with respect to the breadth of the protection, but most will protect a nurse who renders aid, without expectation of compensation, in a competent manner. Gross negligence will usually void the statutory protections.

36. **(1)** A professional appearance boosts your credibility as a witness. Inappropriate attire and gum-chewing detract from the professional demeanor that you will want to project. Preparation is critical before your words are recorded and transcribed as part of the official litigation transcript. Review documents as noted, but refrain from bringing any materials with you to the deposition without your attorney's approval. Always ask for clarification of ambiguous questions. Speculation is not appropriate. Your professional work history is always asked, so a copy of your curriculum vitae (CV) is a useful tool to bring along to a deposition.

37. **(1)** Jousting in the client's medical record is never a good idea. It provides fodder for plaintiffs' lawyers but does not contribute to quality nursing care. If you have a conflict with another provider, deal with the provider directly, preferably in person. Another arena for resolving such disputes is the quality review process.

38. **(4)** All of these factors enter into an analysis of whether it is appropriate to accept a minor's consent to treatment. Another factor to consider is the type of treatment sought. Some states have statutes allowing minors to consent to specific therapies, such as treatment for venereal disease.

39. **(4)** Long-term care is a specialized area with layers of regulatory requirements, most stemming from the federal government. Nurses who work in this environment need to be vigilant about learning the rules and maintaining compliance. Ongoing, effective communication with regulators is essential.

40. **(4)** We have a tendency to get very careless with our information management and the way we interact with clients and their very personal data. The often wide-open and very frantic front-desk atmosphere of an office does little to calm client fears that their information will be too easily accessible to those without a need to know.

41. **(2)** Sexual preference is not a protected classification. The other options refer to groups for whom different federal laws provide varying degrees of protection to those groups. It is prudent to check with your business attorney to determine if the policies you have drafted for your office are in compliance with federal guidelines. The Equal Employment Opportunity Commission (EEOC), which enforces the laws, publishes guidelines about the various statutes. These publications are available, either free or at minimal cost, from the agency. Some may be available on the Internet.

42. **(3)** This seems to fit the criteria for a hostile environment, a form of sexual harassment. The harassment seems to be pervasive and longstanding; the women have complained and apparently no action has been taken. The isolated incident and single date request do not rise to the level of harassment. The participants did not find the actions objectionable, and job performance was not affected. In Option #2, although the potential was there for the nurse to use the prior relationship as a club to either downgrade the employee or deny a benefit, this result did not occur.

43. **(4)** Advance directives are documents crafted by individuals who personally decide how they wish their future health care decisions to be handled. The documents must be prepared while the signer is fully capable of understanding their content and importance. Since the wife in this scenario is already comatose, she has missed her opportunity to prepare advance directives. This does not mean that the spouse is unable to decide on her medical treatment; it just means that a different consent process needs to be employed.

44. **(3)** This option would create liability potential for the nurse practitioner under at least two legal theories (e.g., battery and false imprisonment). Obviously, Option #2 would be the first prong of a planned approach to convince this client that she needs the prescribed medical therapy. Option #4 would be the next choice. Court-ordered treatment is a consideration with a viable fetus.

45. **(1)** This is the overall goal of the ADA. It is not another entitlement program, and it cannot impose wheelchair ramp requirements on every building owner in America. Access ramps and interpreters may be required as a "reasonable accommodation" to qualified people in certain defined circumstances. There is no across-the-board mandate for these types of aid to the handicapped.

46. **(1)** The Supreme Court essentially deferred to the states to legislate on this topic. In most states, the activity is not permitted. In one of the states involved in the high court's case, a statute permitting assisted suicide is being challenged. Nurse practitioners need to look at their states' laws on this topic for guidance. The providers referenced in Options #2, #3, and #4 would act at their peril if their states' laws followed the current majority view.

47. **(1)** The purpose of a medical malpractice action is to make the claimant whole by the awarding of money damages. The award compensates the claimant or plaintiff for the wrong (or tort) he/she has suffered at the hands of the defendant. On the criminal side, the state sues on behalf of society for violations of society's criminal laws. The punishment is fines, imprisonment, or both. Professional liability insurance usually excludes criminal and intentional acts, so coverage for these types of activities is unlikely.

48. **(4)** The full-blown jury trial is what ADR seeks to avoid. Mediation and arbitration are the most well-known forms of ADR. Some jurisdictions use the settlement conference as a technique to attempt settlement after a lawsuit has been filed but before a trial begins. Another type of ADR is called a summary jury trial, which is a private, shortened version where the parties share some evidence and get a sense of the strengths and weaknesses of each side's position. There are also hybrids such as "med-arb" where a proceeding starts out as a mediation but, if the case does not settle, it is referred to an arbitrator for resolution.

49. **(3)** This is the so-called "long tail" of professional liability; there is always a time lag from the date of injury to the date a claimant files a malpractice action. In the case of an infant, that time lag can be many years because of the effect of the statute of limitations. This extends the period of potential risk to the nurse who cares for children. Although there may be a sympathy factor involved when jurors decide damages awards, the judgment is usually proportional to the injury and not the age of the claimant. Insurance coverage for pediatric providers is no less available than for other specialties; insurers adjust premiums to account for the level of risk.

50. **(4)** All clients are entitled to medical information in order to make an informed decision about treatment. Age, in and of itself, is not an exclusionary criterion. Providers may treat in the other circumstances.

51. **(4)** If the Human Resources Department has established guidelines for the handling of references, it would be wise to follow them. It is also an effective mechanism to deflect potentially problematic queries by passing requests to the department most equipped to handle them. Most employers will be very circumspect about the information released, often limiting the data to dates of employment only. Absent some protective state legislation, employers should be prudent about sharing comments on former employees' work histories.

52. **(3)** The purpose is to determine the appropriateness of the applicant for the job. Identifying health problems to prevent hiring an individual is discriminatory. The mental status and disabilities may also be a part of the pre-employment physical but are not the primary purpose.

53. **(3)** OSHA requires that these records must be held for 30 years after termination of employment.

54. **(3)** It is required by law that a report of any work-related injury be filed with the industrial commission of the state in which the injury occurred.

55. **(2)** OSHA requires the report of any injury or illness that requires more than first aid treatment and/or involves loss of work time, limited work status, loss of consciousness, or death.

56. **(1)** The purpose is to record occupational injuries and illnesses, which would also include death reports and lost work days, which would also reveal dangerous working conditions.

57. **(4)** All of the conditions listed would qualify under the ADA and may require accommodation in the workplace.

58. **(4)** The crux of a bioethical dilemma is that the proposed solution(s) are not perfect and therefore create some aspect of moral conflict.